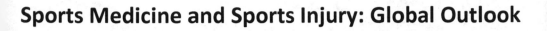

Sports Medicine and Sports Injury: Global Outlook

Sports Medicine and Sports Injury: Global Outlook

Edited by **Pablo De Souza**

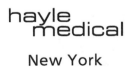

New York

Published by Hayle Medical,
30 West, 37th Street, Suite 612,
New York, NY 10018, USA
www.haylemedical.com

Sports Medicine and Sports Injury: Global Outlook
Edited by Pablo De Souza

© 2015 Hayle Medical

International Standard Book Number: 978-1-63241-359-8 (Hardback)

Contents

Permissions

List of Contributors

Preface

Playing sports regularly can often lead to some distinct injuries. For the last several years, sports medication has been a growing discipline in USA and Western Europe. Immense strides have been made in comprehending the fundamental functioning of work outs, power utilization and the mechanisms of sports damage. Furthermore, a development in minimally invasive surgeries and physical rehabilitation has led to athletes returning to their respective sport quickly after injuries. This book presents some latest information from experts on the epidemiology of sports medicine injuries and diseases. It also includes exceptional summaries of management options for ordinary sports-related injuries to the skeletal structure.

This book is the end result of constructive efforts and intensive research done by experts in this field. The aim of this book is to enlighten the readers with recent information in this area of research. The information provided in this profound book would serve as a valuable reference to students and researchers in this field.

At the end, I would like to thank all the authors for devoting their precious time and providing their valuable contribution to this book. I would also like to express my gratitude to my fellow colleagues who encouraged me throughout the process.

Editor

Part 1

Epidemiology of Sports Medicine Injury and Disease

The Physical Demands of Batting and Fast Bowling in Cricket

Candice Jo-Anne Christie
Department of Human Kinetics and Ergonomics,
Rhodes University
South Africa

1. Introduction

Even though cricket is one of the oldest organized sports, there are very few studies on the physical demands of the game (Woolmer & Noakes, 2008; Christie & King, 2008; Christie et al., 2008). Batting and bowling are intermittent in nature with the demands placed on the players being dictated by the type of match being played. Due to this stop-start nature of cricket, accurate assessments are often difficult and as such, research is sparse (Bartlett, 2003) and as a consequence, there are few scientifically sound training programmes for cricketers. In fact, the idea that cricketers need to be well trained is a relatively new one (Woolmer & Noakes, 2008). Historically cricket players never trained as hard as other sportsmen in team based sports such as rugby and soccer and in fact, many were overweight which dispelled any reason to be trained for their sport (Woolmer & Noakes, 2008). It wasn't until the Australians (cricket) and New Zealanders (rugby) demonstrated that, by focusing on physical training, performance benefits would be derived, that this started to change. This was a direct consequence of more scientifically based physical training programmes prior to their Cricket and Rugby World Cup wins in 1991 and 1987 respectively.

Further, the increased demands being placed on many cricketers now provide further need for them to be in peak physical condition not only for performance, but also for prevention of injury. International cricketers are now exposed to greater demands reflected by more five-and one day matches per season, longer seasons and more frequent touring (Noakes & Durandt, 2000). For example, during the 1998/1999 cricket season, the South African cricket team played eight five-day Test matches, 17 one-day international games and were eligible to play in eight four-day and ten one-day provincial (county) cricket matches – 99 days of playing (Woolmer & Noakes, 2008). In 1970, in contrast, players were asked to play 35 days of cricket (Woolmer & Noakes, 2008). Woolmer & Noakes (2008) therefore argue that only the best physically prepared cricketers will perform better, more consistently and with fewer injuries and, in turn, will enjoy longer and more illustrious careers. Thus, understanding the physiological demands placed on players and in particular batsmen and bowlers is imperative. Having said that, it is important to acknowledge the skills and mental aptitude needed to succeed in the game of cricket and that being physically trained cannot, on its own, fully compensate (Noakes & Durandt, 2000). However, being physically well conditioned will differentiate between two players of equal skill and, as such, enhancing our understanding of the physical requirements of the game can assist in bringing the game forward. Despite the limited data on cricket, teams that have embraced the concept that research in the sport contributes to improved performance, have excelled over the last few decades (Mansigh, 2006). Science and cricket is a fairly new marriage and only now do many of the international teams realize the gap between those who incorporate science and those who rely solely on talent (Mansigh, 2006).

2. Physical characteristics of cricketers

As a generalization, it has been found that batsmen tend to be smaller and lighter than bowlers (Stretch, 1987; Noakes & Durandt, 2000; Bartlett, 2003) but that they have similar morphological profiles with both batsmen and bowlers averaging approximately 12-14% body fat (Figure 2) (Noakes & Durandt, 2000; Bartlett, 2003). Batsmen also have higher predicted maximal oxygen uptake values and faster running (simulated three runs protocol) with quicker turn times than bowlers but have similar strength and 35 m sprint performances (Noakes & Durandt, 2000). When compared to rugby players, cricketers demonstrate similar performance characteristics (Figure 2). This is despite the fact that rugby is typically viewed as more physically demanding requiring players to be well trained. Cricket, in contrast, has tended to be viewed as less physically demanding requiring less training (Fletcher, 1955). Data on South African international rugby and cricket players clearly shows differences in morphology as well as performance with cricketers reaching higher levels on the typical shuttle run test (Figure 1). Further, there are no reported differences in strength measures between the two groups (Figure 2) which is interesting, as rugby players are also viewed as stronger possibly due to the larger size (Figure 2).

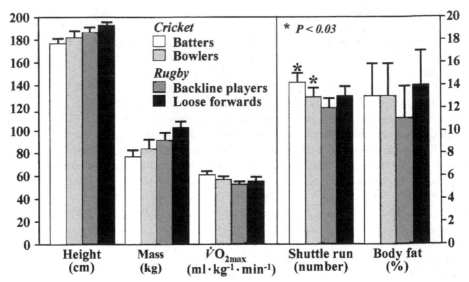

Fig. 1. Comparison of South African international cricket and rugby players (Taken from Noakes & Durandt, 2000).

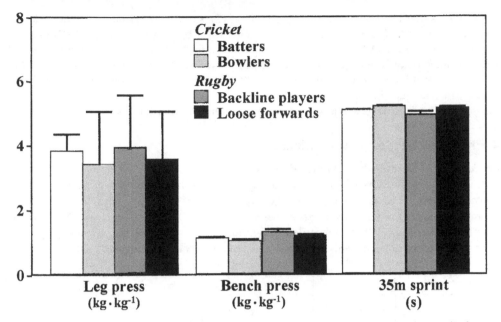

Fig. 2. Strength comparisons between elite South African rugby and cricket players (Taken from Noakes & Durandt, 2000).

3. Most frequent injuries in cricket

There have been many reports on the types of injuries incurred by elite teams worldwide (Orchard et al., 2006; Leary & White, 2000) with a more recent paper reporting on injuries at all levels of play including recreational cricketers (Walker et al., 2010). These latter authors found that of all age groups, the upper (36%) and lower (31%) limbs were most commonly injured. This was higher than that reported by Stretch (1995) who found a 23% occurrence of lower limb injuries in school boys. However, with respect to more adult and elite players, the incidence rate is higher and between 38% and 50% (Leary & White, 2000; Orchard et al., 2002). Walker et al. (2010) reported that contact with the ball or bat was the dominant mechanism of injury for those under age 50 while overexertion, strenuous or repetitive movement, slips and falls were the mechanisms for those over age 50 (Walker et al., 2010). Walker et al. (2010) showed that 35% of injuries to the lower limb areas were as a result of strains and sprains to muscles in the lower limb region. This was the highest percentage of all injuries to the lower limb region and was most obvious in the 30-39 year age group; the typical age at which cricketers 'peak' and are playing at top level. This is important considering the high demands placed on the lower limb musculature when sprinting and turning between the wickets and when sprinting and during the rapid acceleration and deceleration in the run-up and delivery of the ball when fast bowling (Christie et al., 2011b). It is contended that this repeated eccentric loading of the lower limb musculature is the real source of stress for cricket players (Noakes & Durandt, 2000) and which would reflect in more lower limb muscle sprains and strains. Injury research on bowlers has largely focused on low-back injuries in fast bowling and the current thinking is that the mixed technique results in the most injuries (Bartlett, 2003). The loading on the bowler's musculoskeletal system at back-foot and front-foot strike is a potential risk for not only lower back injury (Bartlett, 2003) but also lower limb musculoskeletal strain. Peak vertical forces for back- and front-foot strike are 2.4 and 5.8 times body weight (Hurion et al., 2000). In terms of increasing playing hours and increased risk of injury, surprisingly, despite a 30% increase in player hours over more than a decade, match injury incidence has remained relatively constant (Orchard et al., 2006) which may reflect improvements in injury detection and treatment (Mansigh, 2006).

4. Physiological demands of cricket

One of the first studies which attempted to assess the energy cost of cricket calculated that the mean energy expenditure of cricketers, during a five-match test series, was 86.4 kcal.m^2.h^{-1} (Fletcher, 1955). This equates to an energy expenditure of approximately 650 kJ.h^{-1} for an average cricketer with a body surface area (BSA) of 1.8 m^2 (Christie et al., 2008). These calculations, together with data recorded using indirect calorimetry with cricketers playing in the nets, led to the development of Figure 3 (redrawn by Noakes & Durandt, 2000).

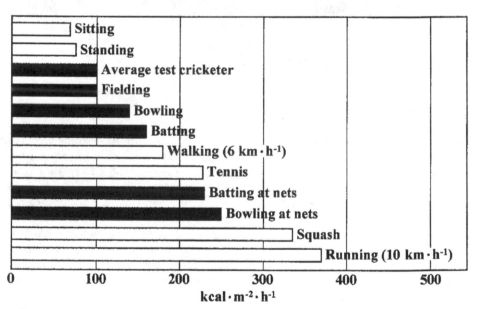

Fig. 3. The energy demands of different cricketing activities compared with other sports and activities. (Redrawn by Noakes & Durandt, 2000 from Fletcher, 1955).

Fletcher's data suggested that the energy demands of cricket are only slightly more than that required to stand (Christie et al., 2008) which led to the understanding that cricket was physically undemanding requiring more skill than "fitness" (Noakes & Durandt, 2000). However, it must be noted, that Fletcher included time spent sitting watching the game in his calculations (Petersen et al., 2010). Despite this, these findings were confirmed more recently by Rudkin and O'Donoghue (2008) who, after analyzing first-class fielding in the United Kingdom, concluded that cricket is physically undemanding. In contrast, studies from our laboratory, simulating one day batting, have estimated much higher energy demands (Christie et al., 2008; Christie et al., 2011a).

4.1 Physiological demands of batting

Noakes & Durandt (2000) estimated that during a one-day game, a hypothetical player scoring 100 runs, made up of 50 singles, 20 twos, 10 threes and 20 fours, would cover a distance of 3.2 km in an activity time of 8 minutes. Average running speed would be 24 km.h[-1] with at least 110 decelerations required (Noakes & Durandt, 2000). From this, these authors deduce that the physiological demands of batting in a one-day game are substantial. Players need to be well trained to do this as they are also required to field for 3.5 hours which adds to the stress placed on them.

The first study done in our laboratory, focusing specifically on the physiological demands of batting, looked at 10 batsmen receiving one delivery every 30 s with a total of 7 overs (42 deliveries) faced (Christie et al., 2008). After every 3rd delivery the player was required to complete one shuttle run at full pace. The two popping creases were set 17.68 m apart. The 2 by 2 singles run per over simulated the high work rate likely to be achieved after the 15th over in a high-scoring one-day match (King et al., 2001). The total distance run by each player was approximately 495 m. The 30 s period of inactivity between deliveries was to account for the bowler walking back to his 'mark'. The 1-minute break between each over was reflective of a change in bowler. The results were that heart rate increased significantly during the first three overs (Figure 4) and then more marginally for the remaining four overs during which mean heart rate was 152 bt.min[-1] (Christie et al., 2008).

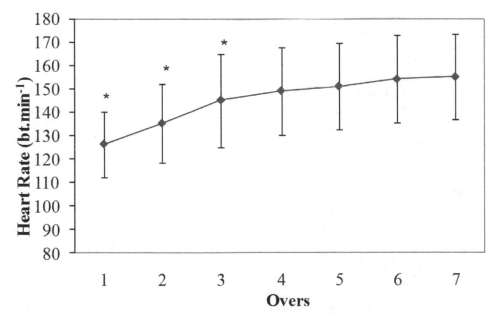

Fig. 4. Mean heart rate responses (bt.min[-1]) from the first to the seventh Over. (* *Denotes a significant increase in heart rate for the first three Overs*)

Oxygen consumption during the first over (23.5 ml.kg^{-1}.min^{-1}) was significantly (P < 0.05) lower than the remaining six overs (mean of 27.3 ml.kg^{-1}.min^{-1}) which demonstrated a 'steady-state' response (Christie et al., 2008). Further, the mean energy cost of the work bout was 2536 kJ.h^{-1} (301 kcal.m^2.h^{-1}) (Christie et al., 2008).

This initial research in our laboratory therefore demonstrated that batting was a lot more physically taxing than previously thought. Further, these findings also contradicted the notion of Gore et al. (1993) that during a ODI a batsman's heart rate rarely rises above 128 bt.min^{-1}.

A subsequent study in our laboratory, with a slightly altered work bout due to more recent time motion analyses (35 second break between balls as well as a 75 second break between overs as well as a single sprint per ball), found even higher responses (Christie et al., 2011a). During the first over, heart rate increased significantly (p<0.01) to 142 bt.min^{-1} and then continued to increase until the end of the third over (161 bt.min^{-1}). Thereafter heart rate stabilised and remained between 161 bt.min^{-1} and 167 bt.min^{-1} (final over). Oxygen consumption and energy expenditure increased significantly (p<0.01) until the end of the second over after which both responses stabilised. VO$_2$ stabilised between 27 and 28 mlO$_2$.kg^{-1}.min^{-1} in the final six overs while energy expenditure remained constant at 11 kcal.min^{-1}. These studies confirmed our belief in the higher physiological demands of batting.

4.2 Physiological demands of bowling

Research on the physiological demands of bowling is sparse with the only studies available being those which included some physiological measures when assessing other aspects of the game. One study found heart rates of between 154 and 158 bt.min^{-1} during a 6-over fast bowling spell (Devlin et al., 2000). This was confirmed by Taliep et al. (2003) who found that heart rates during fast bowling ranged between 73% and 77% HR max. Burnett et al. (1995) reported peak heart rates of between 180 and 190 bt.min^{-1} during a 12-over fast bowling spell. To the author's knowledge, no in-depth physiological studies have been done on bowlers suggesting a need to investigate these demands further. During a 6 to 8-over spell, bowling speed remains unchanged while accuracy has shown some non-significant variation (Portus et al., 2000; Devlin et al., 2000). In contrast, Taliep et al. (2003) found significant reductions in bowling speed after the 6th over in a 12-over bowling spell and no change in accuracy.

5. Musculoskeletal demands of cricket

Noakes & Durandt (2000) speculate that the main cause of stress for cricket players is the repeated eccentric muscle damage resulting from multiple declarations that occur in batting and fast bowling. The stop-start nature of both sprinting between the wickets and fast bowling (during the 'run up' and delivery of the ball), contributes to early-onset fatigue indicators which, over time, results in a specific type of fatigue which negatively impacts performance and increases the risk of injury (Christie et al., 2011b). It has recently been shown that the physiological demands of batting in a one-day game are substantial and that players need to be well trained to optimally maintain this type of workload (Noakes & Durandt, 2000; Christie & King, 2008; Christie et al., 2008; Christie et al., 2011a and b). With respect to bowling, although most of the research has focused on lower back injuries (Stretch et al., 2000), it is the view of Noakes & Durandt (2000), that the repeated eccentric actions during fast bowling are the real source of stress for fast bowlers and that this needs to be followed up and related to speed and accuracy of bowling as well as injury potential. Substantial muscle strength is needed to reduce muscle damage arising from these repeated actions (Thompson et al., 1999). The ability to cope with repeated eccentric loading such as during cricket may require substantial muscle strength in order to reduce the damage (Noakes & Durandt, 2000). Running research has shown that repeated eccentric actions produce a specific form of fatigue that requires substantial recovery time (Nicol et al., 19991). They alter muscle function particularly with respect to a reduction in elastic energy production which results in increased work during the push-off phase (Nicol et al., 1991). Recovery time from this damage can take up to 2 weeks post-marathon.

Although the research on eccentric load placed on cricketers is still in its infancy, a recent pilot study from our laboratory looked specifically at the strength decrements associated with repeated sprints between the wickets (Christie et al., 2011b). The protocol was exactly that of Christie et al. (2011a) but which assessed isokinetic (concentric and eccentric) strength changes.

Leg	Speed (deg.s^{-1})	QUADRICEP DECREASE (%)		HAMSTRING DECREASE (%)	
		Concentric	Eccentric	Concentric	Eccentric
Right	60	14.12	18.68	9.76	12.15
Left	60	7.53	6.07	8.79	13.36
Right	180	3.69	15.65	10.41	14.94
Left	180	7.58	6.66	11.19	9.33
	MEAN	8.23	11.77	10.04	12.45

Table 1. Representing the percentage decrease (%) in peak torque values.

Eccentric strength changes were greater than concentric changes (Table 1). Overall, the strength of the quadriceps decreased by 8.23% concentrically and 11.77% eccentrically while the strength of the hamstrings decreased by 10.04% concentrically and 12.45% eccentrically. This was evident in both legs and in both muscle groups (mean decrement of 11.77% and 12.45% in the quadriceps and hamstrings eccentric strength respectively). While concentric hamstring decrements ranged between 9.76% (Right leg at 60 deg.s^{-1}) and 11.19% (Left leg at 180 deg.s^{-1}) the range was much larger for the quadriceps concentrically. More specifically, there was a 14.12% decrement in concentric quadriceps strength at 60 deg.s^{-1} in the right leg and only a 3.69% in the same leg at 180 deg.s^{-1}.

As with the peak torque changes, there were similar decrements in work over time (Table 2). The greatest decrement in work was to the hamstring musculature eccentrically (decrement of 14.70%). This was followed by the eccentric work of the quadriceps muscle group

(11.13%). With respect to eccentric changes, although the hamstrings were affected similarly in both legs, the quadriceps showed greater decrements in the dominant, right leg and virtually no change in the non-dominant, left leg (Table 2).

Leg	Speed (deg.s⁻¹)	QUADRICEP DECREASE (%)		HAMSTRING DECREASE (%)	
		Concentric	Eccentric	Concentric	Eccentric
Right	60	16.34	21.53	9.65	15.73
Left	60	11.74	1.56	5.65	14.12
Right	180	3.98	14.99	12.73	17.91
Left	180	10.27	6.44	8.47	11.04
	MEAN	10.58	11.13	9.12	14.70

Table 2. Representing the percentage decrease (%) in peak work values.

Strength losses are considered reliable indicators of exercise-induced muscle damage (Warren et al., 1999) which are likely after repeated eccentric muscle actions. When strength losses occur, there is a much higher chance of muscular strain and joint instability. Further, this could impact performance such as reduced ability to accelerate and decelerate when running between the wickets or could lead to more errors, increasing susceptibility to injury (Rhanama et al., 2003). The greater eccentric strength decline of the hamstrings may be due to the greater requirement of the hamstrings to control running actions and for stabilizing the knee joint during foot contact with the ground. If this is the case, then it could lead to less control and lower stability of the knee and greater risk of injury (Rhanama et al., 2003).

5.1 Eccentric loading and fatigue

In their book 'Art and Science of Cricket', Woolmer & Noakes (2008) provide a comprehensive section on what they consider to be the main cause of cricketing fatigue. Basically, they propose that eccentric actions alter muscle recruitment over time resulting in the inability to store the energy of landing and recover energy for the push-off phase of the running stride which follows. The brain must then decide to either recruit more fibres to assist in the push-off phase in order to keep the same speed of running or reduce running speed in order to cope. As the bowling spell or batting innings progresses, the way in which the muscles are recruited will change because of the body's natural desire to protect the vital organs from catastrophic failure, referred to as the 'central governor' (Noakes et al., 2001). Despite this, the player must still produce the same result.

So, according to the central integrative model of exercise regulation (Figure 5), the subconscious brain is making these choices, and altering the way in which it recruits the muscles (St Clair Gibson & Noakes, 2004). It sets the number of motor units activated throughout the exercise bout (1). Sensory feedback from various physiological systems results in an appropriate adjustment in muscle recruitment (2). At the start of the bowling spell or batting innings, the subconscious brain informs the conscious brain (3) of increasing neural effort and this is interpreted as an increased sensation of fatigue (4) which can then also further influence the subconscious (5). Basically, the subconscious influences the conscious brain with sensations of fatigue (commonly seen in ratings of perceived effort) so the bowler or batsmen alters speed in order to ensure they have enough reserve to complete the bowling spell and/or innings.

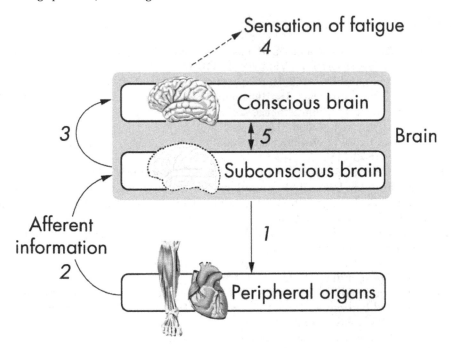

Fig. 5. The central integrative model of exercise regulation. (Taken from St Clair Gibson & Noakes TD, 2004).

If their theory is correct, then the main goal of training programmes should be on the development of eccentric training programmes to assist players in coping with this stress and hopefully reducing their risk of injury by delaying the onset of fatigue (Woolmer & Noakes, 2004).

6. Conclusion

Research on all aspects of the game of cricket is needed in order to better understand the demands being placed on players as well as to link these to fatigue indicators and injury risk. The sport has a long way to go in terms of linking science and practice evident in other sports such as football. Until more is understood of the demands of the game, training programmes will be merely based on trial and error and not grounded in science. This means that it is probable that players are not getting adequately prepared for play and as a result, are becoming injured more frequently. This is particularly the case for injuries which are more avoidable and linked to fatigue, such as sprains and strains. Further, there is a need for more communication and cooperation between sports scientists involved in cricket research and coaches of the game to ensure mutual benefit. This chapter contends that the real source of stress for cricketers is the musculoskeletal demands and associated stressors and that research needs to consider linking appropriate eccentrically based training programmes with fatigue indicators, performance affects and injury risk reduction.

7. References

Bartlett, RM. (2003). The science and medicine of cricket: an overview and update. *Journal of Sports Sciences,* Vol.21, pp. 733-752, ISSN 1466-447X

Burnett, AF.; Khangure, MS.; Elliott, BC.; Foster, DH.; Marshall, RN. & Hardcastle, PH. (1996). Thoracolumbar disc degeneration in young fast bowlers in cricket: a follow-up study. *Clinical Biomechanics,* Vol. 11, No., pp 305-310, ISSN 0268-033

Christie, CJ. & King, GA. (2008). Heart rate and perceived strain during batting in a warm and cool environment. *International Journal of Fitness,* Vol.4, No., pp 33-38, ISSN 0973-2152

Christie, CJ.; Barford, G. & Sheppard, B. (2011b). Concentric and eccentric strength changes in the lower limb musculature following repeated sprints between the wickets. *Proceedings of the 4th World Congress on Science and Medicine in Cricket,* pp. 82, Chandigarh, India, 31 March–01 April, 2011

Christie, CJ.; Pote, L. & Sheppard, B. (2011a). Changes in physiological and perceptual responses over time during a simulated high scoring batting work bout. *Proceedings of the 4th World Congress on Science and Medicine in Cricket,* pp. 83, Chandigarh, India, 31 March–01 April, 2011

Christie, CJ.; Todd, AI. & King, GA. (2008). The energy cost of batting during a simulated batting work bout. *Science and Medicine in Sports and Exercise,* Vol.11, pp 581-584, ISSN 1440-2440

Devlin, L. (2000). Recurrent posterior thigh symptoms detrimental to performance in Rugby Union. *Sports Medicine,* Vol. 29, No.4, pp 273-277, ISSN 0112-1642

Fletcher (1955). Calories and cricket. *Lancet* Vol.1, pp 1165-1166, ISSN 0104-6736

Gore, CJ.; Bourdon, PC.; Woolford, SM. & Pederson, DG. (1993). Involuntary dehydration during cricket. *International Journal of Sports Medicine,* Vol.14, pp 387-395 ISSN 0172-4622

Hurion, PD.; Dyson, R. & Hale, T. (2000). Simultaneous measurement of back and front foot ground reaction forces during the same delivery stried of the fast-medium bowler. *Journal of Sports Sciences,* Vol.18, pp 993-997, ISSN 1466-447X

King, GA.; Christie, CJ. & Todd, AI. (2001). Effect of protective gear on skin temperature responses and sweat loss during cricket batting activity. *The South African Journal of Sports Medicine,* Vol.9, No.2, pp 30-35, ISSN 1015-5163

Leary, T. & White, J. (2000). Acute injury incidence in professional county cricket players (1985-1995). *British Journal of Sports Medicine,* Vol.34 pp 145-147, ISSN 1473-0480

Mansingh, A. (2006). Cricket and Science. Invited Commentary. *Journal of Science and Medicine in Sport,* Vol.9, pp 468-469, ISSN 1440-2440

Nicol, C.; Komi, PV. & Marconnet, P. (1991). Fatigue effects of marathon running on neuromuscular performance. I. Changes in muscle force and stiffness characteristics. *Scandinavian Journal of Medicine and Science in Sports*, Vol.1, pp 10-17, ISSN 0905-7188

Noakes, TD.; Peltonen, JE. & Rusko, HK. (2001). Evidence that a central governor regulates exercise performance during acute hypoxia and hyperoxia. *The Journal of Experimental Biology*, Vol.204, pp 3225-3234, ISSN 1477-9145

Noakes, TD. & Durandt, JJ. (2000). Physiological requirements of cricket. *Journal of Sports Sciences*, Vol.18, pp 919-929, ISSN 1466-447X

Orchard, J.; James, T. & Portus, M. (2006). Injuries to elite male cricketers in Australia over a ten year period. *Journal of Science and Medicine in Sport*, Vol.9, pp 459-467, ISSN 1440-2440

Petersen, CJ.; Pyne, D.; Dawson, B.; Portus, M. & Kellett, A. (2010). Movement patterns in cricket vary by both position and game format. *Journal of Sports Sciences*, Vol.28, No.1, pp 45- 152, ISSN 1466-447X

Portus, M.; Sinclair, PJ.; Burke, ST.; Moore, DJA. & Farhart, PJ. (2000).Cricket fast bolwing performance and technique and the influence of selected physical factors during an 8-over spell. *Journal of Sports Sciences*, Vol.18, pp 999-1011, ISSN 1466-447X

Rahnama, N.; Reilly, T.; Lees, A. & Graham-Smith, P. (2003). Muscle fatigue induced by exercise simulating the work rate of competitive soccer. *Journal of Sport Sciences*, Vol.21, pp 933-942, ISSN 1466-447X

Rudkin, ST. & O'Donogue, PG. (2008). Time motion analysis of first-class cricket fielding. *Journal of Science and Medicine in Sport*, Vol.11, No.6, pp 604-607 ISSN 1440-2440

St Clair Gibson, A. & Noakes TD. (2004). Evidence for complex system integration and dynamic neural regulation of skeletal muscle recruitment during exercise in humans.*British Journal of Sports Medicine*, Vol.38, pp 797-806, ISSN 0306-3674

Stretch, RA. (1987). Anthropometric profile of first-class cricketers. *South African Journal for Research in Sport, Physical Education and Recreation*, Vol.10, pp 65-75, ISSN 0379-9069

Stretch, RA. (2001). Incidence and nature of epidemiological injuries to elite South African cricket players. *South African Medical Journal*, Vol.91, No.4, pp 336–339, ISSN 0256-9574

Stretch, RA.; Bartlett, RM. & Davids, K. (2000). A review of batting in men's cricket. *Journal of Sports Sciences*, Vol.18, pp 931-949, ISSN 1466-447X

Taliep, MS.; Gray, J.; St Clair Gibson, A.; Calder, S.; Lambert, MI. & Noakes, TD. (2003). The effect of a 12-over bowling spell on bowling accuracy and pace in cricket fast bowlers. *Journal of Human Movement Studies*, Vol.45, pp 197-217, ISSN 0306-7297

Thompson, D.; Nicholas, CW. & Williams, C. (1999). Muscular soreness following prolonged intermittent high-intensity shuttle running. *Journal of Sports Sciences*, Vol.17, pp 387-395, ISSN 1466-447X

Walker, HL.; Carr, DJ.; Chalmers, DJ. & Wilson, CA. (2010). Injury to recreational and professional cricket players: Circumstances, type and potential for intervention. *Accident Analysis and Prevention*, Vol.42, pp 2094-2098, ISSN 00014575

Warren, GL.; Lowe, DA. & Armstrong, RB. (1999). Measurement tools used in the study of eccentric contraction-induced injury. *Sports Medicine*, Vol.27, pp 43-59, ISSN 0112-1642

Woolmer, B. & Noakes, TD. (2008). *Art and Science of Cricket*, Struik Publishers, ISBN 978-1-77007-658-7, Cape Town, South Africa

2

Community Options for Outdoor Recreation as an Alternative to Maintain Population Health and Wellness

Judy Kruger
Department of Environmental and Occupational Health
Rollins School of Public Health, Emory University
USA

1. Introduction

Among professional, elite amateur and recreational athletes, having a sports injury can cause physical, social and psychological concern. Individuals with a sports injury may experience a significant challenge due to the reduced ability to participate in regular training. The injury may result in changes to their daily routine, and require time to heal. Regardless of etiology or prognosis, the loss presents a serious challenge to the athlete's health. In order to promote recovery, it is important for the injured person to adopt alternative approaches to remaining active. The injured athlete can engage in a variety of challenging and satisfying activities which will provide assistance in overcoming physical psychological and social concerns associated with being inactive. Outdoor recreation allows injured athletes the opportunity to modify their training activity in order to rest the injured body part, and provide a variety of physical activity opportunities to maintain health and wellness.

2. Health and wellbeing

The health benefits of outdoor recreational physical activity can be attributed to many different dimensions beyond physiological. Researchers have studied the relationship between outdoor recreational physical activity and psychological health and have found improved ratings of quality of life, decreased stress reduction, improved feelings of self-competence, and positive changes in mood and emotions. Thus, the health benefits of outdoor recreational activity are extensive, and outdoor recreation is a viable community alternative for places to participate in sport, exercise and physical activities. The outdoor environment provides an opportunity for people to recover from daily stress and fatigue, and on any given day, ¼ or about 54 million U.S. adults participate in a sport, exercise, or recreational activity. The benefit of many community outdoor recreational locations is that they provide an easily accessible place to maintain an active lifestyle. Community options surround everyone and to name a few, may consist of forests, beaches, parks, and sports fields. There is growing recognition for the value of outdoor recreation in promoting activity options to recover from sports-related injuries.

3. Physical health

Prolonged inactivity is detrimental to recovering from a sports injury. Research has shown that regular physical activity reduces people's risk for heart attack, colon cancer, diabetes, and high blood pressure and may reduce risk of stroke (USDHHS, 2008). Evidence compiled from many decades of research investigating the frequency, intensity and duration of physical activity show that regular physical activity assists in increasing and maintaining muscle strength, balance, and neuromuscular control. Evidence also suggests that moderate physical activity may in part offer some protection against injuries and may mediate tissue repair, the formation of new blood vessels, tissue remodeling and scar tissue healing. Movement also helps to provide a continued supply of nutrients and ensures that the muscles do not atrophy. Current guidelines for physical activity suggest that to prevent repetitive strain on the initial injury site, early movement is important for tissue to repair. The U.S. Department of Human Health and Human Services recommends that all adults should set the goal to accumulate at least 150 minutes per week or more of moderate-intensity physical activity (e.g., brisk walking) to reduce the risk of disease (USDHHS, 2008; USDHHS, 1996). In addition, these guidelines suggest that benefits can also be obtained with 75 minutes per week of vigorous-intensity physical activity (e.g., biking). Those with acute injuries may consider beginning a new activity plan with small amount of moderate- to vigorous-intensity physical activity such as 10 minutes, and gradually build up to the 150 minutes per week goal overtime. To strengthen muscle and bones, this minimal standard may be derived by intermittent or short bouts of activity (such as brisk walking, cycling, swimming and yard work) of at least 10 minutes in duration. The impact of an inactive lifestyle has severe consequences, thus injured athletes are encouraged to engage in a variety of their preferred type of activity. People who perform more formal exercise (e.g., structured exercise program) can accumulate this daily total through a variety of recreational or sports activities. Community outdoor recreation environments provide numerous opportunities such as participation in low impact sports, walking or hiking groups and can accommodate most individual preferences.

Public park settings provide opportunities for a variety of physical activities such as walking, biking, playing sports and games, etc. and oftentimes offer places to engage in hobbies such as boating, gardening, and picnicking. Participation in hobbies of the recreational kind may assist in providing opportunities for more gentle movement of the injured area. Encouraging participation in low-impact sports and recreation activity in the community provides alternative activity options that can help prevent re-injury and recovery from the sports injury. Recreational fitness facilities are also sought out places.

4. Psychological health

Little is known about the mechanism by which physical activity plays in treating mental illness. The most common mental illness is depression. Evidence of reduced depression in populations defined as being clinically depressed, have been noted within 4 to 8 weeks and results have persisted for up to one year. Moreover, studies show that physical activity provides an equally beneficial anti-depressant effect to that of standard psychotherapeutic treatments. One possible explanation is that physical activity reduces anxiety and improves mood. Exercise helps to improve psychological health through the release of neurotransmitters and endorphins. The release of the 'feel-good' brain chemicals may help ease the feelings of depression. Also, physical activity helps to improve the immune system and increase the body temperature, all which have calming effects on the body.

It is also plausible that the environment in which people are active in has an effect on their psychological health. Studies have examined the amount of green space in people's direct living environment and the amount of time they spend walking or bicycling. In the Netherlands, where bicycling for leisure or transportation is very popular, children under age 12 who reported living in a lush green neighborhood had lower levels of anxiety or depression. Researchers found that the environment influences positive mental health (Maas et al., 2008). Physical activity in the outdoors can provide emotional benefits as well. By being active in the outdoors may provide a healthy distraction from negative thoughts, and help individuals take their mind off of their worries. Some adults may choose to 'walk away their worries' as a coping mechanism.

Whether the changing of the environment or being active in a new environment influences psychological health, it is important to do something positive to manage symptoms of distress. Regardless of the outdoor setting, the natural environment has long been thought of as an ideal environment for rest, reflection, and positive mental health. The relationship between an individual's home, work and play life as well as their feelings of mental health, security and calmness will continue to be the subject of much discussion in future years.

A green environment has also been found to reduce stress (Pretty et. al., 2005). In some cities, planting of flowers and trees in the median of the roadways can to reduce accidents as the creation of these aesthetically pleasing surroundings narrows the roads causing drivers to reduce their speed and slow down. The use of aesthetically pleasing road designs such as buried utility cables, improved storm water management (e.g. raising curbs, improving storm water drainage) and pedestrian friendly sidewalks have also helped to reduce accidents among pedestrians and bicyclists. Another successful advancement in urban centers is the expansion of multi-use trails (those that connect residential areas with green spaces), the creation of pocket parks, planting of street trees (those planted along streetscapes) which help to establish green spaces and absorb heat. People who live in environments without viable green spaces may be forced to seek community options for places to participate in sports, exercise and physical activities.

5. Social health

The benefits of recreational physical activity also support social health. Being active outdoors gives people the chance to meet or socialize with others. Just exchanging a friendly smile or a greeting with others can help raise one's mood. The action of strolling around the block by foot or by rollerblade is an activity that can also boost self-confidence and familiarity with the environment and with those who reside in the surrounding area. Research has found that social support from both family and friends are positively associated with wellbeing (Warr et. al., 2009). Being active with a partner or in a group provides social cohesion or support, and this can enhance psychological health as well. Recently it has been found that people who lack a strong network of friends and family are at greatest risk of developing and dying from heart disease. Therefore, a lack of companionship can be a detriment to health.

The social environment can encourage physical activity, which does not need to be strenuous to be beneficial. The outdoor environment allows people to encounter others to make new friends or become acquainted with others who enjoy engaging in the same activity (e.g., biking on a trail). Being part of a team-based activity (e.g., playing softball) can help one develop social skills as team activities require commitment to participating in a weekly practice schedule. Interacting on a team can encourage physical activity among people who tend to be socially isolated. Also selecting activities that require refined skill such as pool, shooting, archery, and so on, can enhance focus and attention. The challenge of these types of activies can increase self-confidence. Successfully developing new skills and builds self-esteem and mastery.

Neighborhood parks provide opportunities for social cohesion within a community. Neighborhood corner parks also provide viable outdoor recreational options to walk or bike to and are great places where people can gather. Access to parks via multi-use trails provide socially responsible communities opportunities to volunteer to assist with trail maintenance. Natural environments also allow local residents to have places to read, relax or view birds or animals. The provision of parks and connective trails in non-urban areas has been found to improve wellbeing for local residents and increase overall physical activity levels (Sugiyama et al., 2008).

6. Physical activity and weight loss and weight maintenance

Research has shown that physical activity helps to control weight, contributes to healthy bones, muscles and joints. The negative consequences of an inactive lifestyle and being obese have resulted in over 300,000 premature deaths a year. Increasing physical activity is one of the cornerstones of a long-term healthy weight management program (USDDHHS, 2008). Physical activity has been effective at helping people to keep from gaining weight and in losing weight when combined with a decrease in caloric intake. Injured athletes may find themselves inactive for the first time after an injury, and as a result, start to gain weight.

Physical activity should be an integral part of a weight control treatment plan since an inactive lifestyle is an important contributor to gradual weight gain and can lead to obesity. Sometimes the reason for being inactive in the first place is because of an acute or re-occurring sports injury. An athlete in this predicament may need to look closely at their activity pattern and select an activity that they can participate in fully without being re-injured. More research on patterns of physical activity among persons trying to lose weight or trying to maintain their weight may provide injured athletes with direction as to how to increase their physical activity levels beyond their preferred form of sport.

The inter-relationship between physical activity and weight maintenance is complex. Research has found that aerobic physical activity alone only produces a modest weight loss of 1-2kg compared to that seen with combined physical activity and diet interventions (USDDHHS, 2008). Research has found that sedentary habits may lead to obesity. In the general population, those trying to lose weight or maintain their weight, compared to those not trying to control their weight are three times more likely to be regularly active than inactive (Kruger et. al., 2008). Pooled data from the 1999-2002 National Health and Nutrition Examination Survey (NHANES) showed that the most common physical activities reported by those trying to control their weight were: yard work, biking, running and weight lifting (Table 1). Walking was the most common activity reported across all weight control categories, although the prevalence of walking was greater among those trying to maintain (45.3%) compared to those trying to lose (38.3%) or not lose/maintain (24.0%).

	Lose weight		Maintain weight only		Not lose/maintain	
Activity	%*	95%CI**	%*	95%CI**	%*	95%CI**
Walk	38.3	(36.1, 40.7)	45.3	(41.1, 49.6)	24.0	(21.4, 26.8)
Yard work	14.5	(11.5, 18.1)	15.9	(11.8, 21.1)	11.9	(9.5, 14.8)
Biking	12.5	(10.9, 14.4)	15.4	(11.8, 19.9)	8.3	(6.9, 9.9)
Run	11.6	(10.3, 13.0)	12.6	(8.6, 18.1)	8.7	(7.1, 10.6)
Weight lifting	10.0	(8.5, 11.7)	11.1	(8.4, 14.5)	6.2	(5.0, 7.6)
Dancing	9.8	(8.5, 11.3)	9.7	(7.7, 12.2)	6.4	(5.5, 7.5)
Aerobics	9.0	(7.6, 10.6)	6.2	(4.7, 8.0)	2.9	(2.3, 3.6)
Basketball	5.2	(4.0, 6.7)	7.3	(5.6, 9.4)	5.2	(4.3, 6.1)

* Percent is weighted.; ** Confidence interval.

Table 1. Prevalence of most common physical activities reported among all adults (≥18 years), stratified by trying to lose weight, maintain weight only or not lose/maintain – National Health and Nutrition Examination Survey, 1999-2002.

Studies have also shown that increases in physical activity can result in reductions in abdominal adiposity (LaMonte et al., 2009) and an increased dose of physical activity can improving overall health. Research shows that increasing the amount of energy expended can result in more calories being burned. Thus persons trying to lose weight or keep from gaining weight should be active at a minimum level of ≥150 minutes on most days through moderate- or vigorous intensity physical activity.

7. Sports injury prevention

Because injury results in days lost from work or training, it is important to promote safe alternatives to protecting joints and muscles while maintaining a physically active lifestyle. Murphy's Law states that "If anything is used to its full potential, something will break". This saying sums up the etiology of overuse injuries. Recovery from a sports injury requires time for the area to heal. Pain often accompanies injury and may occur when starting to be active after a period of rest. That is why it is important set activity goals that are pain-free, promote range of motion and gradual increase in intensity and duration when the area is restored back to normal function. Injury incidence may differ by physical activity level because of the differences in the amount of potential overuse of a specific body part due to repetitive activities. Outdoor recreation is a healthy option for injured athletes to consider because low intensity recreational physical activities can be modified easily in regard to frequency, intensity and duration.

Because recovery requires a change in usual activities (from the original activity which caused the initial injury to occur), community options offer viable solutions to maintaining an active lifestyle. Walking has been shown to produce lower rates of injury than other activities such as running. Walking is also the most common form of physical activity and can be performed in any environment such as an inside or outside track, park, beach or neighbourhood. In general, walking can be performed by most people at varying speed. It has been estimated that' in front of 50% of athletes

50% of athletes who participate in team sports have reported one or more injuries over a season of activity. This is much higher than estimates in the general public (non-athletes)

where 5% those who participate in sport activities report an injury. One reason that injuries are not as common in the general public is because they engage in sports less frequently (they are only occasionally active). Second they may be active at a lower intensity level instead high-intensity activities of sprinting or.

Table 2 reports the distribution of sports injuries by the specific region or site of the injury. Data from the Aerobics Center Longitudinal Study showed the most frequently injured site of the body for both men and women (Hootman et al., 2002). In general for both sexes, the three most common sites of the body are the knee (23.3% men, 22.3% women), the foot (12.9% men, 15.7% women), and the back (10.6% men, 10.3% women). Interestingly, less than one percent of women reported eye injury compared to 12.9% of men.

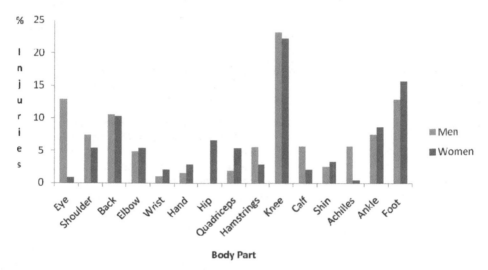

Body Part

Fig. 1. Distribution (percentage) of injuries by body part for men and women — Aerobics Center Longitudinal Study, 1970-1886.

8. Classification of sprains, strains and other injuries

Injuries can be classified by the body part affected, or the site of the injury. Table 2 is a simple classification overview of the anatomical site (includes the area, tissue and anatomical structures affected) and resultant injury (what is wrong with the area). Depending on the nature of the problem and its severity, rest or modified activity may be recommended. The type of injury reported may depend on the sport.

Regardless of the cause of sports injury, general management include restoring function, enhancing the healing of the injury and being comfortable while engaging in activities of daily living. Sprains and strains are the most common form of sports injury. A sprain is defined as damage to a ligament or its attachment due to overstress. A strain is defined as damage to a muscle or tendon due to overstress (acute strain) or over use (chronic strain).

Sprains, when acute require the traditional RICE approach which consists of Rest, Ice, Compression, Elevation, and encouraged movement. The principle is to prevent increased injury by controlling swelling and promoting recovery of function. Rest may require a tensor bandage, and adhesive strap, splint or plaster cast. Sprains can become chronic depending on the severity of the initial injury, and re-occurrence due to additional injuries. Principles for treating chronic sprains require encouraging the individual to get back to regular physical activity as much as possible, localized muscle strengthening activities, pain management to relieve distress, prevention of further ligament lengthening problems (e.g., use of orthotic brace or straps) and in some situations surgery. Self-treatment modes used by injured athletes for musculoskeletal injuries also include the use of bandages, orthotics or change in the model or brands of the shoes they currently wear. Studies have shown that with these adaptations, injured athlete have been able to continue participating in moderate-intensity physical activity for >30 minutes a day.

Acute muscle strains often result from an accidental injury. A single event will cause sudden pain usually due to tears at the muscle-tendon junction. This types of this sports injury often results in localized tenderness at the muscle or tendon due to the violent force acting against great opposition. Chronic muscle strain often results from too much strain overtime on the muscle-tendon junction. In some cases, muscle strain begins as a minor injury (that is often neglected and becomes chronic), or as a poorly treated acute injury. Overtime, micro tears may occur at the muscle-tendon junction or muscle-bone junction, resulting in common problems such as shin-splints, jumper's knee, and Achilles tendonitis.

Anatomical site	Result of injury
Soft tissue	Cut
	Abrasion
	Laceration
	Contusion/hematoma
	Muscle strain
	Ligament sprain
	Tendonitis/bursitis
Bone injury	Bruise
	Fracture: stable, unstable
Joint injury	Dislocation
	Cartilage: contusion/fracture
	Cartilage: bone/ligament sprains
Special areas: head injury	Fracture, concussion, hematoma
Special areas: chest injury	Rib cage, lungs, heart
Special areas: abdominal injury	Various internal organs

Table 2. Classification of Injuries

9. Common sports injuries

The human skin provides a protective cover for the internal body structure and organs. The skin is the largest body organ of the body and accounts for between 15-18% of total body weight. The skin has average thickness of 0.00394 mm and it is the most injured human organ. Injured athletes often sustain abrasions, cuts and lacerations to the skin. The layer of skin that envelopes the body is comprised of three separate components, namely the epidermis (outer shell), the dermis (middle layer) and the sub cutis (lower layer). In general, abrasions and cuts are less serious and affect the more superficial outer shell. A common cause of an abrasion is the friction produced between an athlete's unprotected skin and another surface (e.g., such as gravel or pavement). This type of injury generally heals within a few days after the initial incident. A cut is a penetration of the epidermis and generally results in damage to the circulatory system with blood being drawn to the opening. Contact with a sharp object such as a hockey puck or hockey stick can require stitches to close the opening and a bandage to prevent foreign objects from entering the skin. Generally, once the cut is bandaged and protected, athletic performance is usually not impaired. Lacerations are often regarded a more serious wound and often impact the deeper layers of skin, the fatty tissues or underlying muscles. A laceration is often associated with significant blood loss from a large opening. Repair often requires medical treatment to repair the jagged edges of the skin and may require suturing of the skin. Restricted movement may be required to allow the wound to heal (often 10-14 days).

Sports injuries often do not result in immediate death but may require hospitalization. In Table 3, U.S. data from 2009 are shown. These data provide an overview of the frequency of sports injury. Based on the number of injuries reported, the ten most popular sports injuries are: bicycling, basketball, football, exercise equipment, baseball/softball, playground equipment, soccer, swimming, skateboards and skiing/snowboarding. Of course popularity of these sports will influence the frequency in which these sports injuries are reported.

Estimated Number of Injuries	Sport	Type of Injury
544,470	Bicycling	Feet caught in spokes, head injury, collision
501,251	Basketball	Cut hands, sprained ankles, broken leg, eye and forehead injury
451,961	Football	Fractured wrists, chipped teeth, neck strain, head laceration, dislocated hips, jammed fingers
349,543	Exercise, Exercise Equipment	Twisted ankles and cut chins from tripping on treadmill. Head injury from falling backwards, ankle sprains
286,708	Baseball, Softball	Head injury from bats and balls. Ankle injuries from running or sliding on bases
237,184	Playground Equipment	Fractures from climbers, slides, swings, falls to the surface below playground equipment
208,214	Soccer	Twisted ankles or knees after falls, fractured arms during game
160,542	Swimming	Head injuries from hitting the bottom of pools, leg injuries from accidental falls
144,416	Skateboards	Fractures and cuts from falls
100,359	Skiing, Snowboarding	Head injuries from falling, cut legs and faces, sprained knees or shoulders

Table 3. Estimated Number of Sports Injuries in the 2009 National Electronic Injury Surveillance System.

Sports injuries are very common and can be examined using data from the U.S. Consumer Product Safety Commission's National Electronic Injury Surveillance System (NEISS). Data describing the number of injuries by sport type have been collected during hospital emergency department visits. Although fitness status (e.g., whether one is an athlete or not) is not determined with these data, estimates on the incidence of injury during sport and non-sport activities for the general population are provided. One limitation of these data is that adults who are physically active in general, have a lower incidence of injury compared to those who are inactive. However, data that make up the NEISS surveillance system are obtained from a national probability sample of hospitals of differing sizes and locations.

Unintentional injuries (falling) may happen during performance of a skilled sport such as skiing, which can give rise to a number of injuries such as cuts, sprains, strains or fractures. As the body ages, it takes longer for the body to heal. For example the skin (epidermis) of a 60 year old is 30-80% thinner than that of a 20 year old. Both acute and overuse injuries will take significantly longer for the older athlete to heal.

The growing increase in the number of baby boomers (those born between 1946 and 1964) and the desire of this cohort to remain active in recreation and competitive sports has resulted in an increase in the number of reported sports injuries over time. According to the U.S. Consumer Product Safety Commission, sports injuries among baby boomers (age ≥65) increased slightly from 2007 to 2009 (see Figure 2).

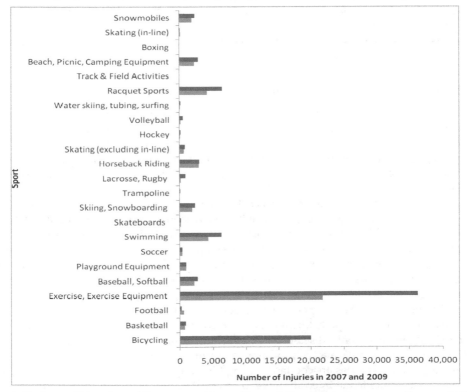

Fig. 2. Estimated Number of Emergency Room Treated Sports Injuries among Persons ≥65 Years of Age – National Electronic Injury Surveillance System, 2007 and 2009.

Figure 2 shows the number of injuries reported for 23 popular sports categories. The number of injuries associated with bicycling, basketball and football continue to rise. Although major advances have been made through the promotion of protective equipment, these data show that exercise equipment are the most popular category responsible for emergency room treated sports injuries among those ≥65 years of age. Educational efforts to assist older athletes to begin low-intensity activity programs and progress gradually to more intense activity levels are needed.

By 2050 the percentage of the population 65 years or older will be 21% (US Census Bureau, 2010). Research shows that baby boomers may appear to be aging actively. Data suggests sports-related injuries among baby boomer have been reported to cost almost $20 billion dollars a year. Therefore, prevention of injuries through education on rehabilitation after injury, early recognition of symptoms of overuse and training principles in addition to the promotion of recreational physical activity is needed.

The rise in chronic disease rates among adults at large requires injured athletes to consider ways to prevent and manage their injuries as they grow older. The growing increase in the baby boomers as a whole will require promotion of sustainable recreational physical activities that encourage lifelong activity patterns. Although medical advances continue to improve recovery from sports injuries, the use of sports protective equipment such as helmets, mouth guards, skin pads and knee pads have been shown to be effective in reducing injury. To date, laws have been developed require the use of protective equipment to protect to protect athletes from injury. These laws require the use of select equipment such as face masks among hockey players, and helmets among bicyclists, have been shown to help reduce head injuries.

10. Implications and future research

Community options for outdoor recreation allow individuals to experience the physical, psychological and social benefits of nature directly as a preventative measure to maintain health and wellness. Participation in outdoor recreational activities offers viable alternative to sports, gyms and community centers and can be a fun way to be physically active. Within this chapter, an overview of activities and sport injuries observed in national surveys has been highlighted.

It is clear from an extensive body of evidence that movement is important for everyone. Given the acceptability of walking among people with and without sports injuries, and the fact that brisk (e.g., fast walking) can improve fitness, walking should be considered a community options for outdoor recreation. Elimination of sedentary behavior is a public health priority and most people can meet the 150 minute/week recommendation by engaging in intermittent walks throughout the day (e.g., such as three 10-minute bouts). This is especially important to athletes with a sports injury who may be unable to sustain prolonged activity.

As adults age, they begin to experience re-occurring aches and pains often as a result of a repetitive unintentional injury. Maintaining or increasing involvement in physical activity with or without a chronic disease has significant implications for health in terms of maintaining balance, muscular control prevention of falls, and offers mental stress relief. Because age-related injuries are common among high impact sports, some athletes will tend to switch to more moderate-intensity types of physical activity over time. Research suggests that participation in several types of recreational leisure activities can meet the functional needs of injured athletes.

Alternative options in the community allow individuals to engage in an active lifestyle by using local parks or nearby places as places to be physically active. As one ages, priorities change and participation in sports declines, community based approaches to obtaining physical activity may play a bigger role. Community engagement through physical activity can provide internal satisfaction for athletes. Outdoor recreational activity can be a forum for developing or maintaining a social support system different from the sports teams previously held.

11. Conclusion

The health benefits of outdoor recreational activity are extensive, and outdoor recreation is a viable community alternative for places to participate in sports, exercise and recreational physical activities. Among professional, elite amateur and recreational athletes, having a sports injury can cause psychological concern. Injuries require time to heal and considerations to adopt a modified training plan may be required. Community options for outdoor recreation can assist injured athletes to overcome functional decline, social isolation and depression. Outdoor recreation allows individuals with a sports injury to modify their activity in order to rest the injured part, and provides social opportunity to maintain health and wellness.

12. Acknowledgement

Thank you to the U.S. Consumer Product Safety Commission for use of the National Electronic Injury Surveillance System (NEISS). NEISS is available online at www.cpsc.gov/library/neiss.html.

13. References

Hootman JM. Macera CA, Ainsworth BE, Addy CL, Martin M, Blair SN. (2002). Epidemology of musculoskeletal injuries among sedentary and physically active adults. *Medicine and Science in Sports & Exercise*, 2002; 34 (5):838-844.

Kruger J, Yore MM, Kohl HW. (2008). Physical activity levels and weight control status by body mass index, among adults in the National Health and Nutrition Examination Survey 1999-2004. *International Journal of Behavioral Nutrition & Physical Activity*, 1 (5):25.

LaMonte MJ, Kozlowski KK, Cerny FJ. Health benefits of exercise and physical fitness. In RJ Maughan (ed), Olympic Textbook of Science in Sport. Hoboken, NJ: Wiley-Blackwell Publishing, 2009, PP. 401-416.

Maas J, Verheij RA, Spreeuwenberg P & Groenewegen PP.(2008). Physical activity as a possible mechanism behind the relationship between green space and health: A multilevel analysis. *BMC Public Health*, 8:206: 1-16.

Pretty J, Peacock J, Sellens M, Griffin M: The mental and physical health outcomes of green exercise. *International Journal of Environmental Health Research* 2005, 15:319-337.

Sugiyama T, Leslie E, Giles-Corti B, Owen N. (2008). Associations of neighborhood greenness with physical and mental health: do walking, social coherence and local social interactions explain the relationship? *Journal of Epidemiology &Community Health*, 62(5): e9.

U.S. Department of Health and Human Services. (1996). *Physical activity and health: report of the Surgeon General.* National Center for Chronic Disease Prevention and Health Promotion: Atlanta.

U.S. Department of Health and Human Services. (2008). Physical activity guidelines for Americans. Hyattsville, MD: US Department of Health and Human Services. Available at http://www.health.gov/paguidelines. U.S. Census Bureau. 2010. Available at http://2010.census.gov/2010census/data

Warr D, Feldman P, Tacticos T, Kelaher M. (2009). Sources of stress in impoverished neighborhoods: insights into links between neighborhood environments and health. *Australia and New Zealand Journal of Public Health.* 33(1):25-33.

3

Prediction of Sports Injuries by Mathematical Models

Juan Carlos de la Cruz-Márquez, Adrián de la Cruz-Campos,
Juan Carlos de la Cruz-Campos, María Belén Cueto-Martín,
María García-Jiménez and María Teresa Campos-Blasco
University of Granada,
Department of Physical Education and Sport,
Spain

1. Introduction

A number of different methodological approaches have been used to describe the inciting event for sports injuries. These include interviews of injured athletes, analysis of video recordings of actual injuries, clinical studies (clinical findings of joint damage are studied to understand the injury mechanism, mainly through plain radiography, magnetic resonance imaging, arthroscopy, and computed tomography scans), in vivo studies (ligament strain or forces are measured to understand ligament loading patterns), cadaver studies and simulation of injury situations, and measurement/estimation from "close to injury" situations. This chapter describes mathematical modeling approach and assesses its strengths and weaknesses in contributing to the understanding and prevention of sports injuries. This chapter demonstrates the relationship between structural measures and lower limb injuries.

Sports injuries can affect any and all parts of the body depending on the particular repetitive movement performed just like any repetitive motion injury. While there are factors that raise the risk of injury, there are also elements that predispose athletes to sports injuries. Rehabilitation and preventative efforts should be centered on a thorough knowledge of risk factor etiology as well as knowledge of how such factors contribute to sports injuries.

In most epidemiological studies directed toward identifying major sports injury causation factors, injured athletes have been compared with uninjured athletes through single variable techniques. However, many of the factors highlighted later in this paper through these analytical techniques either interact or are interrelated.

Multivariable statistical techniques have also been used to detail risk factor interaction (Mechelen, 1992), such as discriminatory analyses and stepwise logistic regression (Dixon, 1993). In this chapter we will identify potential predictive factors that can be used in logistic regression equations, the basic concepts of this mathematical study, and equations that have been developed to what they are today.

2. Predictive factors of sports injuries

Predictive factors of sports injuries are biological variables and the relations between them that can be indicators for creating a health profile or diagnosis. For example, weight can be a predictive factor of diabetes, arteriosclerosis, and other metabolic illnesses. It is even more useful when associated with height, BMI, and waist-hip ratio since it can then be used in predicting hypertension, myocardial infarction, diabetes, and strokes. In order to effectively predict health complications, the WHO recommends using anthropometry to monitor risk factors of chronic diseases and to perform studies that define the association between the aforementioned factors and specific outcomes, such as arterial hypertension. Predicting factors of sports injuries can be grouped into two types of factors: Intrinsic factors and extrinsic factors.

2.1 Extrinsic factors

Sports injuries are most commonly caused by poor training methods; structural abnormalities; weakness in muscles, tendons, ligaments; and unsafe exercising environments. The most common cause of injury is poor training. For example, muscles need 48 hours to recover after a workout. Increasing exercise intensity too quickly and not stopping when pain develops while exercising also causes injury.

The most common cause of sports injuries is improper training whether from a technical or tactical point of view or simply training that is poorly planned and executed (Shaffer, 2006). The athlete exposes him or herself to possible sports injuries without adequate preparation for: exposure to potential danger, the playing position or type of activity, the duration of the competition or league, competition level, time dedicated to training and to rest. These variables can be quantified and turned into predictive factors (Ferrara, 2007). Among such:

2.1.1 Poor physical condition due to inadequate training (Mechelen, 1996).

2.1.2 Abrupt increments of training intensity or training load, resulting from overuse and overstress. These injuries tend to appear in underdeveloped locomotion devices, caused by unvaried and unbalanced sports practice especially after training intensification or excessive training. Aerobic training increments between 55% and 75% do not transmit negative effects and do not result in injury risk (Tate, 1995), although disproportionate increases in intensity can provoke anxiety and states of distress.

2.1.3 Premature competition and quasi-adult training performed by a child or adolescent expose the athlete to injuries from excessive force when pulling or pushing.

2.1.4 Resistance training, specifically in adolescents, without the appropriate battery of tests to identify the actual state of regulating and homeostatic mechanisms.

2.1.5 Performing new or unfamiliar exercises. This is common at the beginning of seasons, as well as upon introducing changes in the overall training regime. The same happens when sessions of active rest are planned in which the athlete reflects on unknown sports activities.

2.1.6 Environmental factors and atmospheric conditions, especially when weather conditions vary unexpectedly or unpredictably, the time of day and the season of the year (Mechelen, 1996).

2.1.7 The type and integrity of the playing surface, playing surface incline.

2.1.8 Game mediation: Judges and referees and the official game mediation. Competition among equals is typically promoted in most sports.

2.1.9 Sports and training equipment. Type and quality of protection, type of footwear, thermal and isothermal clothing. Before using a specific type of shoe, the athlete should know the structural morphology of his or her own feet. Advances in sports injury prevention technology has obligated sports brands to offer a wider variety of models, each model having specific characteristics that complement and correct potential foot dysmorphia.

2.1.10 Equipment protection, as well as player protection such as shin guards, ankle support, orthotic devices, mouth guards, helmets, prophylactic tape, etc...

2.1.11 Methodological training development and the level of physicality. Extrinsic factors associated with exposure to injurious situations are: potential dangers, playing positions, competition length, competition level, training time, training frequency, rest intervals or the frequency of exertion, weekly distance run or the number of jumps, hits, throws and impacts, number of trainings per week, training speed, number of competitions per year, absence of regularity in training, etc. All having to do with requirements for the level of physicality needed for different sports activities.

2.1.12 Prior years of sports training and experience under certain competition and training conditions.

2.1.13 Inadequate warm-up, whether insufficient or excessive. In some sports, the athlete is required to warm up over such a long period of time that he or she loses concentration on his or her movements and they consequently become ineffective.

2.1.14 Mastery of a sports technique, technical ability, skill and quality that contributes to the effectiveness of a movement.

2.1.15 Mental and psychological conditions: Intelligence and creativity, motivation and discipline that influence the precision of technical execution, skill level, previous experiences and the necessity of some athletes to take risks.

2.1.16 Intrinsic characteristics of common movements in sports activities, linked to structural, biomechanical, and functional characteristics of the athlete. In basketball, the height of the players, the number of jumps, sprints, stops, turning jumps, and backwards jumps can be determining factors in the occurrence of injuries (Grubbs, 1997; Shambaugh, 1991).

2.1.17 Nutritional and hydroelectric imbalances. (The most common cause of sudden death in marathons is overhydrating).

2.1.18 The type of sport, notably high-risk and contact sports as well as sports performed when unbalanced or in which unbalancing equipment is used.

2.1.19 Incorrect playing, inattention to game rules with an excess of rough play and the absence of fair play.

2.1.20 And, of course, muscular fatigue that stems from technical errors in execution and leads to injury.

2.2 Intrinsic factors

Everyone's bone architecture is a little different, and almost all of us have one or two weak points where the arrangement of bone and muscle leaves us prone to injury.

2.2.1 Age. There is an increase in the occurrence of injuries in children and adolescents' locomotion devices when they try to perform more ambitiously in hopes of improving their short-term performance. As age and competition level increase, so increases the risk of injury (Inklaar, 1996).

Nonetheless, in many studies, age is not a factor of predisposition, except when it relates to increased speed and distance in training that is significantly greater than that of an older athlete.

In children, the most frequent factors of predisposition to injuries are:

2.2.1.1 Intrinsic causes in children

2.2.1.1.1 Muscle tendon imbalance related to strength deficit, excessive flexibility and scant muscle volume.

2.2.1.1.2 Biomechanical alterations, curved, flat feet, femoral anteversion, and the genu valgum that promotes and increased deviation of the Q angle, lumbar hyperlordosis, and length difference between the lower limbs.

2.2.1.1.3 Abrupt weight modifications from growth, since injuries tend to happen from overexertion in growth zones (epiphisitis) when a sudden increase in bone length occurs without parallel adaptation of muscle tendon units.

2.2.1.2 Extrinsic causes in children

2.2.1.2.1 Derived from training errors, high-intensity and long-duration training involving frequent use of still developing structures.

2.2.1.2.2 Planning children' s training as though it were adult training, modifying only the workload or volume.

2.2.1.2.3 Technopathies derived from incorrect use of footwear, overly large equipment for the child, hard surfaces, accessories and clothing that are generally inappropriate.

2.2.2 Sex. Not a determining risk factor per se, although there are substantial anatomical differences which, in women, are: a wide pelvis, a more pronounced Q angle, greater pelvis anteversion and greater flexibility (Plisky, 2007). Women' s levels of training quality and quantity tend to be less intense than that of men due to women' s lower muscle mass.

2.2.3 Structural, neuromuscular conditions that affect athletic performance. Especially noteworthy conditions are:

2.2.3.1 The alteration of axis lines in the rachis, lumbar curvature, and lower and upper limbs.

2.2.3.2 Lower limb dissymmetry greater than 1 cm.

2.2.3.3 Muscular imbalance: muscular hypotonia and hypertonia.

Genu varum and genu valgum, along with an accentuated Q angle, the genu recurvatum and a smaller intercondylar notch favor the occurrence of injuries in the knees, particularly, cruciate ligaments in women (Shambaugh, 1991). This and the spinal column become real limitations on physical exercise. An excessive Q angle, as well as femoral anteversion favor the occurrence of injuries (Heiderscheit, 1999). The intrinsic causes of jumper's knee, can be sought in the mechanical properties of tendons (resistance, elasticity and extensibility) rather than in morphological or biomechanical abnormalities of the knee extensor mechanism (Ferretti, 1986). Athletes with jumper's knee demon strated better performance in jump tests than uninjured athletes, particularly in ballistic jumps involving eccentric force generation (Lian, 1996). Bilateral patellar tendinopathy may have a different etiology from unilateral pathology (Gaida, 2004).

2.2.3.4 Functional instability and muscular imbalances in the ankle, ligamentous laxity, peronial musculature weakness that can diminish control of excessive ankle inversion (Arnold, 2006)). The arch index is a substitute for quantifying foot structure. High-arched runners are at a greater risk of foot injury. Low-arched runners risk soft tissue damage and knee injury (Howard, 2006). While the pronated foot is implicated as a risk factor for **sports injury** in some studies, others suggest that a supinated foot posture increases the risk of overuse lower limb **injuries**. Athletes in a given **sports** discipline may tend to have a similar foot morphology, which varies from that observed elsewhere. Further, the foot morphology that is beneficial for performance in a **sport** may be detrimental with regard to **injury**. (Cain, 2007). Mark (2006) suggest that there are certain factors, including foot pronation, **sport**, and a history of this condition, that are associated with an increased risk of exercise-related leg pain. However, according Barnes (2008) no definitive conclusions can be drawn relating foot structure or function to an increased risk of tibial stress injuries. Extremes of foot types are likely to pose an increased risk of tibial stress injuries compared to normal arched feet.

2.2.3.5 Joint laxity is still the subject of much debate, although muscular elasticity and flexibility programs are recommended to increase ligaments 'defense. (Barber Foss, 2009; Kraemer, 2009)

2.2.4 Warm-up and stretching before competitions (Herbert, 2002, Andersen, 2005).

2.2.5 Height. Taller males are at risk of injury, using single variable logistic regression adjusted to age (Walter, 1989).

2.2.6 High BMI (<19,5 and > 27) relative to the sports activity in question. Simple anthropometric measurements, weight, and age can be effective indicators of future injuries (Backe, 2009). Rose (2008) was found out that students with body mass index (BMI) in the 50th to 90th percentiles had the greatest risk of sport injury. It is concluded that factors like location of residence, ethnicity, and BMI were predictors of sports injuries in adolescents. Men with a waist girth greater than 83 cm seem to be at greater risk of developing patellar tendon pathology. There may be both mechanical and biochemical reasons for this increased risk (Malliaras, 2007).

2.2.7 Deterioration of the senses, such as reduced peripheral vision, myopia or hyperopia, can increase the risk of injury when mistakenly judging the location of teammates, of opponents, the position of the ball or other obstacles.

2.2.8 Somatotype or constitutional type.

2.2.9 Strength and constitutional resistance achieved through training, as well as muscle tone and joint stability. The right- and left-hand power was higher for injured athletes in some sports (Dane, 2002).

2.2.10 Basic conditional qualities such as balance, agility, speed and coordination.

2.2.11 Reaction time and timing.

2.2.12 Physical maturity and posture alignment.

2.2.13 Previous injuries and incomplete recovery from the same before returning to train or compete at the desired tempo and intensity. In these cases, the causes of the injuries may persist, the healed tissue might not work with the required efficacy or the injury might not completely heal. Through a multiple logistic regression analysis, Walter (1989) demonstrated that previous injuries are one of the most indicative factors.

2.2.14 Previous and persisting systemic illness, general and local inflammation, chronic illness, rheumatic diseases, and connective tissue diseases, as well as dental cavities and tonsil stones.

2.2.15 Mental and psychological conditions: intelligence, creativity, motivation, discipline, level of distress, previous experience in the same sports activity, the need to take risks, excessive bravado, fervor, strict adherence to rules and fair play.

3. Predictive factors of injuries

When an injury occurs, biomechanical, kinematic, and body composition analyses tend to provide more predictive information than the analyses focused on training intensity, resistance, muscle tone, agility, physical maturity, previous injuries or training methods.

Unevenness in the length of lower limbs, misalignments, anatomical abnormalities, club foot, genu valgum, support type, or posture defects are typically factors cited as injury predictors.

Footprints have also been examined: the average arch, the foot' s plantarflexion and dorsiflexion, excessive pronation, as well as the quadriceps' Q angle.

In this chapter we will also delve into constitutional defects in regards to an ideal constitution.

With the exception of the case of athletics, Watson (1987) states that constitutional and postural defects during practice, as opposed to during sports activities, have not received the attention they deserve. Watson points out the clear relation between postural defects and the risk of sports injuries, although it is difficult to prove and establishes a clear relation between foot anomalies and decompensation in the transmission of force in lower limbs, and future repercussions of injury depending on the player' s dysmorphia.

3.1 The relationship between lower limb structure and sports injuries

Common predisposing factor in injuries to the ankles, legs, knees, and hips include:

Bilateral weight and structural symmetry, Quadriceps and calf girth, patella alta, a kneecap that's higher than usual, Q-angle of the knee (high Q angle: kneecap displaced to one side, as with knock knees), Forefoot varus, Rear foot valgus, true and apparent leg length, uneven leg length, excessive pronation (flat feet), cavus foot (over-high arches), bowlegged or knock-knee alignment.

Uneven leg length may lead to awkward running and increases the chance of injury, but many people with equal-length legs suffer the same effects by running on tilted running tracks or along the side of a road that is higher in the centre. The hip of the leg that strikes the higher surface will suffer more strain.

Pronation is the inward rolling of the foot after the heel strikes the ground, before the weight is shifted forward to the ball of the foot. By rolling inwards, the foot spreads the shock of impact with the ground. If it rolls too easily, however, it can place uneven stress on muscles and ligaments higher in the leg.

While an overly flexible ankle and foot can cause excessive pronation, a too-rigid ankle will cause the effects of cavus foot. Although the arch of the foot itself may be normal, it appears very high because the foot doesn't flatten inwards when weight is placed on it. Such feet are poor shock absorbers and increase the risk of fractures higher in the legs.

Bowlegs or knock knees add extra stress through knees and ankles over time, and may make ankle sprains more likely.

Other structural conditions that make sports injuries more common include **lumbar lordosis.**

Having some muscles that are very strong and others that are weak can lead to injury. If your *quadriceps* (front thigh muscles) are very strong, it can increase the risk of a stretched or torn hamstring (rear thigh muscle). Tight iliotibial bands may be the cause of knee pain for many athletes in running sports.

Overuse injuries are caused by repeated, microscopic injuries to a part of the body. Many long distance runners experience overuse injuries even after years of running. For road runners, the surface is hard and sometimes uneven, and the running movements are repetitive. In addition, there are usually both up- and downhill elements, and these increase the stress on tendons and muscles in the lower leg. You will more likely develop running injuries if you wear the wrong shoes or sneakers. You should use footwear that doesn't allow side-to-side movement of the heel, and that adequately cushions the foot.

Barnes (2008) have not found definitive results that can confirm that constitutional defects are risk factors for injury, while Ferretti (1986) demonstrates that 78% of knee injuries and 50% of spinal column and ankle injuries are closely related to anatomical alteration in static and dynamic foot postures. Regarding these constitutional defects, females could consider themselves at risk due to having a greater articular laxity and less muscle tone, although, at the same time possessing greater coordination, laterality and body outline. Women also have certain anatomical aspects that can contribute to a greater disposition to injury: a wider pelvis, a greater femoral anteversion, less muscle development of the vastus internus in the quadriceps, a smaller intercondylar notch, a greater tendency towards genu valgum and ligament laxity, external tibial torsion and a higher number of misalignments in lower limbs.

4. Logistic regression equations

The purpose of regression techniques is two-fold:
1. **To estimate the relation between two variables** while taking the presence of other factors into account
2. **To construct a model that allows for the prediction of the value of the dependent variable** (in logistic regression, the probability of success) for specific values of a predicted group of variables

4.1 The concept of logistic regression
The benefit of logistic regression no doubt comes from its capacity to analyze clinical and epidemiological research data. The primary objective that this technique accomplishes is modeling how the presence, or absence, of diverse factors and their values influence the probability of the, typically dichotomic, occurrence of an event. This technique can also be used to estimate the probability of the occurrence of an event with more than two (polytomous) categories.

These sorts of situations are approached using regression techniques. Nonetheless, lineal regression methodology is not applicable since the outcome variable only provides two values (we will focus on the dichotomic case), such as the presence/absence of a knee sprain, or the presence/absence of injury.

If we classify the value of the outcome variable as 0 when the event does not occur (the absence of a knee sprain) and as 1 when it does occur (the athlete sprains his or her knee), and we look to calculate the possible relation between the occurrence of a sprained knee and, for example, the difference in the thickness of both thighs (considered a possible risk factor), we could fall into the temptation of using a linear regression:

$$\text{Knee sprain} = a + b * [\text{difference in thigh thickness}] \tag{1}$$

And, based on our data, gauge the coefficients a and b of the equation through the normal procedure of least squares. However, although this is mathematically possible, we arrive at nonsensical results; upon calculating the resulting equation for different values of thigh thickness, we will obtain results that generally differ from 0 and 1, while the only results actually possible in this case are 0 and 1. Since this restriction is not imposed in lineal regression, the outcome can theoretically take on any value.

If we use p as the dependent variable of probability that an athlete suffers a knee sprain, we can build the following equation:

$$\text{Ln}\frac{p}{1-p} \tag{2}$$

now we do have a variable that can take on any value, and we can therefore propose a traditional regression equation in order to find that value:

$$\ln \frac{p}{1-p} = a + b \text{ [difference in thigh thickness]} \tag{3}$$

which, with a slight algebraic manipulation, can be turned into:

$$\text{Injury probability} = \frac{1}{1 + e^{\left[-a - b - \left(\text{difference in thigh thickness}\right)\right]}} \tag{4}$$

And this is exactly the kind of equation known as a logistic model, where the number of factors can be greater than one. Therefore, in the denominator exponent, we could have:

$$b1.\text{difference in thickness} + b2.\text{age} + b3.\text{sex} + b4.\text{height} \tag{5}$$

4.2 Logistic model coefficients as risk quantifiers

One of the factors that make logistic regression so interesting is the relation that logistic model coefficients preserve with a risk quantification parameter known in the field as an "**odds ratio**" .

The odds associated with an event is the quotient of the probability of occurrence given the probability that it does not occur:

$$\text{Odds Ratio} = \frac{p}{1-p} \tag{6}$$

with p being the probability of occurrence. Therefore, we can calculate the odds of an injury occurrence when the difference in thigh thickness is equal to or greater than a specific quantity, which determines how much more probable it is that an injury occurs than if it were not to occur in this situation. Likewise, we could calculate the odds of an injury occurrence when the difference in thigh thickness in less than that same figure. If we divide the first odds by the second, we will have calculated an odds quotient, or an odds ratio, which in some way quantifies how probable the occurrence of an injury is when the difference in thickness is greater than a specific figure (first odds) relative to when the difference in thickness is less. The notion being measured is similar to what we find in the **relative risk,** which corresponds to the probability quotient that an injury occurs when a specific factor is present (difference in thickness) compared to when it is not. In fact, when the prevalence of the event occurring is low (<20 %), the odds value ratio and the relative risk are very similar; but such is not the case when the occurrence of the event is quite common, a fact that is often ignored.

$$\text{Relative Risk} = \frac{\text{Probability of Injury the presence of the risk factor}}{\text{Probability of Injury the absence of the risk factor}} \tag{7}$$

$$\text{Absolute risk Increase} =$$
$$\left(\text{post test probability if risk factors is present}\right) \tag{8}$$
$$-\left(\text{post test probability if risk factors is present}\right)$$

If we have a dichotomic factor in the regression equation, for example if the subject is not a jumper, the b coefficient of the equation for this factor is directly related to the odds ratio OR of being a smoker compared to not being one:

$$OR = \exp(b) \tag{9}$$

where $exp(b)$ is a measurement that quantifies the risk presented when the corresponding factor is present compared to when it is not, assuming that the rest of the model' s variables remain constant.

When the variable is numerical, for example, age or body mass index, it is a measurement that quantifies the change in risk when a variable changes its value while the rest of the variables remain constant. Insomuch, the odds ratio that, in theory, moves from age $X1$ to age $X2$, with b being the coefficient that corresponds to age in the logistic model is:

$$OR = \exp[b * (X2 - X1)] \tag{10}$$

This is a model in which the increase or decrease of risk is proportional to the change in one factor' s value to another. In other words, it is proportional to the difference between the two values, but not to the starting point, meaning that the change in risk, in the logistic model, is the same when we move from 20 years old to 30 years old as when we move from 40 to 50.

When the variable' s coefficient b is positive, we obtain an odds ratio greater than 1 that therefore corresponds to a risk factor. On the other hand, if b is negative the odds ratio will be less than 1 and will correspond to a non-risk factor.

$$\text{Pre-test odds} = \frac{\text{pre-test probability of injury}}{1 - \text{pre-test probability of injury}} \tag{11}$$

$$\text{Pre-test odds} = \text{pre-test odds} \times \text{positive likelihood ratio negative-likelihood ratio} \tag{12}$$

Where

$$\text{positive - likelihood ratio} = \frac{\text{sensitivity}}{(1 - \text{specificity})} \tag{14}$$

$$\text{negative-likelihood ratio} = \frac{(1 - \text{specificity})}{\text{sensitivity}} \tag{15}$$

$$\text{Post-test probability} = \frac{\text{post-test odds}}{(\text{post-test odds} + 1)} \tag{16}$$

4.3 Qualitative variables in the logistic model

Given that the employed methodology for calculations with the logistic model is based on using quantitative variables, the same way as in any other regression process, it is incorrect that qualitative variables are used in regression processes, whether nominal or ordinal variables.

Assigning a number to each category does not solve the problem since the physical exercise variable has three possible answers: sedentary, sporadically performing exercise, frequently performing exercise; and we assign the values 0, 1, 2, respectively, to these variables. But then, performing frequent exercise has twice the value of performing exercise sporadically, which makes little sense. Even more absurd would be if a nominal variable, for example civil status, did not have any ordering relation among the outputs. The solution to this problem is to create as many dichotomic variables as the number of outputs. These new variables, artificially created, are called "*dummy*", or indicator, internal, or design variables. Therefore, if the variable in question produces exposure data with the following outputs: *Never ran, Ex-runner, Runs less than 10 kilometers per day, Runs 10 or more kilometers per day*, we have 4 possible answers from which we will construct 3 dichotomic internal variables (values 0,1) with different possibilities for codification that lead to different interpretations. The most frequent of which is the following:

	I1	I2	I3
Never ran	0	0	0
Ex-runner	1	0	0
Runs less than 10 km per day	0	1	0
Runs 10 or more km per day	0	0	1

Table 1. Design variables.

In this type of codification the regression equation' s coefficient for each design variable (always transformed with the exponential function), corresponds to the odds ratio for this category given the reference level (the first output). In our example, it quantifies how the risk changes given the situation of never having run. There are other possibilities, among which we will highlight an example with a qualitative variable and three outputs:

	I1	I2
Output 1	0	0
Output 2	1	0
Output 3	1	1

Table 2. Qualitative variable and three outputs.

With this codification, each coefficient is interpreted as an average of the change in risk upon moving from one category to the next. In the event that a category cannot naturally be considered a reference level, for example blood group, a possible classification system is:

	I1	I2
Output 1	-1	-1
Output 2	1	0
Output 3	0	1

Table 3. Classification system of category not natural.

Where each coefficient of the indicator variables has a direct interpretation as a change in risk regarding the average of the three outputs.

4.4 How to present logistic regression results
It is common to present logistic regression results in a table wherein each variable will be shown with a coefficient value, its standard error, a parameter (labeled *chi² Wald*), which allows us to check if the coefficient is significantly different from 0 and check the p value for this context. It also allows us to check the odds ratio of each variable, together with its confidence interval for 95% reliability.

Term	Coeff.	Stand. Err.	chi²	p	Interpretation
Indepen.	-1.2168	0.9557	1.621	0.2029	NO
Age	-0.0465	0.0374	1.545	0.2138	NO
Race *			* 5.684	0.0583	Almost (p < 0.1)
Race 1	1.0735	0.5151	4.343	0.0372	p < 0.05
Race 2	0.8154	0.4453	3.353	0.0671	Almost (p < 0.1)
Runner	0.8072	0.4044	3.983	0.0460	p < 0.05
Injury	1.4352	0.6483	4.902	0.0268	p < 0.05
Dissymmetry	0.6576	0.4666	1.986	0.1587	NO
Q Angle	0.8421	0.4055	4.312	0.0379	p < 0.05
Thigh Thickness	1.2817	0.4621	7.692	0.0055	p < 0.01

Table 4. Example of Logistic Regression Presentation.

Variable	Odds ratio	OR < 95%	OR > 95%
Age	0.95	0.89	1.03
Race 1	2.93	1.07	8.03
Race 2	2.26	0.94	5.41
Runner	2.24	1.01	4.95
Injury	4.20	1.18	14.97
Dissymmetry	1.93	0.77	4.82
Q Angle	2.32	1.05	5.14
Thigh Thickness	3.60	1.46	8.91

Table 5. Odds Ratio.

4.5 Goodness of fit
As long as we are dealing with a regression model, it is fundamental that the model be checked for an appropriate adjustment to the data used in the calculation before drawing conclusions (Bender, 1996).
In the case of logistic regression, a rather intuitive idea is to calculate the probability of an event, the occurrence of an injury or knee sprain in our case, for all athletes from the sampling. If the goodness of fit is acceptable, one would expect a high probability value to

be associated with the presence of an injury, and vice-versa, if the calculated probability value is low, one would likewise expect the absence of injury.

This intuitive idea is formally realized through the Hosmer-Lemeshow test , that basically consists in dividing the range of probability in deciles of risk (which would be injury probability ≤ 0.1, ≤ 0.2, and so forth up to ≤ 1) and calculating the distribution of both injured athletes as well as uninjured athletes that are calculated in the equation and actually observed. These distributions, both calculated and observed, contrast with each other through a chi^2 test.

In the final presentation of logistic regression data, a goodness of fit test should be included as well as a commented conclusion drawn from the same test. With these, the Hosmer-Lemeshow test would be more illustrative than the mere obtained distribution values.

5. Logistic regression equation and logistic regression analysis

Despite the fact that accidents are unavoidable in sports, injury prediction and prevention is a practical aspect of sports medicine considered to be the best treatment. Regression models encompass mathematical techniques that deal with measuring the relation between an outcome variable and predictive variables. When the outcome variable is continuous, the preferred model is logistic regression. However, when the outcome variable is dichotomic (injured/not injured) and the object of study is the relation between this and one or more predictive variables (right Q angle, left Q angle, the difference in thigh thickness, lower limb dissymmetry, age, sex, hours of training, kilometers run, etc...) the chosen regression model is a simple logistic regression model (for one factor) or a multiple logistic regression model (for more than one factor).

Therefore, the logistic regression analysis technique is used when it is suspected that one of the values of specific categorical variables depends on a series of predictive or independent variables, along with the goal of finding a mathematical function that expresses such a relation.

When the goal is to calculate the relation or association between two variables, the regression models allow for the consideration that there may be other factors that affect this relation.

So, if the possible relation between lower limb dissymmetry and the probability of suffering a knee injury is being studied as a risk factor, that relation can be different if other variables are taken into account such as age, sex, or body mass index. Because of this, these factors could be included in a logistic regression model as independent variables in addition to dissymmetry. In the resulting equation when considering *DISYMMETRY, AGE, SEX*, and *BMI* as independent variables, the *exp* (coefficient of the equation for *DISYMMETRY*) gives us the **adjusted or controlled odds ratio for the rest of the factors**, given the data for DISSYMETRY.

The other variables, in addition to the interest factor (in this example *AGE, SEX, BMI*), are called by several names: control variables, external variables, covariants, or **confounding variables**.

Interaction

When the relation between the factor being studied and the dependent variable is modified by the value of a third variable, we are then dealing with interaction. In our example, we assume that the probability of suffering **a sports injury** increases with age when there is lower limb dissymmetry. In this case we decide that there is an interaction between the variables of *AGE* and *DISSYMETRY*.

If we focus only on the logistic model exponent, without considering interaction, we would have:

$$-b_0 - b_1 * DISSYMETRY - b_2 * AGE \qquad (17)$$

If we want to consider the interaction between INJURY and AGE, the model changes:

$$-b_0 - b_1 * DISSYMETRY - b_2 * AGE - b_3 * DISSYMETRY * AGE \qquad (18)$$

If the variable for *DISSYMETRY* is dichotomic (values 0 and 1), the relation between *INJURY* and *DISSYMETRY* will end up quantified by b1 in the first model while in the second...

$$-(b_1 + b_2 * AGE) * DISSYMETRY \qquad (19)$$

In other words, the relation is modified in function of the value of *AGE*.

5.1 Precautions

The wide availability of programs that allow access to sophisticated statistical tests can lead to the improper and merely mechanical usage of these tests. Regression models require that the model constructor possess at least a minimal knowledge of the model's underlying philosophy, as well as not only a knowledge of the advantages of this technique, but also of its problems and shortcomings. The use of mathematical processes often convinces us that we are observing "objective" results, and to an extent this is true. However these techniques also carry an intrinsic subjectivity from the selection of a mathematical model to the selection of the variables inserted in that model

5.1.1 Independent variable and probability direction

One of the first considerations we must take into account is that the relation between the independent variable and the event probability doesn't change direction. In such a case, the logistic model doesn't work for us. This is something that does not typically occur in clinical studies, but because of that same fact, it is easier to ignore when it does occur.

A very clear example of this situation arises when we evaluate the probability of an athlete's sports injuries in relation to the age when he or she first began sports competitions. Up to a certain age, the probability can increase as the age at which the athlete began competing is earlier. And starting from a mature age, the likelihood of injury also increases compared to the older age at which an athlete competes. In this case, a logistic model would be inadequate.

5.1.2 Collinearity

Another problem that may arise in regression models, and not only logistic models, is that the variables involved may be correlated, which would lead us to a nonsensical model and therefore to some values of the coefficients that cannot be interpreted. This situation, with correlated independent variables, is called collinearity.

In order to understand it, let's look at an extreme case in which the same variable is introduced in the model twice. We would then have:

$$\exp(-b0 - b1 * X - b2 * X) \qquad (20)$$

or

$$\exp\left[-b0 - (b1 + b2) * X\right] \tag{21}$$

Where the sum of b1+b2 allows infinite possibilities when the value of a coefficient is divided into two addends, and therefore the calculation obtained from b1 and b2 doesn't make sense.

An example of this situation could be given if we include variables such as the length of the lower limbs and the length of the calves in the equation, two variables that are closely correlated.

5.1.3 Sample size

As a basic rule, it is necessary to have at least 10 participants, or $(k + 1)$ cases to estimate a model with k independent variables; in other words, at least 10 cases for each dependent variable (the probability of the event).

It is useful to point out that the qualitative variables appear as $c - 1$ variables in the model, when constructing the corresponding internal variables based on the qualitative variables.

5.1.4 Model selection

When talking about models that can be multivariable, an interesting topic is how to choose the best set of independent variables to include in the model (Tsigilis, 2005)

The definition of the "best" model depends on the type and objective of the study. In a case where something will be predicted, the best model would be one that produces the most reliable predictions. And in a case where the relation between two variables is being calculated (correcting the effect of other variables), the best model will be one that obtains the most precise calculation of the coefficient of the variable in question. This is often forgotten and leads to completely different model strategies. Therefore, in the second case a covariant with a statistically significant coefficient, but whose inclusion in the equation does not modify the value of the coefficient of the variable in question, will be excluded from the equation since it doesn't deal with the confounding factor: the relation between the variable in question and the probability are not modified if that variable is taken into account. However, if the outcome of a predictive model is included in the equation, then we look for more reliable predictions.

5.1.5 Types of differences

Whenever data in analyzed, it is important to distinguish between numerical differences, statistically significant differences, and clinically relevant differences. These three concepts do not always coincide.

5.1.6 Number of variables

The first thing one must consider is the **maximum model,** or the maximum number of independent variables that can be included in the equation, while taking their interactions into account when appropriate.

Although there are different processes for choosing a model, there are only three basic mechanisms for doing so: start with only one independent variable and, one by one, add more according to the pre-established criteria (forward-moving process). Or also, starting with the maximum model, eliminate the variables one by one according to a pre-established criteria (reverse-moving process). The third method, called "*stepwise*", combines the two previous mechanisms and, in each step, a variable already present in the equation can be eliminated or another can be added.

In the case of logistic regression, the criteria for deciding if we should choose a new model or stay with the currently used one at each step is established by the **models' likelihood ratio logarithm**.

5.1.7 The likelihood equation

A model's likelihood equation is a measurement of how compatible the model is with the actual outcome data. If upon adding a new variable to the model, the likelihood does not increase in a statistically significant way, then that variable will not be included in the equation.

To evaluate the statistical significance of a particular variable within the model, we will focus on the Wald chi2 value corresponding to the variable's coefficient and on its level of probability.

5.1.8 Sports monitoring

To develop this equation it is necessary to perform a prior monitoring of a representative group of athletes taking into account their age, sex, and sport during a sufficiently long observation period that could be called a season. During this period it is crucial to differentiate the subjects into two groups: injured and non-injured.

Consequently, the relation between the different measured variables and the final outcome of injury or no-injury is established.

In order to determine the predictive variables, we should identify those that show significant differences among the two groups, thus establishing the relation between the injury/no injury dependent variable given the distinct anthropometric and sports variables (activity time, training time, team position, etc...).

5.1.9 Sensitivity, specificity, positive predictive value and negative predictive value

It is useful to use control techniques to evaluate the fit of the outcome results. With the mathematical equations defined in the logistic regression analysis. The results should be analyzed in all studied subjects, for the studied group of athletes in question, and for a control group of both sexes and differentiating the success rate by sex.

5.1.9.1 Sensitivity

Proportion of injured subjects in relation to how many the equation predicted would be injured.

$$Sensitivity\,(Sn) = \frac{True\,Positive}{(True\,Positive + False\,Negative)} \qquad (22)$$

The following table summarizes these calculations:

	POSITIVE TEST (T+)	NEGATIVE TEST (T-)
INJURY PRESENT (I+)	TRUE POSITIVE (TP)	FALSE NEGATIVE (FN)
INJURY ABSENT (I-)	FALSE POSITIVE (FP)	TRUE NEGATIVE (TN)

Table 6. Sensitivity.

$$Sn = P\,[T^+ \text{ if } D^+]\tag{23}$$

$$Sn = \frac{TP}{(TP + FN)}\tag{24}$$

5.1.9.2 Specificity

Proportion of uninjured subjects in relation to how many the equation predicted would not be injured.

$$Specificity(Sp) = \frac{True\ Negative}{(True\ Negative + False\ Positive)}\tag{25}$$

You can think of specificity as 1- the false positive rate. Notice what the denominator for specificity is the number of healthy players. Using conditional probabilities, we can also define specificity as:

$$Sp = P[Test\ is\ negative\ if\ Patient\ is\ healthy]\tag{26}$$

$$Sp = P\left[T^- if\ I^-\right]\tag{27}$$

The following table summarizes these calculations:

	POSITIVE TEST (T+)	NEGATIVE TEST (T-)
INJURY PRESENT (I+)	TRUE POSITIVE (TP)	FALSE NEGATIVE (FN)
INJURY ABSENT (I-)	FALSE POSITIVE (FP)	TRUE NEGATIVE (TN)

Table 7. Specificity.

$$Sp = P\,[T^- \text{ if } D^-]\tag{28}$$

$$Sp = \frac{TN}{(TN + FP)}\tag{29}$$

5.1.9.3 False positives

Proportion of uninjured subjects in relation to how many the equation predicted would be injured.

5.1.9.4 False negatives

Proportion of injured subjects in relation to how many the equation predicted would not be injured.

In order to know the probability of whether or not a subject injures him or herself in relation to the outcome injury ratio, we must know the positive predictive values (PPV) and the negative predictive values (NPV) that should be defined as the following:

Positive predictive values: The probability of an athlete injuring him or herself when predicted by the equation. To calculate this we use the equation:

$$PPV = \frac{(S*PL)}{(S*PL)(FL*PNL)} \qquad (30)$$

Where S: Sensitivity. PL: Probability of injury. FP: False Positives. PNL: Probability of non-injury.

The following table summarizes these calculations

	POSITIVE TEST (T+)	NEGATIVE TEST (T-)
INJURY PRESENT (I+)	TRUE POSITIVE (TP)	FALSE NEGATIVE (FN)
INJURY ABSENT (I-)	FALSE POSITIVE (FP)	TRUE NEGATIVE (TN)

Table 8. False negatives.

$$PPV = P\,[I^+ \text{ if } T^+] \qquad (31)$$

$$PPV = \frac{TP}{(TP + FP)} \qquad (32)$$

Negative predictive values: The probability that the athlete does not injure him or herself when the model has predicted a situation of non-injury. To calculate this we use the equation:

$$NPV = \frac{(E*PNL)}{(E*PNL)+(FN*PL)} \qquad (33)$$

	POSITIVE TEST (T+)	NEGATIVE TEST (T-)
INJURY PRESENT (I+)	TRUE POSITIVE (TP)	FALSE NEGATIVE (FN)
INJURY ABSENT (I-)	FALSE POSITIVE (FP)	TRUE NEGATIVE (TN)

Table 9. Negative predictive values.

$$NPV = P\,[I^- \text{ if } T^-] \qquad (34)$$

$$NPV = \frac{TN}{(TN + FN)} \qquad (35)$$

Where S: Sensitivity. PL: Probability of injury. FP: False Positives. PNL: Probability of non-injury.

It is always necessary to find false negatives and positives beforehand, as well as the probability of injury or non-injury for each athlete before determining the positive and negative predictive values.

In order to perform this type of calculation, the probability that an individual exhibits the characteristic in question (suffering an injury) is expressed in function of the predictive variable or variables; if we make P the probability, the model is expressed as follows:

$$P = \beta_0 + \beta_1 X \qquad (36)$$

Where β_0 y β_1 are the model parameters and X is the predictive variable. The probability (P) is equal to a constant β_0 plus the product of the other constant β_1 multiplied by the value of the predictive variable X.

The coefficient β_0 is an independent or constant term and it is the value of the outcome variable's average. The coefficient β_1 is the regression coefficient and it is interpreted as the change in the outcome variable's average by the unit of increase of the predictive variable. The change will be an increase if the regression coefficient value is positive and it will be a decrease if the value is negative.

It is possible that once the model parameters are calculated, the substitution of some values of the predictive variable gives way to values that aren't allowed for a probability. This is why one should perform a probability transformation for the probability of showing the characteristics in question. This logit transformation that consists in the logarithmic odd $\dfrac{p}{1-p}$ that a characteristic will present itself, is modeled by the following formula:

$$Log \left[\frac{p}{1-p} \right] = \beta_0 + \beta_1 X \tag{37}$$

$$The\ Log \left[\frac{p}{1-p} \right] is\ called\ logit\ (P) \tag{38}$$

In the logistic regression model, the coefficient $\beta 1$ is the logarithm of the odds ratio (OR) between two individuals that are differentiated in a unit in terms of the predictive variable. Likewise, by raising e to β_1, we obtain the OR value between those two individuals.

$$Log\ (O.R.) = \beta_1 \tag{39}$$

Or:

$$O.R. = e^{\beta 1} \tag{40}$$

where e is the number that serves as the base of the Napierian logarithm, approximately 2.72.

In the logistic regression model, β_1 is the OR logarithm between two individuals that are differentiated in a unit in terms of the predictive variable, or likewise, by raising e to β_1, one obtains the OR value between these two individuals. In the case where $\beta_1=0$, it is implied that the logit(P)= β_0 + (0) X= 0, in other words, it does not change with X. Or equally, O.R. = e^0 = 1, which indicates that the two variables are independent and there is no relation between them. The calculation of β_1 is called the logistic regression coefficient.

If we have several predictive variables and we try to study the relation between the outcome variable and the whole set of predictive variables simultaneously, a multiple logistic regression model will be used.

$$Log \left[\frac{p}{1-p} \right] = \beta_0 + \beta_1 X + ... + \beta p\ Xp \tag{41}$$

where P is also the probability of presenting the characteristic in question.

An alternative form of presenting the same model is:

$$P = \frac{e^{\left(\beta_0 + \beta_1 + \ldots + \beta_p X_p\right)}}{1 + e^{\left(\beta_0 + \beta_1 + \ldots + \beta_p X_p\right)}} \tag{42}$$

Which allows the calculation of the probability that an individual with certain predictive values will exhibit the characteristic in question.

5.2 Logistic regression equations applied to sports
5.2.1 Shambaugh injury score

Shambaugh (1991) proposed the first logistic regression equation that would predict injuries occurring within a season with 91% accuracy. The variables initially proposed were the diameter of the thigh, diameter of the calf, the Q angle, ankle dorsiflexion, genu varum and valgum, the difference in supported weight, and the length of the legs. Ankle dorsiflexion and varum were more elevated in uninjured players, and therefore we reject them in the final equation.

When the outcome of the equation was positive, the subject was predicted to be at risk for injury. But one equation with so many relative coefficients and too many collateral effects was, aside from being difficult to design, too complicated to be reliable.

Shambaugh determined that there should only be three dependent variables selected, and since one of the fundamental goals was to find structural asymmetries or imbalances, he opted for the Q angle of the knees and the difference in supported weight between both legs, resulting in the following equation, applicable only to males:

SHAMBAUGH injury score (1991) =

$$\left(\begin{array}{l}\text{imbalance in bilateral weight* .36+right abnormal Q angle*0.48+} \\ \text{left abnormal Q angle*0.86}\end{array}\right) -7.04 \tag{43}$$

considering the weight imbalance between the right and left leg to be an absolute value and the abnormality of the Q angle for males beginning at $10°$.

The value of the Shambaugh score would be directly proportional to the possibility of injury; the higher the score was, the greater the probability of including the athlete in the injury category. There was a 95% success rate. The player that obtained a higher score was also the one who incurred the most serious injury.

Grubbs (1997) studied the Shambaugh score in relation to its predictive value, calculating the statistical values of sensitivity, specificity and positive and negative prediction in men as well as women. Its results were less outstanding, upon inclusion of results for women, the abnormality value of the Q angle in women was set at $15°$.

In 2000 he proposed a modification to his injury score, introducing 4 variables instead of the three original ones in his logistic regression equation. The new variable was the squared value of the difference between thigh thickness:

SHAMBAUGH Injury Score (2000) =

Weight Imbalance * 0.27 + 1.46 * $\left(\text{Difference in thigh thickness}\right)^2$

+ 0.22 * Difference in the Q angle of both knees

+ 0.94 * Right abnormal Q angle - 6.46. \hfill (44)

5.2.2 Salazar injury score (Salazar, 2000)

Salazar (2000) expanded on the Shambaugh injury score by including data from exposure to injury at practice, training time, and game play time. He used the control sheets created by DeLee (1992):

$$\text{SALAZAR INJURY PROBABILITY SCORE} = \frac{1}{1 + e^{(0.1621 - 0.06344 * average\ Shambaugh\ score)}} \quad (45)$$

5.2.3 Fernández-de la cruz injury score (Fernández-Martínez, 2008)

$$\text{FERNANDEZ} - \text{DE LA CRUZ DE INJURY PROBABILITY SCORE} = \frac{1}{1 + e^{-\left(0.757 * AQI - 0.647 * DGM^2\right)}} \quad (46)$$

where AQI is the left knee Q angle and DGM^2 is the squared value of the difference in thigh thickness, demonstrating a 72.9% success rate for injury prediction (positive prediction at 75.68%; negative prediction at 70.73%). This equation is applicable to men as well as to women. The overall percentage of correct classification was 68.6%. The cutoff point (0.5) indicates that the subjects with values equal to or greater than 0.5 would be placed in the "at risk" category, while a value less than the cutoff point would place them in the "reduced risk for injury" category.

6. Conclusion

Logistic regression equations allow injury prediction for athletes, risk calculation, and the opportunity for establishing the most effective and appropriate measures to be taken. Its versatility and capacity for being applied to specific sports groups allows personalized attention for each group.

This chapter shows that the logistic regression analysis can be used as a valid method in determining anthropometric parameters related to sports injuries, while providing a reliable and simple method that can be used in the common practice of sports medicine.

7. References

Andersen, J. C. (2005). Stretching Before and After Exercise: Effect on Muscle Soreness and Injury Risk. *Journal of Athletic Training*, Vol. 40 Issue 3, 218-220. ISSN 1062-6050.

Arnold, Brent L.; Doherty, Carrie L. (2006). Low-Load Eversion Force Sense, Self-Reported Ankle Instability, and Frequency of Giving Way. *Journal of Athletic Training*, Vol. 41 Issue 3, 233- 239. ISSN 1062-6050.

Backe, S.; Ericson, L.; Janson, S.; Timpka, T. (2009). Rock climbing injury rates and associated risk factors in a general climbing population.. *Scandinavian Journal of Medicine & Science in Sports*, Vol. 19 Issue 6, 850- 856. ISSN 0905-7188

Barber Foss, Kim D.; Ford, Kevin A.; Myer, Gregory D.; Hewett, Timothy E. (2009). Generalized Joint Laxity Associated With Increased Medial Foot Loading in Female Athletes. *Journal of Athletic Training*, Vol. 44 Issue 4, 356- 362. . ISSN 1062-6050.

Barnes, A.; Wheat, J.; Milner, C. (2008) Association between foot type and tibial stress injuries: a systematic review. *British Journal of Sports Medicine*. Vol. 42 Issue 2, 93- 98. ISSN 0306-3674.

Bender, R.; Grouves, U. (1996) Logistis regression models used in medical researchare poorly presented. *British Medical Journal*. 313, 628 ISSN: 0959- 8138.

Bowers, Andrea L.; Spindler, Kurt P.; McCarty, Eric C.; Arrigain, Susana (2005). Height, Weight, and BMI Predict Intra-articular Injuries Observed During ACL Reconstruction: Evaluation of 456 Cases From a Prospective ACL Database. *Clinical Journal of Sport Medicine*: Vol. 15 Issue 1. p. 9-13. ISSN 1536-3724.

Cain, L.; Nicholson, L.; Adams, R.; Burns, J. (2007) Foot morphology and foot/ankle injury in indoor football. *Journal of Science & Medicine in Sport* . Vol. 10 Issue 5. p. 311-319. ISSN 1440-2440.

Dane, S.; Can, S.; Karsan, O. (2002). Relations of body mass index, body fat, and power of various muscles to sport injuries. *Perceptual & Motor Skills*: Vol. 95 Issue 1. p. 329-334. ISSN 0031-5125.

Dixon, W.J. Brown,M.B.; Engelman, L. and Jennerich, R.I. (1993). *BMDP Statistical Software Manual, 1992 Edition, 3 Volume set*. pp 1105- 45. University of California Press. ISBN 978-05-2008-141-3. Berkeley.

Fernández, A.; De la Cruz-Márquez, JC.; Cueto-Martín,B.; Salazar Alonso, S.; De la Cruz-Campos, J.C. (2008). Predicción de lesiones deportivas mediante ecuaciones de regresión logística. Apunts Medicina de l`sport, 157- 41-44. ISSN: 1886- 6581.

Ferrara, C.M.; Hollingsworth, E. (2007) Physical Characteristics and Incidence of Injuries in Adult Figure Skaters. *International Journal of Sports Physiology & Performance*, Vol. 2 Issue 3, 282- 291. ISSN 1555-0265.

Ferretti , A. *(1986) Epidemiology of jumper's knee. Sports Medicine.; 3:289–95.* ISSN: 1179-2035.

Finkelstein, E.A.; Hong Chen; Prabhu, M; Trogdon, J.G.; Corso, P.S. (2007) The Relationship Between Obesity and Injuries among U.S. Adults. *American Journal of Health Promotion*, Vol. 21 Issue 5, 460- 468. ISSN 0890-1171.

Gaida J, Cook J, Bass S, *Austen S.; Kiss, Z.S. (2004)* Are unilateral and bilateral patellar tendinopathy distinguished by differences in anthropometry, body composition, or muscle strength in elite female basketball players? *British Journal of Sports Medicine*. 38:581–5. ISSN 0306-3674.

Gissane, Conor; White, John; Kerr, Kathleen; Jennings, Deanna (2001) An operational model to investigate contact sports injuries. *Medicine & Science in Sports & Exercise*: Vol 33 - Issue 12 - pp 1999-2003. ISSN 0195-9131.

Grubbs, N.; Nelson, R.T.; Bandy, W.D. (1997) Predictive validity of an injury score among high school basketball players.., *Medicine & Science in Sports & Exercise* Oct 1997: Vol. 29 Issue 10. 1279-1285. ISSN 0195-9131.

Heiderscheit, B.C.; Hamil, J.; Van Emmerrik, R (1999) Q-angle influences on the variability of lower extremity coordination during running. *Medicine Science and Sport Exercise*, 31, 1313- 1319 ISSN: 1530- 0315.

Herbert RD, Gabriel M. (2002) Effects of stretching before and after exercise on muscle soreness and risk of injury: systematic review. British Medical Joutnal.325:468. ISSN 0959-8138.

Howard, J.S.; Briggs, D. (2006) The Arch-Height-Index Measurement System: A New Method of Foot Classification. *Athletic Therapy Today*, Vol. 11 Issue 5, 56-57. ISSN 1078-7895.

Kraemer, R.; Knobloch, K. (2009) A Soccer-Specific Balance Training Program for Hamstring Muscle and Patellar and Achilles Tendon Injuries: An Intervention Study in Premier League Female Soccer., American Journal of Sports Medicine, Vol. 37 Issue 7, 1384- 1394. ISSN 0363-5465.

Inklaar, E.; Bol, E.; Schmikli, S.L.; Mosterd, W.L. (1996) Injuries in male soccer players: team risk analysis. International Journalof Sports Medicine, 17, 229- 234. ISSN: 0172- 4622.

Lian O, Engebretsen L, Ovrebo RV, Bahr, R. (1996) Characteristics of the leg extensors in male volleyball players with jumper's knee. American Journal of Sports Medicine; 24:380–5. ISSN 0363-5465.

Lian O, Refsnes P, Engebretsen L, Bahr, R. (2003) Performance characteristics of volleyball players with patellar tedinopathy. American Journal of Sports Medicine, 31:408–13. ISSN 0363-5465.

Lowry, R.; Lee, S. M.; Galuska, D. A.; Fulton, J. E.; Barrios, L. C.; Kann, L. (2007) Physical Activity-Related Injury and Body Mass Index Among US High School Students. Journal of Physical Activity & Health. Vol. 4 Issue 3, 325- 342. ISSN 1543-3080.

Malliaras, P.; Cook, J.L.; Kent, P.M. (2007) Anthropometric risk factors for patellar tendon injury among volleyball players. British Journal of Sports Medicine. Vol. 41 Issue 4. 259-263. ISSN 0306-3674.

Mark F. (2006) Exercise-Related Leg Pain in Female Collegiate Athletes The Influence of Intrinsic and Extrinsic Factors. American Journal of Sports Medicine: Vol. 34 Issue 9. pp. 1500-1507. ISSN 0363-5465.

Mechelen, V. (1999). Lesiones en el atletismo. In: Prácticas clínicas sobre asistencia y prevención de lesiones deportivas. Renströn, P.A. Paidotribo Publisher. pp: 479- 506. ISBN: 978- 84- 8019- 420-4. Barcelona.

Meyers, M.C. and Barnhill, B.S. (2004). Incidence, Causes, and Severity of High School Football Injuries on FieldTurf Versus Natural Grass. A 5-Year Prospective Study. American Journal of Sports Medicine., 32, 1626-1638. ISSN 0363-5465.

Plisky, M. S.; Rauh, M. J.; Heiderscheit, B.; Underwood, F.B.; Tank, R.T. (2007) Medial Tibial Stress Syndrome in High School Cross-Country Runners: Incidence and Risk Factors.. Journal of Orthopaedic & Sports Physical Therapy, Vol. 37 Issue 2, 40- 47. ISSN: 0190-6011.

Rose, M. S.; Emery, C.A.; Meeuwisse, W.H (2008) Sociodemographic Predictors of Sport Injury in Adolescents. Medicine & Science in Sports & Exercise. Vol. 40 Issue 3, 444- .450. ISSN: 0195-9131

Salazar, S. (2000). Aplicación del Índice de Shambaugh en jugadores/as de baloncesto cadetes y júnior en relación con la exposición práctica. Doctoral Thesis. University of Granada. Spain.

Shaffer, S.W.; Uhl, T. L. (2006) Preventing and Treating Lower Extremity Stress Reactions and Fractures in Adults. Journal of Athletic Training. Vol. 41 Issue 4, 466- 470. ISSN: 1062-6050.

Shambaugh, J.; Klein, A.; Herbert, J. (1991). Structural measures as predictors of injury in basketball players. Medicine & Science in Sports & Exercise , 23, 522- 527. ISSN 0195-9131.

Tate, A.; Petruzello, S (1995). Varying the intensity of acute exercise: implications for change in affect. Journal of Sports Medicine and Physical Fitness, 35, 295- 302. ISSN 0022- 4707.

Tsigilis, N.; Hatzimanouil, D. (2005) Injuries in handball: Examination of the risk factors. European Journal of Sport Science. Vol. 5 Issue 3, 137- 142. ISSN: 1536-7290.

Walter, S.D.; Hart, L.; McIntosh, J. (1989) The Ontario cohort study of running related injuries. Archives of Internal Medicine, 149, 2561- 64. ISSN 0003- 9926.

Watson, M. Paul, P. (1987) Incidence of injuries in high school track and field athletes and its relation to performance ability. American Journal of Sports Medicine, 15, 251-54. ISSN 0363-5465.

4

Intervention Strategies in the Prevention of Sports Injuries From Physical Activity

Luis Casáis and Miguel Martínez

Faculty of Education and Sport Sciences, University of Vigo
Spain

1. Introduction

Injuries are a serious problem in the training-competition process, since their occurrence leads to the modification or interruption of the activity. Any injury alters training plans and is an important factor in training monitoring. Within the sports community, the most common intervention focuses on recovering from injuries in order to return to previous performance levels; a process that is expensive from both the economic and sporting points of view. However, in many sports, strategies aimed at injury prevention have not been systematically implemented, despite their proven effectiveness. The present chapter reviews some of preventive programs that must be incorporated in training schedules to minimize the impact of injuries. With regard to the introduction of intervention strategies in sport, through preventive measures from physical activity, it is necessary to review the power of the proposed measures and assess their effectiveness. There are numerous published papers on the subject, although it requires a careful study of them, both from the standpoint of methodology as adequacy of proposals, so as to adequately inform such interventions.

2. Multifactorial analysis of the model for injury prevention

One of the most important aspects of training and competition would be the control of the process and its development. The control of training comprehends all the aspects that permit the adaptation of the contents and the training load. One of the reasons why the modification of training programs becomes necessary is sports injuries, as they generate a partial or total interruption of the training process. It is a fact that is practically usual in the majority of sports, as a great number of sportsmen and women injury themselves at least once a season (Bahr & Krosshaug, 2005; Van Mechelen et al., 1992). The injuries constitute set-backs, which cannot be totally avoided, as the mere practice of sports carries with it the risk of injury happening. However, their impact could be lessened through the monitoring, controlling and analysing of the factors and their evolution by using adequate means of control.

The objective would be to ensure that the risk is lessened (prevention) or that its evolution is more favourable, and to ensure the incorporation of the sportsperson in as little time as possible (functional recuperation). Until a few years ago, efforts were centred on treating injure, paying special attention to the therapeutic process from a clinical perspective. However, in the last few years interest has become directed towards the development of strategies and multidisciplinary proposals related to the prevention of and the recovery from sports injuries. Therefore, the intervention performed presents a model of general control, which includes a global evaluation of the specific sporting context (sport, characteristics of the sportsperson, training conditions, etc.), an adequate prevention in the face of multiple factors of injury predisposition (multifactorial model), and a systematic effort in case of the injure appearing, guaranteeing a full recovery.

2.1 Sequence of prevention

To establish a plan of prevention one must begin with Van Mechelen et al.´s proposal (1992) in a sequence of four steps: establishing the extent of the injury, identifying the factors and mechanisms of injury, introducing preventive measures and, lastly, evaluating their effectiveness (Figure 1). The last few decades have seen a significant increase in the epidemical studies contributing information on the first two steps: identifying injury incidence in each sport, along with the factors and mechanism involved in the production of the injuries, as well as establishing the possible factors provoking the injury, upon which to act in a preventive manner. To understand the importance of the problem it is necessary to know the injury profile for the different sports: injury frequency (number of injuries per 1,000 hours of training or competition), location of the different body structures, severity, typology and the rest of relevant aspects (Fuller et al., 2006). Meeuwisse (1994) developed a model to explain the different risk factors involved in producing sports injuries, rejecting approaches involving an only factor.

Model/Stage	TRIPP (Finch, 2006)	Van Mechelen et al. (1992)
1	Injury surveillance	Establishing extent of the problem
2	Establishing aetiology and mechanisms of injury	Establishing aetiology and mechanisms of injury
3	Developing preventive measures	Introducing preventive measures
4	"Ideal conditions"/scientific evaluation	Assessing their effectiveness by repeating stage 1
5	Describing intervention context to inform implementation strategies	
6	Evaluating effectiveness of preventive measures in implementation context	

Fig. 1. The "sequence of prevention" of sports injuries (Van Mechelen et al., 1992) and The Translating Research into Injury Prevention Practice, TRIPP (Finch, 2006)

Later, this proposal is completed by showing the complex interaction of the internal and external risk factors and the mechanisms that cause sports injuries (Parkkari et al., 2001). In recent years, the theoretical framework of research has been expanded with contributions from Finch (2006), increasing the number of steps in the sequence of prevention to the implementation and evaluation of injury prevention in a real context.

These injuries are associated to a series of risk factors that need to be identified so as to introduce preventive measures in training (Figure 2). This factors are classified in intrinsic factors (predisposal of the sportsperson) and extrinsic factors (exposal to factors of risk), although in reality the process indicates that these factors are produced in a complex manner and they interact between them (Larson et al., 1996; Murphy et al., 2003; Peterson & Renström, 1988).

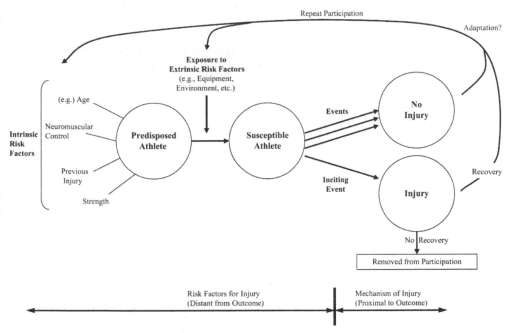

Fig. 2. Recursive model of aetiology in sport injury (Meeuwisse, 2007).

Among the most important intrinsic factors would be the existence of a previous injury and inadequate rehabilitation, age, the sportsperson's state of health, psychological state and aspects, etc. With regard to extrinsic factors, these are: type of activity and motive gestures specific to the sport, dynamics of the training load, training and competition exposition time, material and equipment, type of surface of the playing, environmental conditions and anatomic fatigue (Galambos et al., 2005; Junge & Dvorak, 2000).

Once the most frequent injuries of each modality and their risk factors are known, preventive measures can be introduced (Figure 3). The efficiency of these measures and their suitability from the methodological point of view (Finch, 2006; Shepard, 2005) are known beforehand. The prevention programs should be evaluated through more rigorous designs, with not only random experimental designs of group control, but also quasi-experimental designs that permit more representative samples (professional sportspeople) and more realistic practice contexts (training – competition processes), with truly ideal intervention programmes. Only in this way can the efficiency of the preventive intervention in sports be evaluated (Junge & Dvorak, 2004).

2.2 Different levels of sports injury prevention
2.2.1 Primary Level
The objective of the Primary Level of prevention is to avoid injury before it happens. It consists of a general preventive intervention taking into account the general factors and

mechanisms characteristic of a given person and their effect on a sportsperson with an injury risk. This level implies a change in beliefs, attitude, habits and behaviour towards prevention, and their training by both coaches and sportspeople.

The main measures are of an indirect type: they will control the type, quality and state of the training grounds and competition surfaces; the type of footwear that respects cushioning, traction and rotation upon the field; the use of protective elements; the organization of travel; sleeping and eating habits; the use of tapping as a possible factor in reducing ligamentous affectations; or hydration, controlling the number and quantity of liquid intake and the combination with other sports drinks.

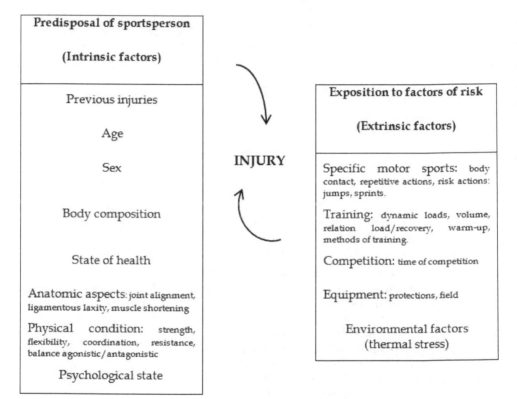

Fig. 3. Factors related to the occurrence of sports injuries (adapted from Bahr & Krosshaug, 2005; Meeuwisse, 1994; Parkkari et al, 2001; San Román, 2005).

2.2.2 Secondary Level

The Secondary Level of prevention constitutes an early level of detection in which intervention takes place in the stages immediately previous to injury or when it has already happened. At this level, one must be in contact with the sportsperson in risk of injury with the objective of diagnosing and detecting the injury once it has occurred by means of the appearance of signs and symptoms. Through the analysis and the discovery of the different risk indicators, there is the possibility of intervening by organizing programmes of intervention at an individual or group level (Muir & Fowler, 1990).

The tendency nowadays entails identifying risk values by means of an exhaustive process of evaluating and monitoring of the sportsperson. Clinical, physical and motor tests will be used to obtain risk indicators, as well as registering and analysing the clinical history of said sportsperson and his/her injuries in previous seasons. Age, competition experience, fatigue and overtraining will be taken into account with regard to exposal to training and competition, as well as psychological factors, reducing or controlling those situations which are potentially stressing for the sportsperson.

2.2.3 Tertiary Level
The Tertiary Level of prevention is the prediction and treatment of possible complications during the post-injure phase. This constitutes an individual level of prevention that involves reducing the grade of injury incidence by eliminating all those contents and work means that could worsen the injury or its consequences and executing programmes directed towards developing the elements of protection from a specific injury.

The elements of intervention at this level should be directed towards regulating and reducing mechanical, muscular, articular, ligament or tendon imbalance that a sportsperson may be exposed to after a specific injury.

3. Review of the basics of preventive measures through physical activity

3.1 Warm up
The efficiency of warm up in the training-competition process is explained by the change of the viscoelastic properties of tissues with increasing temperature or the improvement of metabolic conditions. Content such as joint mobility, jogging, stretching, and proprioceptive technical training (Figure 4) prior to the main activity provide an important preventive security (Fradkin et al., 2006).

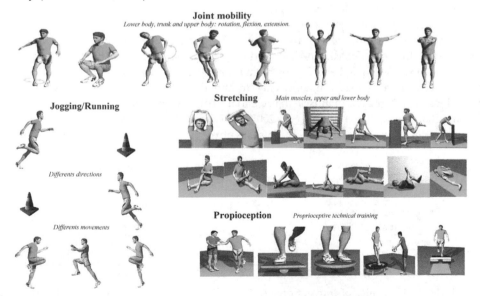

Fig. 4. Examples of exercises with preventive content in warm-up.

Different studies have found a relation between the absence or deficient execution of warm-up and posterior injury in specific actions of the sport (Agre & Baxter, 1987; Ekstrand, 1983; Hopper, 1986; Seward & Patrick, 1992) and, in contrast, proposed tactics that introduce preventive contents, which include the previously mentioned elements, manage a decrease of the number of injuries (Dvorak & Junge, 2000; Ekstrand, 1983; Hewett et al., 1999; Olsen et al., 2005; Wedderkopp et al., 1999).

3.2 Strength

Strength plays an important role in the stabilisation of different bodily structures through the normal functioning of passive stabilizers (articular: ligamental structures and meniscus) and active stabilizers (muscles), as well as the interaction between both (Gleeson et al., 1998). The bibliography argues the protective factor that muscle can provide by contributing active stability to the different articular structures, as well as the correct balance between the different muscular groups, developing a fixative and balancing function which allows the individual to develop specific actions with the greatest safety possible, without risk of injury. The main goal of working strength as a means of prevention is to ensure the correct balance between the different bodily structures, thus permitting the safe development of the different actions specific to each sport (Árnason, 2008; Askling et al., 2003; Brooks et al., 2006; Croisier et al., 2005, 2008; Domínguez & Casáis, 2005; Hölmich et al., 2010; Mjølsnes et al., 2004; Parkkari et al., 2001; Thacker et al., 2003, 2004; Tyler et al., 2002).

3.2.1 The right artromuscular balance as preventive tool

The practice of sports implies the practice of certain structures in a repetitive manner, which generates a muscular imbalance between antagonistic/agonistic groups. Maintaining a correct artromuscular balance, permitting a lessening of the effects of muscle shortening and weakening, and maintaining the integrity of articulations would be the main preventive objective of strength work.

With this goal in mind, there are different evaluation measures, such as isokinetic appreciation, that can determinate the grade of functional balance between agonistic and antagonistic muscle (Table 1 and 2). The main investigations about this topic establish a ratio that connects both values, fundamentally in the thigh muscle (hamstrings/quadriceps) whose incidence is related to muscle injure and a protective function of the knee articulation (Aagard et al., 1995, 1996; Askling et al., 2003; Croisier et al., 2005, 2008).

Main investigations place adequate ratio values at the following reference values:

Kannus et al. (1988)	0.31 – 0.80 (recommended> 0.50)
Orchard et al, (1997)	< 0.61 larger injury risk
Clanton & Coupe (1998)	0.50-0,60
Brockett et al. (2004)	0.55
Benell et al. (1998)	0.59 – 0.69
Newton et al. (2006)	0.72 – 0.77
Holcomb et al. (2007)	0.78 (PD) – 0.92 (PND)
Lehance et al. (2008)	0.60

Table 1. Reference values of conventional ratio: H CONC/Q CONC < $60°/s^{-1}$ and H EXC/Q CONC >$60°/s^{-1}$ – $240°/s^{-1}$ (Naclerio, 2007).

The value of functional ratio that discriminates the probability of injury is between 0.60 and 0.70 (Aagaard et al., 1995; Croisier et al., 2005). This same value is the one shown for an imbalance bearing a muscular recurrence.

Aagard et al. (1998)	$1 - 1.4$ ($240°/ s^{-1}$)
Tourney-Chollet et al. (2003)	0.8 ($60°/s^{-1}$) $- 0.88$ ($240°/ s^{-1}$)
Holcomb et al. (2007)	0.94 (PD) $- 1.11$ (PND) ($120°/ s^{-1}$)
Lehance et al. (2008)	>1.4 ($240°/ s^{-1}$)

Table 2. Functional ratio values: H EXC/Q CONC $>60°/s^{-1} - 240°/ s^{-1}$ (Naclerio, 2007).

Besides, recent investigations (Árnason et al., 2004; Hewett et al., 1999; Impellizeri et al., 2007; Newton et al., 2006) highlight the relationship between the balance of strength values between a dominant and non-dominant leg. It is established that a good balance should not exceed 10% between them, and in case of exceeding this percentage, the probability of injury would increase, and risk limit of bilateral asymmetry in the strength is at 15%.

In other muscle groups also involved in many sports, the normal ratios between agonist and antagonist muscles are in: adduction/abduction of hip, with hand-held dynamometer, between 0.96 and 1.4 depending on the rating, side lying position and supine position respectively (Hollman, 2006; Thorborg et al., 2010); and, concentric isokinetic $60°/s^{-1}$ and $120°/s^{-1}$are between 0.68 and 0.76, also depending on the position in which the test is performed (Alexander, 1990; Pontaga, 2004). Concerning the shoulder joint, the ratios measured with isokinetic vary depending on the sport practiced so for the rotation ratio internal / external rotation, $60°/s^{-1}$ and $120°/s^{-1}$, between 1 and 1.3, but can reach a value of 2 for specialists sports pitches, both team sports and individual sports; and, for adduction/abduction and extension/flexion, normal values are 30% higher than for adduction to abduction, and 50% higher for extensors than for flexors (Codine et al., 2005).

Functional jump tests are also used to determine possible asymmetries associated to bilateral strength deficits. The majority of them are taken from evaluations of the functional state of the lower extremity after anterior cruciate ligament (ACL) injury, and many studies show their usefulness. Although jump distance tests do not contribute with the sophisticated analysis of the working of the lower extremity that can be obtained from studies of running and strength platforms, jump tests seem useful as an evaluation of early detection that does not require a specialised equipment, it can be done in a short time and uses opposite extremity as control. The highly specific nature and low number of false positives makes these tests useful in confirming asymmetries of lower extremities. By associating them with other clinical evaluating tools, they confirm the magnitude of functional limitations (Noyes, 1991).

It seems that both the progressive test (Shuttle Run) and the vertical jump have a low sensibility to detect functional limitations of the lower extremity (Noyes, 1991). Cates & Cavanaugh (2009), in their revision of lower extremities evaluation during rehabilitation, introduce different types of horizontal jumps (Figure 5) that imply a large coordinative component as a measure of evaluating dysmetrias, comparing the values established between one leg and the other, determining a symmetry index obtained after dividing the result of one extremity by the other and multiplying by 100.

One of the latest technologies applied to the analysis of muscle properties of the superficial muscles of each individual is Tensyomiography (TMG), which is a diagnostic method that observes the time parameters and the maximum displacement of muscles during contraction.

Its analysis could direct the strength work to be done on bodily structures (Dahmane et al., 2005). The evaluation permits a muscular symmetry or asymmetry to be established, Tc Time (the time that a muscle takes to contract) and Dm (muscular tone or volume), that adopts as lateral and functional symmetry between two muscles or muscle groups above 85%, although in certain muscle groups it can tolerate up to 30% Dm and 15-20% Tc (Table 3).

The implementation of preventive programs directed both at reforcing artromuscular structures as well as the tendinous have proved themselves as extremely efficient (Árnason et al., 2008; Askling et al., 2003; Croisier et al., 2005; Mjølsnes et al., 2004; Öhberg et al., 2004; Young et al., 2005).

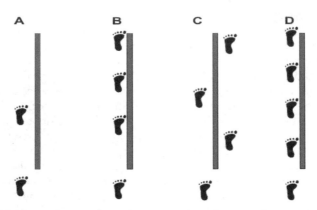

Fig. 5. Example of functional tests of one foot jumps in order to evaluate asymmetric functions; A: Single-leg hop for distance, B: Triple hop for distance, C: Crossover triple hop for distance, D: One-legged timed hop (Cates & Canavaugh, 2009).

VL (Vastus Lateralis)	Dm: 3 - 8 mm Tc: 17ms – 24ms
VM (Vastus Medialis)	Dm: 5-10mm Tc: 22ms – 28ms
RF (Rectus Femoris)	Dm: 3-10mm Tc: 22-30ms
BF (Biceps Femoris)	Dm: 2 – 6 mm Tc: 17-30 ms

Table 3. Range of Tc and Dm in TMG in the main high thigh muscle groups.

3.2.2 Eccentric work as preventive measure

In the last few years, numerous publications that establish the benefits of eccentric strength work with a double objective have appeared: improving the muscular strength values developed by the individual, and exerting a protective function for the prevention of sports injuries (Askling et al., 2003; Brockett et al., 2001). The positive effects of eccentric work on sports injuries are: the increase of the capacity to absorbe muscle tension, a higher hypertrophic level, a protective effect upon the tension-length parameters and the increase of sarcomeres in series (Brockett et al., 2001; Hortobagyi et al., 2001; Proske, 2001).

Taking into account that a great number of muscular injuries take place after eccentric contractions have been done (Thacker et al., 2003), it seems advisable to adapt muscle and tendinous structures to these requests that are produced during the specific actions of each sport, in order to avoid or minimize their seriousness. With the publications of Fyfe & Stanish (1992), the histological modification was established by observing the implications of eccentric training in the rehabilitation of tendinopathy. Later publications (Hortobagyi et al., 2001; LaStayo et al., 2003), confirm that the main effects of eccentric work on tissues allow an increase in elasticity, bringing about an increase in strength and in resistance of the tendon-muscle complex, as well as re-educated the proprioceptive sensibility.

In the last decade, studies by Alfredson et al. (1998) and by Young et al. (2005) have reaffirmed the proposals of Fyfe & Stanish (1992). They have suggested slight modifications, with more aggressive training, going from 10 to 15 repetitions, working on slow speeds, doing the program twice a day for at least 12 consecutive weeks, through "painful exercises".

One of the main biomechanical characteristics of eccentric muscle work is that muscular stretching is obtained whilst producing tension, which implies the stretching of the tendon – muscle, while increasing the levels of muscle strength and improving functional muscle properties at high speed movements. This basis is used in diverse published studies about the prevention of muscle injure in sportspeople, above all, directed at the hamstrings (Árnason et al., 2007; Askling et al., 2003; Croisier et al., 2005; Mjølsnes et al., 2004).

3.2.3 Scientific evidence of the work strength as preventive work

It is necessary to approach this section distinguishing those experiences centred on the protection of tendon structures and those directed towards muscle function.

At a tendon level, the main references to apply preventive work in sport to tendinopathy Achilles and patellar are by Mafi et al. (2001), Silbernagel et al. (2001) and by Young et al., 2005, with adaptations, following the steps indicated by Fyfe & Stanish (1992). The obtained results indicate that eccentric work improved the state of the tendon significantly in comparison to concentric work, especially if the eccentric work is done on inclined plane with 25° degrees overload.

The main studies that deal with eccentric work applied to muscular structures are centred mainly on the hamstrings (Árnason et al., 2008; Askling et al., 2003; Brooks et al., 2006; Dadebo et al., 2004; Mjølsnes et al., 2004), combining the flexibility exercises with FNP modalities and even using isoinertial devices, Yo-yo Technology (Figure 6).

3.3 Flexibility

The lack of muscle extensibility or the high tone of the antagonist muscle, are factors that enhance sports injuries, especially muscle injure.

3.3.1 Improved flexibility as preventive tool

Muscular injure where no external agent is involved generally occurs during the eccentric phase of muscle contraction. In this case, the muscle develops tension whilst increasing in length. Weakness and fatigue make muscle structures more susceptible to injure (Garret, 1996) when at a specific moment they are incapable of absorbing the generated tension.

When overstretching occurs in a muscle during a quick motor action, its ideal stretching tolerance may be surpassed, jeopardizing its integrity and allowing a possible injury (Askling et al., 2000, 2006). An imbalance in the level of flexibility in a muscular group, or in the adequate range of movement for the normal actions in the sport , could predispose to injury (Knapik et al., 1991).

Achieving a correct balance of artromuscular and the structures that make up the locomotor system, as well as achieving an adequately wide level of movements will allow a more fluid movement and coordination in the execution of technical actions and displacements.

3.3.2 Scientific evidence of the use of flexibility
The use of flexibility as a prevention method has been a topic of much controversy in the last few years. There are two fundamental strategies that the studies follow to be able to determine the influence of flexibility levels on injuries and, on the other hand, whether improving flexibility could act as an element protective of and preventive from injuries (Thacker et al., 1999, 2003; Petersen & Hölmich, 2005).

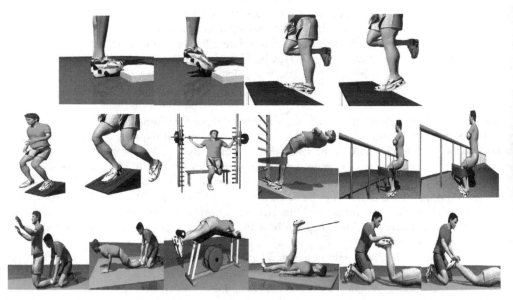

Fig. 6. Examples of eccentric work exercises.

Diverse authors have found a predisposition to injury in sportspeople with low flexibility levels. Low flexibility levels put hamstrings and quadriceps muscles at risk; therefore, it would be interesting to find this type of deficiency to establish adequate prevention programmes (Ekstrand & Gillquist, 1983; Liemohn, 1978; Witvrouw et al., 2000; Worrell, 1991). The use of standard stretching programs, the stretching technique used, and the stretching maintenance time are probably involved in a complex synergism that can reduce muscle injure, modifying the patterns of modern training in professional sportspeople (Dadebo et al., 2004). In opposition to these authors, Orchard et al. (1997) and Hannessey & Watson (1993) found no correlation between flexibility levels and muscle injure.

Training and better flexibility are programmed to preserve sportspeople from possible muscular injuries through a stretching superior to the usual range required in the sport. It seems appropriate to achieve a good residual level of flexibility, to have a range of articulate and muscular reserve, in case an unexpected or unusual gesture is superior to the flexibility or mobility of work. As an important part of muscular injuries in physical sport activities is found in the myotendinous junction, it would be advisable to improve the mechanical properties of this area. Kubo et al. (2001) has shown how repeated training of flexibility can alter the viscoelastic properties of the myotendinous junction, increasing its capacity to absorb to traction force especially in eccentric actions, a typical mechanism, in muscular injure (Witvrouw et al., 2004). In this sense, the stretching work with an eccentric dynamic phase or stretching in active tension or some modalities of FNP would be an interesting stimulus to allow the contractile component to better absorb these types of contractions so common in sports activities.

Witvrouw et al. (2007) and Mahieu et al. (2007) argue that the use of repeated dynamic stretching can improve the properties of the tendon just as eccentric training can, being an important weapon in the prevention of tendon injuries.

Stretching as part of a warm-up is one of the most extended practises in training, and permits the achievement of a series of adaptations that help in the performance and minimise the risk of injury, which is why they are a clear recommendation of the most prestigious associations of exercise prescription (Franklin et al., 2000; Holcomb, 2000). In the same way, it has been confirmed that stretching as part of warm-up content can prevent possible muscular injuries due to overstretching (Shellock & Prentice, 1985). Although there are contradicting opinions, perhaps due to the type of stretching techniques used (static stretching, FNP, rebounds) or to doing the same in different conditions (with or without previous increase of muscle temperature) (Shrier, 2002).

Nowadays, many studies are being published that fuel this important controversy about the type of stretching that should be done in warm-up of sports such as football, with explosive and velocity predominance (Cramer et al., 2004; Fletcher & Jones, 2004; Cometti, 2007). It is being pointed out that passive or static stretching have a contra productive effect, whilst the dynamic one would generate it in a positive way.

The majority of the existing investigation about static stretching focused on its application previous to exercise, reporting negative effects on explosive force when done 60 minutes before training or competition (Shrier, 2004), as well as an increase in time in a 20 meter sprint both in track runners and cross country runners who compete in power events (Nelson et al., 2005), making them inadequate for activities where the production of elastic-explosion and reactive power are decisive, as in the case of football, resulting inappropriate in their short-term effect (Barnett, 2006).

Static stretching reduces power peak, inhibiting the explosive properties of muscle, reducing reaction times and movement, and in some cases jumping capacity (Fowles et al., 2000; Cornwel et al., 2001; Young & Elliot, 2002; Behm et al., 2004; Cramer et al., 2004; Power et al., 2004; Mahieu et al., 2007). Therefore, it is not advisable as previous activity when preceding physical sporting activities dependant on rapid muscle tension or on explosive-elastic or reactive regime (Young & Behm, 2001; Cornwell et al., 2002; Cramer et al., 2004; Fletcher & Jones, 2004; Wittmann et al., 2005; Little & Williams, 2006; Cometti, 2007; Yamaguchi et al., 2007). In these cases, the practice of dynamic or ballistic stretching beforehand improves muscular provision, providing an increase in race speed, or agility actions.

3.4 Proprioception
A normal joint is dependent on the proper functioning of the neuromuscular control to avoid injury, as this allows dynamic control of the loads applied to it. Several authors have

highlighted the role of proprioception in the prevention and treatment of sports injuries. Work towards a better neuromotor control of movement has been shown to be effective, specially, in view of an articular injure, and there are very interesting proposals in this regard.

3.4.1 Fundamentals of proprioception as method of preventive work

Sherrington (1906, as quoted in Hewett et al., 2002) defined this concept as the culmination of the neural inputs originated in the different proprioceptors of the human body. However, this term has evolved, and as years have gone by the interaction between the sensorial, to which more importance was given before, and the motor, which is the formation of this somatosensorial system, has been included and studied and is a central theme of this section.

Actually, the present definitions of proprioception do not only include sensorial information but also position conscience and articular movements, speed and the detection of movement strength (Saavedra et al, 2003). We are therefore speaking of a source of sensorial information that anticipates information for intervening in the neuromuscular control with the objective of improving the functional articular stability (Lephart et al., 2003).

Proprioception consists of a ringlet from the stimulation of the sensorial receptors (cutaneous, articular, muscular) that are found in the visual, vestibular, and auditory systems that translates the mechanic event into a neurological signal (Saavedra et al., 2003) that goes through the spinothalamic tract.

The concept of proprioceptive training based on what has been explained, was initially introduced in the area of rehabilitation, with the objective of restoring the "neurological alteration" produced in the receptors when injury occurs (Freeman, 1965, as cited in Ergen & Ulkar, 2008), as it causes a destruction of proprioceptive of the injured tissue, these are not completely recovered (Griffin, 2003).

An injury produces a proprioceptive altercation, which reduces the neuromuscular control of this structure and those adjacent to it, which in turn causes general functional instability. The proprioceptive work in the field of rehabilitation restores the deficit caused by the injury incidence to values that do not generate functional instability. After recovering from it, the prevention work improves stability and neuromotor control and avoids a possible posterior relapse.

Parallel to previous investigations and in the last few decades, the advances in proprioceptive work in the prevention of injury were also aimed at achieving quicker reaction of the fixative musculature of the articulations after an imbalance. Because of this "anticipation" of the movements, a sportsperson can improve his/her performance by putting into action faster than their physical capabilities, such as strength.

The bibliography explains this phenomenon as anticipatory postural adjustments programmed beforehand without following the usual response steps, which predict possible disorders that can occur during the execution of said movement, acting as a "trigger" of the preparatory adjustments before even doing the movement, avoiding a loss of balance (De Guez, 1991, as cited in Del Abril, 2001). The proprioceptive work, as a learning process requiring repetitive practice and systematic movements, is capable of anticipating voluntary movement and do the bodily adjustments, which requires a previous muscular activation so as not to lose balance.

3.4.2 Scientific evidence as a preventive proprioceptive work

Over the last three decades this form of work has been introduced in the field of injury prevention, being one of the first studies published by Tropp et al. (1985). From the moment when this study was published and the following two decades, more studies were done showing that the most effective prevention of injury was by means of a prevention plan that had as principal content proprioceptive and neuromuscular training. Diverse studies have shown that there is a reduction of injury incidence when exercises on a stable and unstable plan are done, increasing the difficulty in balance within stability as a methodological progression, causing bipodal and unipodal support combining these with jumps (Bahr et al., 1997; Caraffa et al., 1996; Eils et al., 2001; Hewett et al., 2006; Knobloch et al., 2005; McGuine et al., 2006; Mohammadi et al., 2007; Myklebust et al., 1998; Paterno et al., 2004; Wedderkopp et al., 1999). In the same way, there are also some studies that find no significant differences in their results (Söderman et al., 2000; Petersen & Hölmich, 2005; Verhagen et al., 2004).

The publications related to proprioceptive training aimed at injury prevention that have obtained results present two different work angles (Figure 7):

1. Authors who emphasize "static" proprioceptive work (balance and rebalancing), mainly on unstable plan in bipodal and monopodal support, which at times is combined with technical elements (Tropp et al., 1985; Bahr et al., 1997; Caraffa et al., 1996; Eils et al., 2001; Knobloch et al., 2005; McGuine et al., 2006, Mohammadi et al., 2007; Vergahen et al., 2004; Wedderkopp et al., 1999).

2. Authors who emphasize dynamic proprioceptive work (neuromotor control) through specific actions which require a great control of the different bodily structures, like jumps and receptions, on bipodal and monopodal support, and on the stable and unstable plan (Heidt et al., 2000; Hewett et al., 1999, 2002, 2006; Myklebust et al., 1998; Paterno et al., 2004; Petersen & Hölmich, 2005; Zebis et al., 2008).

Proprioceptive work has shown itself useful for the decrease of injuries in sport, especially in the case of those of articular character in knees and ankles, particularly ACL (Caraffa et al., 1996; Hewett et al., 1999; Knobloch et al., 2005; McGuine et al., 2006; Mohammadi et al., 2007; Myklebust et al., 1998; Paterno et al., 2004; Wedderkopp et al., 1999); the common aspects of training load in the studies show (Table 4) that the positive results are:

Hewett et al. (1999, 2002, 2006) also suggest that for knee injury prevention, concretely ACL, proprioceptive work based on "static balance" was not effective, and that it needed to be combined with other techniques to obtain significant results in lessening ACL injuries (combining sports technique exercises, dynamic proprioception and/or plyometric, postural control and/or "core").

Surface	Stable and instable
Type of support	Monopodal and bipodal
Neuromuscular implication	Jumps and receptions
Number of weekly sessions	Season: 1-3 trainings/Preparatory period: 3-5 trainings
Session time	Between 15 – 20 minutes
Number of exercises	Between 2 and 12 exercises
Work time for each exercise	Between 15 and 45 seconds
Sensorial information	Without sensorial privation (SP) (eyes open)/with SP (eyes shut)

Table 4. Common elements of training load in proprioceptive work.

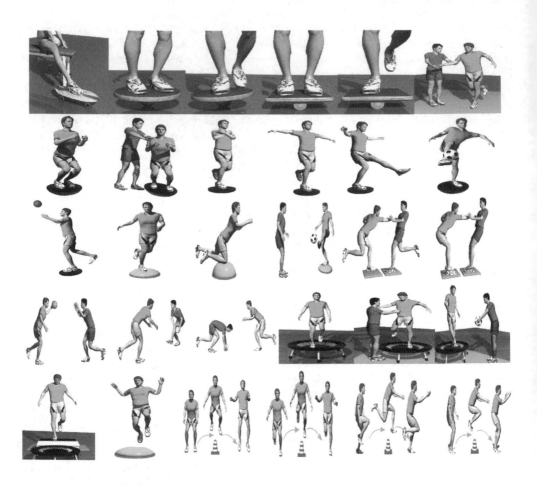

Fig. 7. Examples of proprioceptive exercises on different surfaces.

4. General protocols for injury prevention in sports, intervention strategies: Group vs. individual

The measures successfully introduced in sports to prevent injuries and mentioned previously, allow adequate preventive programs to be designed for each context. This design and its application demand a profound prior reflexion regarding the specific needs of the sportsman/woman with whom the program is to be developed and the best way of tackling the problem.

When introducing a preventive program, one can organise the session or apply the contents of the preventive program in two ways: the first one more generally directed towards dealing with problems generated in each sport, data that will be extracted from the injury profile of the activity and the team sports, being able to organise these programs as parts of the session (warm-up, main part and return to calm) in a group manner. The other direction is more specific and for its organization the individual needs of the sportsperson will be required. It can be done before training with individualised sessions, or reduced group sessions, so as to better attend to their needs.

4.1 Implementation of team sports prevention programs

Currently there are numerous published proposals that seek to encompass different prevention protocols in general, studying their effects in complex ways. The main general preventive published proposals based them on "multistation" work, putting together exercises that present scientific evidence directed towards the protection of muscular-tendon structures and the articular of the lower body.

One the most extended preventive programs in sport, directed towards ACL prevention is the Prevent Injury and Enhance Performance Program (PEP Program), designed by the Santa Monica Sports Medicine Foundation (SMSMF), and which i will be summarised below.

In terms of popularity, another programme by the Fédération Internacionale de Football Association (FIFA) is the F-MARC or "The 11", referring to the number of exercises designed in the program directed to reducing injuries in the lower body in football. One of the last programmes to appear, develop and be promoted by the Mayor Soccer League (MLS) and the SMSMF, the MLS Groin Injury Prevention Protocol, is directed at preventing injuries in the groin, through a protocol.

The programs directed towards general preventive aspects in sport, which try to influence the imbalances particular to the specialty, can be developed in training directed in a group or individual manner and can be developed in parts of the session or in complete sessions with the objective of prevention. The work could be organized in form of a circuit, with different work stations or organising the group in such a way as to have everyone doing the same task at the same time, during a warm-up session, for example.

Such programmes have been developed in elite sportspeople of different team sports such as football, handball and volleyball (Söderman et al., 2000; Myklebust, 2007; Olsen et al., 2005; Steffen et al., 2008). Besides, in schools there are models such as the iPlay Study, where they develop a school-based physical activity injury prevention programme (Collard et al., 2009; Emery et al., 2006).

4.2 Implementation of individual prevention programs

Individual prevention programs are those directed towards particular preventive aspects taking into account the characteristics of each individual, their injury history, previous evaluation and reports about sports life. They are developed in an individual manner, although it allows a greater grade of control by club technicians, a great implication of the player is necessary so that the proposed session has the necessary quality and brings about the desired effects.

The work contents must be individual and adjusted to the individual's injury history, with contents including one or various of the following aspects: rebalance of the strength values in the concentric and/or eccentric work, strengthening of the "core", adjustment of the levels of work flexibility to the specific sport, improving the postural stability through the neuromuscular control and proprioceptive work.

5. Conclusion

The measures indicated have been contrasted in terms of efficiency in different studies. Currently, there are numerous published proposals which aim to encompass them in different ways in protocols of general prevention, studying their effects in a complex way. In conclusion, it can be stated that the preventive measures that have greater scientific evidence are the use of functional bandaging, flexibility and strength training (with special attention paid to eccentric work), and proprioceptive work.

However, the programmes should be evaluated by more rigorous designs, not only with randomised experimental designs control group, but also quasi-experimental designs to use more representative samples (professional athletes) and more realistic practice contents (competition-training process), and intervention programs with really powerful measures. In this way, they must be valued with the rigour required of different preventive measures, thus usually refuting works quoted and taken as reference samples using insignificant and limited prevention protocols.

The next challenges in injury prevention should be to use the opportunities we have to implement methods of preventive work in a real context through programmes that take into account the evaluation of its effectiveness, in order to offer the sportsperson an anticipatory care, considering that the gain in injury prevention is given by the interaction of different changes in behavior and beliefs in all levels of sport. The future of intervention strategies in the prevention of injury from physical activity overcomes barriers to implementation and at each level should be designed in a different programme, adapted to each context.

6. References

Aagaard, P., Simonsen, E., Trolle, M., Bangsbo, J. & Klausen, K. (1995). Isokinetic hamstring/quadriceps strength ratio: influence from joint angular velocity, gravity correction and contraction mode. *Acta Physiologica Scandinavica*, No. 154, pp. 421–427.

Aagaard, P., Simonsen, E., Trolle, M., Bangsbo, J. & Klausen, K. (1996). Specificity of training velocity and training load on gain in isokinetic knee joint strength. *Acta Physiologica Scandinavica*, No. 156, pp. 123–129.

Agre, J. & Baxter, T. (1987). Musculoskeletal profile of male collegiate soccer players. *Archive of Physical Medicine and Rehabilitation*, Vol. 68, No. 3, pp. 147-150.

Alexander, M. (1990). Peak torque values for antagonist muscle groups and concentric and eccentric contraction types for elite sprinters. *Archives of Physical Medicine and Rehabilitation*, Vol. 71, No. 5, pp. 334-339.

Alfredson, H., Pietila, T., Jonsson, P. & Lorentzon, R. (1998). Heavy-load eccentric calf muscle training for the treatment of chronic achilles tendinosis. *The American Journal of Sports Medicine*, Vol. 26, No. 3, pp. 360-366.

Árnason, A., Andersen, T., Holme, I., Engebretsen, L. & Bahr, R. (2008). Prevention of hamstring strains in elite soccer: an intervention study. *Scandinavian Journal of Medicine & Science in Sports*, Vol. 18, No. 1, pp. 40-49.

Árnason, A., Sigurdsson, S., Gudmundsson, A., Holme, I., Engebretsen, L. & Bahr, R. (2004). Risk Factors for Injuries in Football. *The American Journal of Sports Medicine*, Vol. 32 No. 1, pp. S5-S16.

Askling, C., Karlsson, J. & Thorstensson, A. (2003). Hamstring injury occurrence in elite soccer players after preseason strength training with eccentric overload. *Scandinavian Journal of Medicine & Science in Sports*, Vol. 13, No. 4, pp. 244-252.

Askling, C., Saartok, T. & Thorstensson, A. (2006). Type of acute hamstring strain affects flexibility, strength, and time back to preinjury level. *British Journal of Sports Medicine*, Vol. 40, No. 1, pp. 40-44.

Askling, C., Tengvar, M., Saartok, T. & Thorstensson, A. (2000). Sport-related hamstring strains: 2 cases with different etiologies and injury sites. *Scandinavian Journal of Medicine & Science in Sports*, Vol. 10, No.5, pp. 304-307.

Bahr, R. & Krosshaug, T. (2005). Understanding injury mechanisms: a key component of preventing injuries in sport. *British Journal of Sports Medicine*, No. 39, pp. 324-329.

Bahr, R., Lian, O. & Bahr, I. (1997). A twofold reduction in the incidence of acute ankle sprains in volleyball after the introduction of an injury prevention program: a prospective cohort study. *Scandinavian Journal of Medicine and Science in Sports*, Vol. 7, No. 3, pp. 172-177.

Barnett, A. (2006). Using recovery modalities between training sessions in elite athletes: does it help? *Sports Medicine*, No. 36, pp. 781-796.

Behm, D., Bambury, A., Cahill,F. & Power, K. (2004). Effect of acute static stretching on force, balance, reaction time, and movement time. *Medicine & Science in Sports & Exercise*, Vol. 36, No. 8, pp. 1397–1402.

Brockett, C., Morgan, D. & Proske, U. (2001). Human hamstrings muscles adapt to eccentric exercise by changing optimum length. *Medicine & Science in Sports & Exercise*, Vol. 33, No. 5, pp. 783-790.

Brooks, J., Fuller, C., Kemp, S. & Reddin, D. (2006). Incidence, risk and prevention of hamstring muscle injuries in professional rugby union. *The American Journal of Sports Medicine*, Vol. 34, No. 8, pp. 1297-1306.

Caraffa, A., Cerulli, G., Projetti, M. & Aisa, G. (1996). Prevention of anterior cruciate ligament injuries in soccer. A prospective controlled study of proprioceptive training. *Knee Surgery of Sports Traumatology Arthroscopy*, Vol. 4, No. 1, pp. 19-21.

Cates, W. & Canavaugh, J. (2009). Advances in rehabilitation and performance testing. *Clinical Journal of Sports Medicine*, Vol. 28, No. 1, pp. 63-76.

Codine, P., Bernard, P., Pocholle, M. & Herisson, C. (2005). Isokinetic strength measurement and training of the shoulder: methodology and results.*Annales de Réadaptation et de Médecine Physique*, No. 48, pp. 80-92.

Collard, D., Chinapaw, M., Van Mechelen, W. & Verhagen, E. (2009). Design of the iPlay study: systematic development of a physical activity injury prevention programme for primary school children. *Sports Medicine*, Vol. 39, No. 11, 889-901.

Cometti, G. (2007). In : *Les limites du stretching pour la performance sportive. 1ère partie: Intérêt des étirements avant et après la performance.* http://www.u-bourgogne.fr/expertise-performance/stretchingfin.pdf

Cornwell, A., Nelson, A., Heise, G. & Sidaway, B. (2001). Acute effects of passive muscle stretching on vertical jump performance. *Journal of Human Movement Studies*, No. 40, pp. 307-324.

Cramer, J., Housh, T., Johnson, G., Miller, J., Coburn, J. & Beck T. (2004). Acute effects of static stretching on peak torque in women. *Journal of Strength Conditioning Research*, Vol. 18, No. 2, pp. 236-241.

Croisier, J., Ganteaume, S., Binet, J., Genty, M. & Ferret, J. (2008). Strength Imbalances and Prevention of Hamstring Injury in Professional Soccer Players. A Prospective Study. *The American Journal of Sports Medicine*, No. 36, pp. 1469-1475.

Croisier, J., Ganteaume, S. & Ferret, J. (2005). Pre-season isokinetic intervention as a preventive strategy for hamstring injury in professional soccer players. *British Journal of Sports Medicine*, Vol. 39, No. 29, pp. 379.

Dadebo, B., White, J. & George K. (2004). A survey of flexibility training protocols and hamstring strains in professional football clubs in England. *British Journal of Sports Medicine*, Vol. 38, No. 4, pp. 388-394.

Dahmane, R., Djordjevic, S., Simunic, B. & Valencic, V. (2005). Spatial fiber type distribution in normal human muscle histochemical and tensiomyographical evaluation. *Journal of Biomechanics*, Vol. 12, No. 38, pp. 2451-2459.

Del Abril, A. (2001). *Fundamentos biológicos de la conducta* (2ª ed.). Sanz y Torres, Barcelona.

Domínguez, E. & Casáis, L. (2005).*Metodología de la Fuerza en el Fútbol*. Master de Preparación Física en el Fútbol. Real Federación Española de Fútbol-Universidad de Castilla- La Mancha, Madrid.

Dvorak, J. & Junge, A. (2000). Football injuries and physical symptoms. A review of the literature. *The American Journal of Sports Medicine*, No. 28, No. 5, pp. S3-S9.

Eils, E. & Rosenbaum, D. (2001). A multiestation propioceptive exerscice program in patients with ankle inestability. *Medicine & Science in Sports & Exercise*, Vol. 33, No. 12, pp. 1991-1998.

Ekstrand, J. (1983). Prevention of soccer injuries: supervision by a doctor and a phisioterapist. *The American Journal of Sports Medicine*, Vol. 11, No. 3, pp. 116-120.

Ekstrand, J. & Gillquist, J. (1983) Soccer injuries and their mechanisms: A prospective study. *Medicine & Science in Sports & Exercise*, No. 15, pp. 267-270.

Ergen, E. &Ulkar, B. (2008). Propioception and ankle injuries in soccer. Clinical Journal of Sport Medicine, No. 27, pp.195-217.

Finch C. (2006). A new framework for research leading sports injury prevention. *Journal of Sports Science & Medicine*, Vol. 9, No. 1-2, pp. 3-9.

Fletcher, I. & Jones, B. (2004). The effect of different warm-up stretch protocols on 20-m sprint performance in trained rugby union players. *Journal of Strength Conditioning Research*, Vol. 18, No. 4, 885–888.

Fowles, J., Sale, D. & Macdougall, J. (2000). Reduced strength after passive stretch of the human plantar flexors. *Journal of Applied Physiology*, No. 89, pp. 1179–1188.

Fradkin, A., Gabbe, G. & Cameron, P. (2006). Does warming up prevent injury in sport? The evidence from randomised controlled trials? *Journal of Sports Science & Medicine*, Vol. 9, No. 3, pp. 214-220.

Franklin, B., Whaley, M. & Howley, E. (2000). *General principles of exercise prescription. ACSM's Guidelines for Exercise Testing and Prescription.* Williams & Wilkins, Baltimore.

Fuller, C., Ekstrand, J., Junge, A., Andersen, T., Bahr, B., Dvorak, J., Hägglund, M., McCrory, P. & Meeuwisse, W. (2006). Consensus statement on injury definitions and data collectionprocedures in studies of football (soccer) injuries. *Scandinavian Journal of Medicine & Science in Sports,* No. 16, pp. 83–92.

Fyfe, I. & Stanish, M. (1992). The use of eccentric training and stretching in the treatment and prevention of tendon injuries. *Clinics in Sports Medicine,* Vol. 11, No. 3, pp. 601-624.

Galambos, S., Terry, P., Moyle, G. & Locke, S. (2005). Psychological predictors of injury among elite athletes. *British Journal of Sports Medicine,* No. 39, pp. 351-354.

Garrett, W. (1996). Muscle strain injuries. *The American Journal of Sports Medicine,* Vol. 24, No. 6, pp. S2–S8.

Glesson, N., Reilly, T., Mercer, T. & Rakowski, S.(1998). Influence of acute endurance activity on leg neuromuscular and musculoeskeletal performance. *Medicine & Science in Sports Exercise,*Vol. 30, No. 4, pp. 596-608.

Griffin, L. (2003). Neuromuscular Training and Injury Prevention. *Clinical Orthopedics and Related Research,* No. 409, pp.53-60.

Hannessey, L. & Watson, A. (1993). Flexibility and posture assessment in relation to hamstring injury. *British Journal of Sports Medicine,* Vol. 27, pp. 243–246.

Heidt, R., Sweeterman, L., Carlonas, R., Traub, J. & Tekulve, F. (2000). Avoidance of Soccer Injuries with Preseason Conditioning. *The American Journal of Sports Medicine,* Vol. 28, No. 5, pp. 659-662.

Hewett, T., Lindenfeld, T., Riccobene, J. & Noyes, F. (1999). The effect of neuromuscular training on the incidence of knee injury in female athletes: a prospective study. *The American Journal of Sports Medicine,* Vol. 27, No. 6, pp. 699-706.

Hewett, T., Paterno, M. & Myer, G. (2002). Strategies for enhancing proprioception and neuromuscular control of the knee. *Clinical Orthopaedics and related research,* No. 402, pp. 76-94.

Hewett, T., Ford, K. & Myer, G. (2006). Anterior Cruciate Ligament Injuries in Female Athletes: Part 2, A Meta-analysis of Neuromuscular. Interventions Aimed at Injury Prevention. *The American Journal of Sports Medicine,* Vol. 34, No. 3, pp. 490-498.

Holcomb, W. (2000). Stretching and warm-up. In Baechle, T. & Earl, R., Essentials of Strength Training and Conditioning. Human Kinetics, Champaign, Illinois.

Hollman, J., Kolbeck, K., Hitchcock, J., Koverman, J. & Krause, D. (2006). Correlations between hip strength and static foot and knee posture. *Journal of Sport Rehabilitation,* No. 15, pp. 12-23.

Holmich, P.; Larsen, K.; Krogsgaard, K.; Gluud, C. (2010). Exercise program for prevention of groin pain in football players: a cluster-randomized trial. *Scandinavian Journal of Medicine & Science in Sports,* Vol. 20, No. 6, pp. 814-822.

Hopper, D. (1986). A survey of netball injuries and conditions related to these injuries. *The Australian Journal of Physiotherapy,* Vol. 32, No. 4, pp. 231-239.

Hortobagyi, T., Houmard, J., Fraser, F., Dudek, R., Lambert, J. & Tracy, J. (1998). Normal forces and myofibrillar disruption after repeated eccentric exercise. *Journal of Applied Physiology,* Vol. 84, No. 2, pp. 492-498.

Impellizzeri, F., Rampinini, E., Maffiuletti, N. & Marcora, S. (2007). A Vertical Jump Force Test for Assessing Bilateral Strength Asymmetry in Athletes. *Medicine & Science in Sports & Exercise*, Vol. 39, No. 11, pp. 2044-2050.

Junge, A. & Dvorak, J. (2000). Influence of Definition and Data Collection on the Incidence of Injuries in Football. *The American Journal of Sports Medicine*, Vol. 28, No. 5, pp. S40-S46.

Junge, A. & Dvorak, J. (2004). Soccer Injuries. A review on Incidence and Prevention. *Sports Medicine*, Vol. 34, No. 13, pp. 929-938.

Knapik, J., Bauman, C. & Jones, B. (1991). Preseason strength and flexibility imbalances associated with athletic injuries in female collegiate athletes. *The American Journal of Orthopaedic & Sports Medicine*, Vol. 19, No. 1, pp. 76-81.

Knobloch, K., Martin-Schmitt, S., Gösling, T., Jagodzinski, M., Zeichen, J. & Krettek, C. (2005). Prospective proprioceptive and coordinative training for injury reduction in elite female soccer. *Sportverletz Sportschaden*, Vol. 19, No. 3, pp. 123-129.

Kubo, K., Kanehisa, H., Kawakami, Y. & Fukunaga, T. (2001). Influence of static stretching on viscoelastic properties of human tendon structures in vivo. *Journal of Applied Physiology*, Vol. 90, No. 2, pp. 511-519.

Larson M, Pearl, A., Jaffet, R. & Rudawnsky, A. (1996). *Epidemiology of sport injuries*. Human Kinetics, Champaign, Illinois.

LaStayo, P., Woolf, J., Lewek, M., Snyder-Mackler, L., Reich, T. & Lindstedt, S. (2003). Eccentric muscle contractions: their contribution to injury, prevention, rehabilitation and sport. *Journal of Orthopaedic in Sports & Physical Therapy*, Vol. 33, No. 10, pp. 557-569.

Lephart, S.; Myers, J.; Riemann, B. (2003). *Role of proprioception in functional joint stability*. In: DeLee, Drez & Miller. Orthopaedic Sports Medicine: Principles and Practice (2ª ed.). Saunders, Philadelphia.

Liemohn, W. (1978). Factors related to hamstring strains. *Journal of Sports Medicine & Physical Fitness*, No. 18, pp. 71-76.

Little, T. & Williams. A. (2006). Effects of differential stretching protocols during warm-ups on high-speed motor capacities in professional soccer players. *Journal of Strength and Conditioning Research*, Vol. 20, No. 1, pp. 203-207.

McGuine, T. & Keene, J. (2006). The Effect of a Balance Training Program on the Risk of Ankle Sprains in High School Athlete. *The American Journal of Sports Medicine*, Vol. 34, No. 7, pp. 1103-1111.

Mafi, N., Lorentzon, R. & Alfredson, H. (2001). Superior short-term results with eccentric calf muscle training compared to concentric training in a randomised prospective multicenter study on patients with chronic Achilles tendinosis. *Knee Surgery Sports Traumatoloty Arthroscopy*, Vol. 9, No. 1, pp. 42-47.

Mahieu, N., Mcnair, P., De Muynck, M., Stevens, V., Blanckaert, I., Smits, N. & Witvrouw E. (2007). Effect of static and ballistic stretching on the muscle-tendon tissue properties. *Medicine& Science in Sports & Exercise*, Vol. 39, No. 3, pp. 494-501.

Meeuwisse W. (1994). Assessing causation in sport injury: a multifactorial model. *Clinical Journal of Sports Medicine*, Vol. 4, No. 3, pp. 166-70.

Meeuwisse, W., Tyreman, H., Hagel, B., Emery, C. (2007). A dynamic model of etiology in sport injury:the recursive nature of risk and causation. *Clinical Journal of Sport Medicine*, Vol. 17, No. 3, pp. 215 – 219.

Mjølsnes, R., Arnason, A., Osthagen, T., Raastad, T. & Bahr, R. (2004). A 10-week randomized trial comparing eccentric vs. concentric hamstring strength training in well-trained soccer players. *Scandinavian Journal of Medicine & Science in Sports*, Vol. 14, No. 5, pp. 311-317.

Mohammadi, F. (2007). Comparison of 3 Preventive Methods to Reduce the Recurrence of Ankle Inversion Sprains in Male Soccer Players. *The American Journal of Sports Medicine*, Vol. 35, No. 6, pp. 922-926.

Muir, J. & Fowler, G. (1990). *Fundamentos de medicina preventiva*. Díaz de Santos, Madrid.

Murphy, D., Connolly, D. & Beynnon, D. (2003). Risk factors for lower extremity injury: a review of the literature. *British Journal of Sports Medicine*, Vol. 37, No. 1, pp. 13-29.

Myklebust, G., Engebretsen, L., Braekken, I., Skølberg, A., Olsen, O. & Bahr, R. (2007). Prevention of noncontact anterior cruciate ligament injuries in elite and adolescent female team hand ball athletes. *Instructional Course Lectures*, No. 56, pp. 407-418.

Myklebust, G., Haehlum, S. & Holm, I. (1998). A prospective cohort study of anterior cruciate ligament injuries in elite. *Norwegian Team Handball*, No. 8, pp. 149-153.

Naclerio, F. (2007). *Entrenamiento de fuerza y prevención de lesiones en el deporte*. Universidad Europea de Madrid y Escuela de Estudios Universitarios Real Madrid: Madrid.

Nelson, A., Driscoll, N., Landin, D., Young, M. & Schexnayder, I. (2005). Acute effects of passive muscle stretching on sprint performance. *Journal of Sports Sciences*, No. 23, pp. 449-454.

Newton, R., Gerber, A., Nimphius, S., Shim, J., Brandon, K., Robertson, M., Pearson, D., Craig, B., Häkkinen, K. & Kraemer, W. (2006). Determination of functional strength imbalance of the lower extremities. *Journal of Strength and Conditioning Research*, Vol. 20, No. 4, pp. 971–977.

Noyes, F., Barber, S. & Mangine, R. (1991). Abnormal lower limb symmetry determined by functional hop tests after anterior cruciate ligament rupture. *The American Journal of Sports Medicine*, Vol. 19, No. 5, pp. 513-518.

Öhberg, L, Lorentzon, R. & Alfredson, H. (2004). Eccentric training and patients with chronic Achilles tendinosis: normalised tendon structure and decreased thickness at follow up. *British Journal of Sports Medicine*, Vol. 38, No. 1, pp. 8-11.

Olsen, O., Myklebust, G., Engebretsen, L., Holme, I. & Bahr, R. (2005). Exercises to prevent lower limb injuries in youth sports: cluster randomised controlled trial. *British Journal of Sports Medicine*, No. 330, pp. 449.

Orchard, J., Marsden, J. & Lord, S. (1997). Preseason hamstring muscle weakness associated with hamstring muscle injury in Australian footballers. *The American Journal of Sports Medicine*, Vol. 25,No. 1, pp. 81–85.

Parkkari, J, Urho, M., Kujala, U. & Kannus, P. (2001). Is it possible to prevent sports injuries? Review of controlled clinical trials and recommendations for future work. *Sports Medicine*, Vol. 31, No. 14, pp. 985-95.

Paterno, M., Myer, G., Ford, K. & Hewett, T. (2004). Neuromuscular Training Improves Single-Limb Stability in Young Female Athletes. *Journal of orthopaedic and sports Physical Therapy*, Vol. 34, No. 6, pp. 305-316.

Petersen, J. & Hölmich, P. (2005). Evidence based prevention of hamstring injuries in sport. *British Journal of Sports Medicine*, Vol. 39, No. 6, pp. 319–323.

Peterson, L. & Renström, P. (1988). *Lesiones deportivas. Prevención y tratamiento*. Jims: Barcelona.

Pontaga, I. (2004). Hip and knee flexors and extensors balance in dependence on the velocity of movements. *Byology of Sport*, Vol. 21, No. 3, pp. 261-272.

Powers, M., Buckley, D., Kaminski, C., Hubbard, J. & Oritz, C. (2004). Six Weeks of Strength and Proprioception Training Does Not Affect Muscle Fatigue and Static Balance in Functional Ankle Instability. *Sport Rehabilitation*, No. 13, pp. 201-227.

Proske, U. & Morgan, D. (2001). Muscule damage from eccentric exercise: mechanism, mechanical signs, adaptation and clinical applications. *Journal of Physiology*, Vol. 537, No. 2, pp. 333-345.

Saavedra, M.; Coronado, Z.; Chávez, A. & Díez, G. (2003) Relación entre fuerza muscular y propiocepción de rodilla en sujetos asintomáticos. *Revista Mexicana de Medicina Física y Rehabilitación*, Vol. 15, No. 1, pp. 17-23.

San Román, Z. (2005). *El papel del preparador físico en la prevención de lesiones*. Master de Preparación Física en el Fútbol. Real Federación Española de Fútbol-Universidad de Castilla- La Mancha, Madrid.

Seward, H. & Patrick, J. (1992). A three year survey of Victorian Football League injuries. *Australian Journal of Science and Medicine in Sport*, No. 24, pp. 51–54.

Shepard, R. (2005). Towards an evidence based prevention of sports injuries. *Injury Prevention*, Vol. 11, No. 2, pp. 65-66.

Shellock, F. & Prentice, W. (1985). Warming-up and stretching for improved physical performance and prevention of sport-related injuries. *Sport Medicine*, No. 2, pp. 267-278.

Shrier, I. (2002). Does stretching help prevent injuries? In MacAuley, D. y Best, T. (Eds.), *Evidence-based sports medicine*. BMJ Publishing, London.

Shrier, I. (2004). Does stretching improve performance? A systematic and critical review of the literature. *Clinical Journal of Sport Medicine*, No. 14, pp. 267-273.

Silvernagel, K., Thomée, R., Thomée, P. & Karlsson, J. (2001). Eccentric overload training for patients with chronic Achilles tendon pain – a randomised controlled study with reliability testing of the evaluation methods. *Scandinavian Journal Medicine & Science in Sports*, Vol. 11, No. 4, pp. 197-206.

Söderman, K., Werner, S., Pietilä, T., Engström, B. & Alfredson, H. (2000). Balance board training: prevention of traumatic injuries of the lower extremities in female soccer players? A prospective randomized intervention study. *Knee Surgery of Sports Traumatology and Arthroscopy*, Vol. 8, No.6, pp. 356–363.

Steffen, K., Bakka, H., Myklebust, G. & Bahr, R. (2008). Performance aspects of an injury prevention program: a ten-week intervention in adolescent female football players *Scandinavian Journal Medicine & Science in Sports*, Vol. 18, No. 5, pp. 596-604.

Thacker, S., Stroup, D., Branche, C., Gilchrist, J., Goodman, R.., & Weitman, E.. (1999). The prevention of ankle sprains in sports. A systematic review o the literature. *The American Journal of Sports Medicine*, Vol. 27, No. 6, pp. 753-760.

Thacker, S., Stroup, D., Branche, C., Gilchrist, J., Goodman, R. & Kelling, E. (2003). Prevention of knee injuries in sports: A Systematic review of the literature. *Journal of Sports Medicine and the Physical Fitness*, Vol. 43, No. 2, pp. 165-179.

Thacker, S.; Gilchrist, J.; Stroup, D.; Kimsey, C. (2004). The impact of stretching on sports injury risk: a systematic review of the literature. *Medicine & Science in Sports & Exercise*, Vol. 36, No. 3, pp. 371-378.

Thorborg, K., Petersen, J., Magnusson, S. & Hölmich, P. (2010). Clinical assessment of hip strength using a hand-held dynamometer is reliable. *Scandinavian Journal of Medicine & Science in Sports*, Vol. 20, No. 3, pp. 493-501.

Tropp, H., Askling, C. & Gilquist, J. (1985). Prevention on ankle sprains. *The American Journal of Sports Medicine*, Vol. 13, No. 4, pp. 259-262.

Tyler, T.; Nicholas, S.; Campbell, R.; Donellan, S. & McHugh, M. (2002). Effectiveness of a Preseason Exercise Program to Prevent Adductor Muscle Strains in Professional Ice Hockey Players. *The American Journal of Sports Medicine*, Vol. 30, No. 5, pp. 680-683.

Van Mechelen, W., Hlobil, H. & Kemper, H. (1992). Incidence, severity,etiology and prevention of sports injuries. *Sports Medicine*, Vol. 14, No. 2, pp. 82-99.

Verhagen, E., Van der Beek, A., Twisk, J., Bouter, L., Bahr, R. & Van Mechelen, W. (2004). The effect of a proprioceptive balance board training program for the prevention of ankle sprains. *The American Journal of Sports Medicine*, Vol. 32, No. 8, pp.1385-1393.

Wedderkopp, N., Kaltoft, M., Lundgaard, B., Rosendahl, M. & Froberg, K. (1999). Prevention of injuries in young female players in European team handball. A prospective intervention study. *Scandinavian Journal of Medicine and Science in Sports*, Vol. 9, No. 1, pp. 41-47.

Wittmann, M., Babault, N. & Kouassi, B. (2005). Static stretch and warm-up: effects on the lower limb flexibility and jumping ability. *Medicine & Science in Sports & Exercise*, Vol. 37, No. 5, pp. S192-S193.

Witvrouw, E., Mahieu, N., Danneels, L. & McNair, P. (2004). Stretching and injury prevention: an obscure relationship. *Sports Medicine*, Vol. 34, No. 7, pp. 443-449.

Witvrouw, E., Mahieu, N., Roosen, P. & McNair, P. (2007). The role of stretching in tendon injuries. *British Journal of Sports Medicine*, No. 41, pp. 224–226.

Witvrouw, E., Lysens, R., Bellemans, J., Peers, K. & Vanderstraeten, G. (2000). Open versus close kinetic chain. Exercise for patellofemoral pain: a prospective, randomized study. *The American Journal of Sports Medicine*, Vol. 28, No. 5, pp. 687-694.

Worrell, T., Perrin, D., Gansneder, B. & Gieck, J. (1991). Comparison of isokinetic strength and flexibility measures between hamstring injured and noninjured athletes. *Journal of Orthopaedic & Physical Therapy*, No. 13, pp. 118-125.

Yamaguchi, T., Ishii, K., Yamanaka, M. & Yasuda, K. (2007). Acute effects of dynamic stretching exercise on power output during concentric dynamic constant external resistance leg extension. *Journal of Strength Conditioning Research*, Vol. 21, No. 4, pp. 1238–1244.

Young, M., Cook, J., Purdam, C., Kiss, Z. & Alfredson, H. (2005). Eccentric decline squat protocol offers superior results at 12 months compared with traditional eccentric protocol for patellar tendinopathy in volleyball players. *British Journal of Sports Medicine*, Vol. 39, No. 2, pp. 102-105.

Young, W. & Elliott, J. (2001). Acute effects on static stretching, proprioceptive neuromuscular facilitation stretching, and maximum voluntary contractions on explosive force production and jumping performance. *Research Quarterly in Exercise & Sport*, No. 72, pp. 273–279.

Zebis, M., Bencke, J., Andersen, L., Døssing, S., Alkjaer, T., Magnusson, S., Kjaer, M. & Aagaard, P. (2008). The effects of neuromuscular training on knee joint motor control during sidecutting in female elite soccer and handball players. *Clinical Journal of Sports Medicine*, Vol. 18, No. 4, pp. 329-337.

Part 2

Orthopedic and Skeletal Aspects of Sports Medicine

5

Physical Management of Pain in Sport Injuries

Rufus A. Adedoyin and Esther O. Johnson
Department of Medical Rehabilitation,
Obafemi Awolowo University, Ile-Ife,
Nigeria

1. Introduction

The number of people both young and old engaging in sporting activities has increased in the recent times. Apart from the economic benefits of sports which drive youths to engage in competitive sports, adults and seniors are now aware of the health benefits of recreational sports. Inactivity has been linked to many chronic diseases including cardiovascular disease which is leading cause of death worldwide. Health educators are now encouraging the public to be involved in physical activities in order to promote their health. Unfortunately sports are associated with injuries whether it is for leisure or competition. Those who overdo or who are not properly trained are prone to sports injuries. Many sports injuries can be prevented if proper precautions are taken (Lachmann 1989).

If injuries are not properly managed, it could reduce the optimal performance or inability of an athlete to continue participation in sports. Nowadays many sports injuries can be treated effectively and most people who suffer injuries can return to a satisfying level of physical activity after an injury due to advancement in medical management. However, many athletes tend to ignore minor injuries or result into self-management. This always led to more damage to the body structures and makes the injury worse.

Majority of injuries sustained during sporting activities involve musculoskeletal system which include; bones, joints, tendons, ligaments and tendons (Ebnezar, 2003). The injury may be as a result of trauma from external force as it is in contact sports. This is direct trauma also known as macro trauma. Indirect trauma is due to pathology resulting from repeated sub maximal loading. Fracture of bones is less common but not unlikely (Kisner and Colby, 2007).

Signs and symptoms that follow injuries include; pain (from the chemicals released by damaged cells), swelling (from an influx of fluid into the damaged region), loss of function (because of increased swelling and pain), redness (from local vasodilation) and heat (from increased blood flow to the area), which are features of inflammatory reaction.

Pain is the major reasons why many people seek medical attention. International Association for the Study of Pain defined pain as an unpleasant sensory and emotional experience associated with actual or potential tissue damage, or described in terms of such damage (IASP, 1994). Pain experienced from soft tissue injuries is usually related to the extent and type of trauma sustained as well as to the structures involved and an individual's perception and expression of it (O'Sullivan and Schmitz, 1994). Pain and inflammation continue into the sub-acute phase and may fade out in the chronic stage subsiding with healing in 1 to 3 months (Schnedler, 1990).

Management of soft tissues injury is patterned along with the phases of injury.

Inflammatory phase (acute): It can last up to 72 hours. Where there are musculotendinous injuries, there is myofilament reaction and peripheral muscle fiber contraction within the first two hours.

Regeneration and repair phase (sub-acute): This fibro-elastic and collagen-forming phase lasts from 48 hours up to 6 weeks. During this time structures are rebuilt and regeneration occurs. Fibroblasts begin to synthesize scar tissue. These cells produce type iii collagen, which appears in about four days, and is random and immature in its fiber organization. Capillary budding occurs, bringing nutrition to the area, and collagen cross-linking begins. As the process proceeds, the number of fibroblasts decreases as more collagen is laid down. This phase ends with the beginning of wound contracture and shortening of the margins of the injured area.

2. Remodeling phase (Chronic stage)

This phase lasts from 3 weeks to 12 months. There is evidence of cross-linking and shortening of the collagen fibers promote formation of a tight, strong scar. It is characterized by remodeling of collagen so as to increase the functional capabilities of the muscle, tendon, or other tissues. Final aggregation, orientation, and arrangement of collagen fibers occur during this phase (Kisner and Colby, 2007).

Sports injuries are usually treated with pharmacological and non-pharmacological methods. Non pharmacological methods involve conservative methods such as physical therapy and surgery.

Physical therapy is most essential in managing the majority of the soft tissue injuries. Physical therapy should commence early so as to speed up the healing of damaged tissues and to prevent complications that could develop during chronic stage. The athlete may return to full functional activities if the treatments commence early.

3. Cryotherapy

Cryotherapy also known as cold therapy has been reported to be one of the least expensive and most used therapies recommended in the immediate treatment of the skeletal muscle injury. Among chiropractic practitioners it is the most often utilized passive adjunctive therapy.

Cryotherapy is capable of reducing effects related to the damage process, such as pain, edema, haemorrhage and muscle spasm after soft tissue injuries. Although cryotherapy may not reduce edema once it is formed but when used immediately after injury, it can prevent formation of edema. Cold is capable of diminishing secondary hypoxic injury, so there is less free protein in the tissues decreasing the tissue oncotic pressure leading to tissue swelling by decreasing metabolism and lowering permeability rate (Enwemeka et al, 2002).

The mechanism of pain relief after application of ice is not clear. The prevailing theories such as decreased nerve transmission in pain fibres, reduction of the activity of free nerve endings, increase in the pain threshold, release of endorphins and cold sensations which over-ride the pain sensation are plausible reasons provided in the literature.

One of the physiological effects of ice is vasoconstriction. When the blood vessels narrow, the amount of blood delivered to the injured area is reduced thereby reducing bleeding during injuries. Muscles always respond to injury through spasm to protect itself and prevent further damage. Ice, is also beneficial in reducing muscle spasms (Chesterton et al, 2002).

There are several procedures of application of cryotherapy ranging from gel, spray, ice packs, and immersion. Among these ice packs are most popular and safe as it prevent frost bite because of the protection of body tissue by the plastic bag (Martinez et al, 1996).

3.1 Methods of application of cryotherapy

Ice packs: Ice in this method are crushed, shaved, or chipped and put in a plastic bag applied directly to the injured area. Several authors agree that some form of protection be used to prevent frostbite. Ice pack with temperature at 0 o C (32 o F) can be applied directly to the skin to maximize the effectiveness of the cold application.

Cold-gel packs: A gelatinous substance enclosed in a vinyl cover containing water, and antifreeze (such as salt).

Chemical cold packs: These consist of two chemical substances, one in a small vinyl bag within a larger bag. Squeezing the smaller bag until it ruptures and spills its contents into the larger causes a chemical reaction producing the cold. They are ideally utilized for emergency use.

Ice immersion: A container is filled with ice and water, and the body part is immersed in it. Immersion is recommended for extremities.

Ice massage: A cube of ice is rubbed over and around the underlying muscle fiber until numb.

Ice should be used for a period of 5 minutes if being used as first aid. Prolong period of application could cause blood vessels dilation resulting into increase in hemorrhage.

At chronic stage of injury, ice may be used for 10 minutes. An individual experiences cold-burning sensation-aches-numbness during the application of ice (Erith et al, 2002).

When an exercise or manual therapy is to be used for a patient, ice are usually applied to serve as local anesthesia to reduce pain.

4. Reduction of bleeding

By cooling the surface of the skin and the underlying tissues, ice causes the narrowing of blood vessels, a process known as vasoconstriction. This leads to a decrease in the amount of blood being delivered to the area and subsequently lessens the amount of swelling. After a number of minutes, the blood vessels dilate allowing blood to return to the area. This phase is followed by another period of vasoconstriction- this process of vasoconstriction followed by dilation is known as the Hunting Response.

Although blood still flows into the injured area the amount of swelling is significantly reduced if ice is not applied. Decrease in swelling allows more movement in the muscle and so lessens the functional loss associated with the injury (Eston and Peters, 1999). The swelling associated with the inflammatory response also causes a pressure increase in the tissue and this leads to the area becoming more painful. The effects of ice causing vasoconstriction after application led to decrease in pain. Equally the conduction velocity of the nerve is reduced, thereby limiting the pain transmission of the peripheral nerves (Goodall and Howatson, 2008).

5. Reduction of muscle spasm

By reducing the cells metabolic rate, ice reduces the cells oxygen requirements. Thus when blood flow has been limited by vasoconstriction then the risk of cell death due to oxygen demands (secondary cell necrosis) will be lessened.

6. Transcutaneous electrical nerve stimulation

Electrical currents are generated by stimulating the device of transcutaneous electrical nerve stimulation (TENS) and delivered it across the skin through electrodes Figure 1. TENS is a non-invasive treatment modality that involves the application of a low-voltage electrical current for pain relief. TENS is now a popular modality in the field of physical therapy and sport medicine for managing pain.

There are much available clinical evidence concerning the use of TENS for various types of conditions relating to musculoskeletal disorders and other type of pain, such as sympathetically mediated pain, bladder incontinence, neurogenic pain, visceral pain. Although this claim has been challenged by many experts about the degree to which TENS is more effective than placebo in reducing pain (Adedoyin et al, 2005).

Melzack and Wall in 1965 provided the explanation on the mechanism of the analgesia produced by TENS in their pain gate-control theory.—Their explanation was that gate is usually closed, inhibiting constant nociceptive transmission via C fibers from the periphery to the T cell. When painful peripheral stimulation occurs, however, the information carried by C fibers reaches the T cells and opens the gate, allowing pain transmission centrally to the thalamus and cortex, where it is interpreted as pain. The gate-control theory postulates a mechanism by which the gate is closed again, preventing further central transmission of the nociceptive information to the cortex. The proposed mechanism for closing the gate is inhibition of the C-fiber nociception by impulses in activated myelinated fibers.

The Pain Gate can also be shut by stimulating the release of endogenous opioids (endorphins, enkephalins, and dynorphins), which are pain-relieving chemicals naturally released by the body in response to pain stimuli. Opioids are a naturally occurring hormone in the body. They are released in response to an injury or physical stress to reduce pain and promote a feeling of wellbeing. Much like Morphine, and related medications, opioids have a similar chemical structure, which explains their strong painkilling effects.

TENS has not only been found to be indicated for relieving both acute and chronic pain following sports injuries but also found to be enhancing tissues healing. TENS machine is very simple to use. It can be used at home by the athletes without special training. It could be applied to the painful site between 30 to 60 minutes; the machine could also be attached to the body during the performance of daily activity.

One of the main benefits of a TENS machine is that it can be used at home. Unlike most analgesic drugs TENS has little or no side effects. Pain relief drugs are effective but they can lead to several complications including: nausea, headaches, liver damage, and erosion of cartilage, stomach bleeding and stroke. Drug addiction and abuse can also be associated with the use of drugs. This is the reason why conservative treatments such as TENS are becoming more popular. TENS should not be used for people who are on pacemaker and those that develop arrhythmia of the heart.

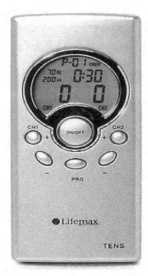 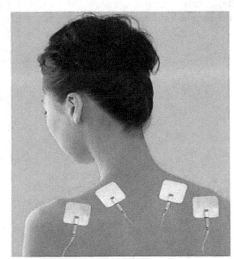

Fig. 1. TENS Machine with electrodes placement

7. Interferential current therapy

In recent past faradic current has been used in the treatment of sport injuries for muscle re education. It is usually prescribed at early stage of injuries and when active contraction of muscles is hindered (Goats, 1990). Faradism is believed to increase muscle bulk and muscular strength especially when the muscle is made to work against resistance. Faradic current is capable of stimulating the motor nerves and cause tetanic contraction of muscles. Contraction of muscles when maintain for a period of time is capable of increasing the metabolism, with a consequent increase in the oxygen demands and nutrients and an increase of waste products, including metabolites. By the action of contraction and relaxation of muscles, there is increase in the pumping action of the veins and lymphatic vessels lying within the muscles. This mechanism is helpful in enhancing good venous and lymphatic return.

However, faradic currents like other direct and low frequency alternating currents (<1 KHz to <10 KHz) usually encounter a high electric resistance in the outer layers of the human skin. This makes the treatment of deep structures painful because a large transcutaneous current passes deeply (Adedoyin et al, 2002). Interferential current (IFC) was therefore designed to overcome this problem. Interference current is a medium-frequency current that delivers currents to deep-seated structures in order to relief pain. The machines are designed to generate an amplitude-modulated interferential wave, called beat frequency. The wave is created by two out-of-phase currents that collide with each other to generate an interferential wave with frequency between 1Hz and 250Hz.

Inferential current is primarily used to relief pain in musculoskeletal injuries. The mechanism of pain relief is similar to that of TENS. The duration of treatment should be between 30-60 minutes. Inferential currents can be applied via 2 or 4 electrodes. Quadripolar application of IFC is claimed to be created deep within the tissues whereas bipolar application is said to be distributed similarly to conventional electrical stimulation with maximal current intensities underneath the electrodes, progressively decreasing with distance (Goats, 1990).

Interferential current has been reported to be liked with stimulation of muscles, reduction of swelling and improved blood circulation and healing process. Many experts believed that TENS and IFC produced analgesic effects in a similar manner while few believed the IFC is better than TENS.

Interferential Currents should be avoided over the trunk or pelvis during pregnancy; and should be placed over the carotid sinuses and epiphyseal region in children. It should not be used for patient with pacemakers.

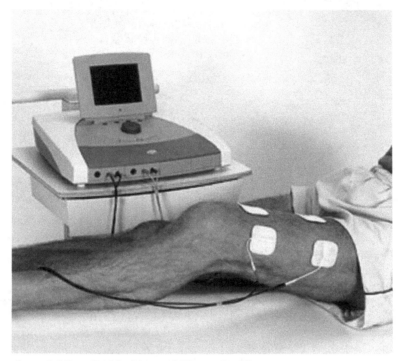

Fig. 2. Interferential Current Machine and Electrodes Placement

8. Therapeutic exercise

There is strong evidence for the use of exercise in the management of soft tissue injuries. In fact other physiotherapeutic modalities such as electrotherapy (Faradism, TENS), thermotherapy (Short wave diathermy), Actinotherapy (Ultrasound) are considered adjunct treatments. Exercise should be encouraged as soon as possible to prevent complications such as reduced range of motion, contractures, adhesions, muscles wasting and reduced strength.

Active movement can improve the integrity of joints and enhance good scar formation in muscles, tendons and ligaments, and improve the tensile strength of the mature scar.

Resisted exercise training would improve muscular strength, muscular hypertrophy, muscular endurance and power. It could also improve dynamic postural stability as related to standing balance and mobility. Resisted exercise is based on overload principle which states that for a muscle or muscle group to increase in strength, it must, on regular basis, be challenged to overcome resistances that are greater than those that are usually encountered (Nyland, 2006).

Where a joint is immobilized, isometric exercise may be encouraged in order to protect the integrity of the joints. By contracting the muscle fibres without moving the joint, the muscle fibres are stimulated. This improves blood supply to the joint and also prevents intra articular and peri articular adhesions

Balance and coordination could also be impaired during musculoskeletal disorder because of deviation of gait especially injuries involving ankle joints. Exercise on wobble board is usually encouraged to improve static balance and strength of the lower extremities. Figure 3. Apart from being useful in stimulating the proprioceptive system and re-educate reflex posturer control, wobble board may improve the symmetry of weight distribution on the lower extremities of individuals (Adedoyin et al, 2009).

All these exercises have been found to bring about relief of pain with or without any other therapeutic analgesic modalities (Adedoyin et al, 2009).

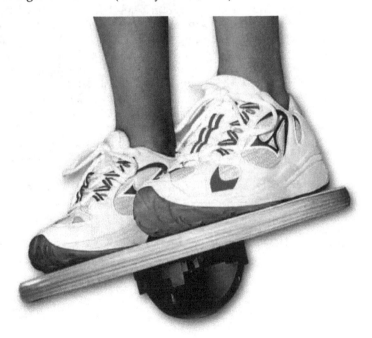

Fig. 3. Wobble Board

9. Ultrasound

Therapeutic ultrasound is one of the most common treatments used in the management of soft tissue injuries. Ultrasound therapy is widespread in sports physiotherapy and physical therapy practice (Khanna et al, 2009).

Ultrasound consists of inaudible high frequency vibrations created when a generator produces electrical energy that is converted to acoustic energy through molecular collision and vibration. It undergoes a progressive loss of intensity of the energy during passage through the tissue (attenuation) (Tee Haar, 1987). Ultrasound frequency, wavelength, intensity, amplitude, continuous/pulsed therapy, coupling medium, movement and angle of transducer and frequency, tissue composition and duration of treatment affect the dosage of ultrasound delivered to target tissue (Tee Haar, 1987, Speed 2001).

Ultrasound produces thermal and non-thermal physical effects (Low and Reeds, 2000). Thermal effects lead to increased blood flow, reduction in muscle spasm, increased extensibility of collagen fibres and pro-inflammatory response. Non-thermal effects of ultrasound including stable cavitation and acoustic streaming and micro massage; which are more important than thermal effects in the treatment of soft tissue lesions (Dyson and Suckling, 1978).

The sound waves are capable of penetrating into the skin and surface layers and cause tendons and soft tissues to vibrate, producing gentle healing vibrations within the affected area that soothe inflammation and relieve pain. Ultrasound waves also cause tendons and tissues to relax and increase blood flow to help reduce local swelling and chronic inflammation (Khanna et al, 2009).

The choice of parameters depends on the condition being treated. Continuous ultrasound therapy is used to treat muscle spasms, pain and to relax tense muscles. In this type of ultrasound, the sound waves transmitted create friction as they pass through muscle fibers, which in turn produce heat in the injured area. The body increases blood circulation to that area to cool it down, and this increased blood flow speeds up the healing process.

Whereas pulse ultrasound is used treat inflammations such as tendinitis and bursitis. This method of ultrasound therapy works through cavitation by transmitting vibrations that stimulate cell membranes, resulting in more rapid repair. No adverse effects have attributable to the use of appropriate therapeutic doses of ultrasound in literature. However, people with pacemakers and other electronic implants should not use ultrasound.

Other hear modalities that commonly used at chronic stage include infra-red, short wave diathermy and hot packs. Many experts believed that heat therapy can reduce pain and muscle spasm following some types of injury. Heat is sometimes recommended prior to exercise for athletes with 'stiff' muscles or in the treatment of chronic conditions in which restricted muscle or joint motion may interfere with recovery. Heat has also been found to enhance stretching of tissues by applying it to the muscles before the stretching is carried out. However, the application of heat to injured parts of the body has also been linked with increases in tissue swelling (oedema), and heat can spur metabolic activity and increase capillary blood flow, effects which may be counterproductive in the early treatment of some injuries.

10. Massage

Massage is the systematic, mechanical stimulation of the soft tissues of the body by means of rhythmically applied pressure and stretching using hands. It's performed to produce mechanical or reflexive effects such as improved range of motion, to increase circulation and lymphatic drainage, to induce general relaxation and reduce pain (Johnson, 2000). Massage has been used in managing athletes since the first Olympic games up until now. In sports, it is usually used in achieving and maintaining peak performance and to support healing of injuries (Fritz, 2004). Massage techniques include effleurage or stroking, petrissage or kneading, tapotement or percussion. Massage techniques involving effleurage, and kneading are used before sport. Massage can also be used after sport to improve the athlete's psyche and during sport in treatment of injuries. In treatment of muscle strain, massage is facilitates healing at the sub-acute and chronic stage. Controlled soft tissue massage of scar tissue along fiber direction towards injury will promote development of mobile scars at the sub-acute stage of healing, while cross-fiber friction of scar tissue coupled with directional stroking along the lines of tension away from injury will increase strength and alignment of scar tissue at the chronic stage (Fritz, 2004).

If properly applied massage therapy can provide pain relief, Improves the flow of nutrients to muscles and joints, accelerating recovery from fatigue and injury, soothe stiff sore muscles, reduce inflammation and swelling. Massage and gentle stretching can help to maintain range of motion of joints.

The choice of the massage is specific to the athlete's sport of choice and is often focused on area prone to injuries. Sport massage is gaining popularity as useful components in a balanced training regimen. Sports massage can be used as a means to enhance pre-event preparation and reduce recovery time for maximum performance during training or after an event. There is evidence that specially designed massage promotes flexibility, removes fatigue, improves endurance, helps prevent injuries, and prepares athletes to compete at their absolute best.

11. Orthotic devices

Orthotic devices are needed during early onset of sport injuries in order to provide rest and support for the damaged structures especially joints. The devices provide support, or correct deformities and improve the movement of joints, spine, or limbs. They also provide stability of joints by limiting abnormal or excessive joint mobility. Excessive movement can worsen the injured parts and increase the pain. Knee and Ankle joints are more prone to injury than any other joints in the body. Ankle foot orthosis is commonly used to protect the ankle joints at acute stage (Figure 4).

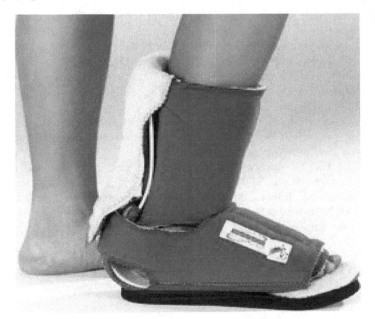

Fig. 4. Ankle Foot Orthosis

For injuries involving the lower limbs, full weight bearing is usually discouraged as this could lead to more tissue damage. Physical therapists usually prescribe cane or crutches for non-weight or partial weight bearing during ambulation.

12. Conclusion

Individuals who engage in regular sporting activities or exercise could be involved in injuries. Injuries can have serious negative impact on athletes in their sport performance as they are affected physically, mentally and emotionally. Pain is one of the major complaints after injuries and it is the reason why athletes seek medical attention. Effective management however depends on correct diagnosis based on history and evaluation. Relieve of pain could restore function and enhance fitness, health and quality of life. Injured athletes can be effectively managed through pharmacological and non pharmacological approaches. Non pharmacologic means involve surgery and conservative managements. Surgery is usually considered when other treatments have failed. Non steroidal anti-inflammatory drugs (NSAIDs) are most commonly prescribed with success. However, these drugs have been reported to have deleterious effects on some body structure especially cartilage. Athletes are enjoined to seek physical therapy, as it plays major roles in pain management of sport injuries with little or no side effects.

13. References

Adedoyin R. A., Olaogun, M.O.B. and Fagbeja, O.O. (2002) Interferential Current Stimulation for the treatment of Osteoarthritis of the knee pain. *Physiotherapy*. 88, 8; 493-499.

Adedoyin R.A. Olaogun M.O.B. Onipede T.O. Ikem IC (2005) Effects of Different Swing patterns of Interferential Current in Managing Low back Pain: A Single Control Trial Turkish Journal of Physiotherapy Rehabilitation. 16,2 :61-66.

Adedoyin R.A, Olaogun MOB, Oyeyemi AL (2005): Interferential Current & Trancutaneous Electrical Nerve Stimulation and Interferential Current Combined with exercise for the treatment of knee Osteoarthritis: a randomized controlled trial. Hong Kong Physiotherapy Journal 2:13-19.

Adedoyin RA, Olaogun MOB, Omotayo K, Olawale OA (2009): Effects of Wobble Board Training on Weight Distribution on the Lower Extremities of Sedentary Subjects. *Journal of Health and Technology.*

Barnett, A. (2006) Using recovery modalities between training sessions in elite athletes. *Sports Medicine*, 36 (9), 781-196

Chesterton LS, Foster NE, Ross L(2002) Skin temperature response to cryotherapy. *Archives of Physical Medicine and Rehabilitation*, 83 (4), 543-549

Dyson m (1987) Mechanisms involved in therapeutic ultrasound. *Physiotherapy*, 73:116-20

Dyson M, Suckling J (1978) Stimulation of tissue repair by ultrasound: a survey of the mechanisms involved. *Physiotherapy* 64:105-8

Ebnezar J (2003) Essentials of orthopaedics for physiotherapists. 1st Ed. New Delhi, Jaypee Brothers Medical Publishers (p) Ltd., 52-59

Enwemeka CS, Allen C, Avila P, Bina J, Konrade J, Munns S (2002). Soft tissue thermodynamics before, during, and after cold pack therapy. *Med Sci Sports Exerc.* 34(1):45-50.

Erith, SJ, Bailey, DM, Grant, N, Hupton, J, Thomas, A and Williams, C. (2007) Influence of cold-water immersion on indices of muscle damage following prolonged intermittent shuttle running. *Journal of Sports Science.* 25 (11), 1163-70

Eston, R. and Peters, D. (1999) Effects of cold water immersion on the symptoms of exercise induced muscle damage. *Journal of Sports Sciences,* 17, 231-238.

Fritz S (2004) Fundamentals of therapeutic massage. 3rd. Ed., Quebecor World Dubuque, Mosby, 513-514, 654.

Goats GC. Interferential Current Therapy. *Br J.Sp. Med* 1990; 24 (20): 87-91.

Goodall, S and Howatson, G. (2008) The effects of multiple cold water immersions on indices of muscle damage. *Journal of Sports Science and Medicine* 7, 235-241.

Hawkins JR, Knight, KL (2007) Rate of Cryotherapy Temperature Change – A Function of Adipose Thickness Or Thermocouple Depth? *Journal of Athletic Training* S-65 42 (2)

International Association for the study of pain (1994) Classification of Chronic Pain Descriptions of Chronic Pain Syndromes and Definitions of Pain Terms. Second Edition

Johnson MI (2001) Transcutaneous electrical nerve stimulation (TENS) and TENS like devices: do they produce pain relief? *Pain Review,* 8:122-158.

Johnson MI. (1999) The mystique of interferential currents when used to manage pain. *Physiotherapy* 85(6): 294-297.

Johnson P H (2000): Massage:physical therapist's clinical companion. United States of America, Springhouse Corporation, 364-365

Khanna A, Nelmes RT, Gougoulias N, Maffulli N, Gray J. (2009). The effects of LIPUS on soft-tissue healing: a review of literature. *Br Med Bull.* 89:169-182

Kisner C, Colby LA (2007) Therapeutic exercise: foundations and techniques 5th Ed. Philadelphia, FA Davis Company, 296-298,305-307.

Lachmann S (1989) Soft tissue injuries in sport. Blackwell Scientific publications

Low J, Reed A (2000): Electrotherapy explained principles and practice. 3rd Ed. New Delhi, Butterworth Heineman, 185-186

Martínez FC, Nohales CP, Canal, CP, Martín MJL, Catalán, MH and G. Cañadas, GO (1996) Dermatological cryosurgery in primary care with dimethyl ether propane Spray in comparison with liquid nitrogen Atención Primaria 18; (5) : 211, 216.

Melzack R, Wall PD (1965). Pain Mechanisms: a new theory. Science 150; 971-979.

Nyland J (2006) Clinical Decisions in Therapeutic Exercise-Planning and Implementation. *Julie Levin Alexander* 171-229.

O'sullivan SB, Schmitz TJ (1994) Physical rehabilitation: assessment and treatment.3rd Ed. Philadelphia, FA Davis Company, 423.

Schneider FJ (1990) Traumatic Spinal cord injury. In Umphred DA (ed)Neurological rehabilitation, ed 2. CV Mosby, st louis, 423.

Sparrow KJ, Finucane SD, Owen JR, Wayne JS. (2005) The effects of low-intensity ultrasound on medial collateral ligament healing in the rabbit model. *Am J Sports Med,* 33, 1048–1056.

Speed CA, (2001) Therapeutic ultrasound in soft tissue lesions. *Rheumatology,* 40: 1331-1336

Sullivan, J. & Anderson, S. (Eds.). (2000). Care of the Young Athlete. American Academy of
    Orthopaedic Surgeons *Source?*

Ter H G, Dyson M, Oakley E M. (1985) the use of ultrasound by physiotherapists in Britain.
    Ultrasound Med Biol, 13 : 33-7

Ter H C (1987) Basic physics of therapeutic ultrasound. *Physiotherapy*, 73 : 110-3

6

Pilates Based Exercise in Muscle Disbalances Prevention and Treatment of Sports Injuries

Sylwia Mętel, Agata Milert and Elżbieta Szczygieł
¹Institute of Physiotherapy Faculty of Health Care,
Jagiellonian University Medical College in Krakow
²Department of Physiotherapy, Faculty of Health and Medicine,
Andrzej Frycz Modrzewski Krakow University,
³Department of Physiotherapy, Faculty of Motor Rehabilitation,
The University School of Physical Education in Krakow
Poland

1. Introduction

The Pilates method has today become more popular than ever. As a form of movement it serves as a basis for fitness, complements sports training and is also one of the methods of physiotherapy. Pilates method combines features typical both for Eastern systems (mind control during exercises, relaxation, increasing of elasticity, movement starting from body center, balance) and Western systems (forming strength, endurance, exercises having both global and local effects). The primary goals in muscle-strain rehabilitation include not only recovery of muscle strength and flexibility but also correction of muscle imbalances. In prevention of sports injuries complementary training regarding body awareness, economical breathing, neuromuscular coordination by executing fluent and precise movement starting from a strong core is suggested. The Pilates based exercise, performed under the supervision of a certified instructor serve these needs and can be part of prophylaxis and kinesitherapy in sport medicine.

2. Joseph H. Pilates – A sportsman and kinesitherapist

Joseph Humbertus Pilates (1880-1967) was born in Germany with poor health. The medicine at that time could not offer any antibiotics nor other modern cures. Human health depended mostly on being able bodied. Regular physical exercises were regarded as a prime method of prevention and treatment of many illnesses.

From his parents Pilates learnt how to run sport activities and incorporate physical exercises in the healing process to stimulate it.

In the 19th century there were two main gymnastic systems. The first one was developed by the German Friedrich Jahn. His system derived from ancient Greek gymnastics and was mostly focused on improvement of strength and fitness, which, according to Jahn, were directly connected with well being. The second system, created by the Swede Per Henrik Ling, emphasized rhythm and fluidity of movements. The purpose of these exercises was to improve the endurance, strength and flexibility of muscles and joints, thereby improving the efficiency of the circulatory system. In Ling' exercise system it was breathing and movement coordination as well as conscious body control during practising were emphasised (Latey 2001). In his early youth J. Pilates gymnastic systems and some common elements can be found in his later invented system of fitness exercises. Since childhood, Pilates was dedicated to practising various physical exercises and developed his interest in human anatomy. As a role model, Pilates took the antic model of beauty, based on the harmonious development of body, mind and spirit. By practising reasonable and balanced sports Pilates became a perfect model for anatomy charts (Mętel & Milert, 2007).

As a young man, Pilates ran many sport activities, e.g. diving and skiing. He was interested in other gymnastic systems (e.g. Yoga) and martial arts (karate). In 1912 he moved to England, earning a living through boxing and as a self-defence trainer. During the World War I he was interned in a prison camp on the Isle of Man, where he organized conditioning exercises for fellow prisoners. It was during this period this Pilates formed his idea on health and healthy lifestyle. Pilates believed that the only way to health is to keep the balance of body and mind, whilst the modern, sedentary lifestyle, bad posture and inefficient breathing were the roots of poor health. Pilates dubbed this philosophy "Contrology", as described in 1934 in his book "Your Health".

Unable to keep practising floor exercises with his fellow camp interns, Pilates used bed springs in resistance exercises, whereby the war wounded could regain their health and fitness while still bed-bound (Sparrowe, 1994, as cited in Latey, 2001). The apparatus Pilates designed during this time served as forerunners of the exercise machines such as „Universal Reformer" and „Cadillac" (Trapeze table); spring-based equipment used in Pilates' exercise method.

Pilates returned to Germany after World War I, but in 1926 emigrated to the USA. In New York, together with his wife Clara, he opened his exercise studio. His clients were mostly dancers, with boxers and gymnasts also embracing his method. One of the reasons the method was enthusiastically welcomed by dancers was its similarity to dance in its pursuit of extreme range of movement with precision and control; something a dancer is always attempting to achieve (Latey, 2002). Pilates taught mat and apparatus classes, which required high physical fitness from trainees (McNeill, 2011). In his second book, "Return to Life Through Contrology" (1945), he included selected exercises to follow and practise at home and the development of his philosophy (Latey, 2001). By the time of his death Pilates had extended his system of fitness exercises, describing the principles of correct performance. Pilates stated that his physical exercises could prevent coronary heart disease, increase muscle power and reduce the risk of respiratory ailments. He claimed the efficacy of his method to be scientifically proven, but at the time no such investigation was performed (Lange et al., 2000).

Nowadays, many new Pilates exercises are created based on the elementary ones. They are modified and adapted to various levels of physical fitness, and to the health and age of the practitioner – including those with trauma and elite athletes. In "Traditional" or "Repertory" Pilates, the exercises are vigorous with a fast, dynamic rhythm and even with high level of concentration are not easy to perform properly. They rely on the client having a fairly healthy body with good level of flexibility and to achieve some of the desired positions or range of motion, some muscle groups are obliged to work very hard. This fact contradicts Joseph Pilates' belief in working all the muscles of the body evenly. However, Pilates' ability to keep the rest of an injured body strong and flexible, while allowing the injured body part to heal enables the client to return to work almost as soon as the injury is repaired. This method of kinesitherapy remains highly relevant today and can be applied to people of all fitness levels (Lately, 2002).

Nowadays, applied Pilates based exercises have been influenced by other body-mind methods and improved by an improved understanding of the human body, new perspectives on illness, advances in medical treatment, new understandings in stress management, developments in psychology and teaching skills. We also support the statement of Lately (Lately, 2002) that updating the principles of the Pilates method has given physiotherapy a new direction, and influenced exercise prescription in many body work fields, including sports medicine. We mainly concentrate on the prevention of injury caused by muscle imbalances and post-acute rehabilitation.

3. Methodology and equipment in Pilates' system

Pilates' exercise system can be divided into two categories: floor mat exercises and professional Pilates' devices. Originally, J. Pilates invented a system of stretching and strengthening mat exercises. Later this was extended to include exercises designed using specially designed apparatuses, e.g. Universal Reformer, Cadillac (Trapeze Table), Wunda (Combo) Chair.

The basis of the Pilates system are mat exercises. Postural muscles are mainly strengthened and stretched in low positions, using gravity and the exercised parts of the body. Balanced development of these muscles promotes proper body posture during various activities of daily living and decreases the effects of long-lasting burden, caused by practicing diverse sport disciplines. This makes the Pilates method similar to spine stabilization exercises. It assumes that weakness or fatigue of postural muscles can lead to disturbances of stability in the lumbar spine, which in turn can lead to strain injuries and chronic back pain. A critically important element of this type of training is conscious activation of the profound muscles of abdomen - transversus abdominis (TrA) and pelvic floor muscles (PV), which should fire first for pre-movement stability, and recovering elasticity and eccentric work of superficial muscles.

Exercises on professional Pilates' devices are mainly resistance exercise performed with the aid of springs and pulleys, but also stress relief of certain parts of the body can be achieved. The machines can be customized to the needs of the practitioner. The resistance during the exercise allows movement to be isolated and performed in the proper plane. Additional resistance prevents automatic movements being responsible for injuries. The exercises using professional Pilates' devices can be performed in post-acute state of sports injuries.

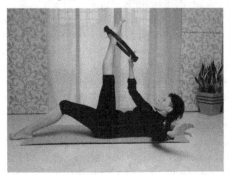

Fig. 1. Multidimensional exercise with Pilates circle

Pilates method also utilises small equipment (balls, foam rollers, Pilates circle, balance boards, Thera-bands etc.). They can be used in intralimb and interlimb coordination exercises, or as an element making exercises more attractive. They can also help transferring the learnt exercises to the movement required to run particular sport activities. (e.g. catching or kicking the ball).

In physiotherapy praxis Pilates based exercises are also performed with a gymnastic stick, a gym ladder and a stool. Pilates based exercises using a Swiss ball are also very popular, as is sensoric massage with this tool.

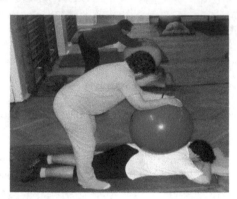

Fig. 2. Sensoric massage with Swiss ball

Exercises are performed from low (lying prone, supine, side-lying, quadriped, sitting) medium and high (kneeling, standing) postures. Low postures ensure better stability during the exercises, used particularly at the early stage of movement learning. Such positions facilitate proper performance of complex movements of upper and lower limbs, aiding concentration on other aspects of exercises (e.g. breathing, precision, flow). In case of complaint such as after injuries or with chronic low back pain, low position stabilisation of the trunk prevents additional unwanted movements that could cause more pain during exercising. For this reason low positions are more often used in early stages of after-injury rehabilitation excluding exercises exerting long lever on the spine. The upper positions can be used at the later stages of rehabilitation. Regardless of the exercise type and position, the movements are performed slowly and deliberately, beginning by correcting the starting position using physical or verbal instructions.

The number of repetitions is usually limited to 5-10. Pilates claimed that the lesser the number of repetitions of the movement performed properly the better the therapeutic effect was. Excessive number of repetitions performed without concentration and awarness can be harmful and lead to injuries. From approximately 500 mat or device exercises that have been developed in Modern Pilates the training programs should be tailored to the practitioner on an individual basis, taking into account his movement abilities and needs (elasticity of tissues, muscle strength and endurance, coordination and concentration ability). The best results can be achieved when practicing one-on-one or in small groups.

The implementation of this method for sports training should start with introducing the so-called pre-Pilates exercises, which allows a moderate degree of difficulty to implement all the principles of this technique from the three-dimensional breathing, slowly adding body alignment, concentration, control, stamina and fluency in performing movement. Moreover, in modern Pilates based exercise it is not recommended to start each session with an exercise called "The Hundred", as it used to be in traditional Pilates method. According to Lately (Lateley, 2002) this exercise is particularly arduous as an initial exercise, might be extremely dangerous for someone new to the method, and even under supervision can result in severe injury. The authors concur with Lately on this issue.

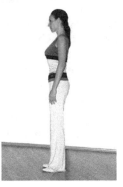

Fig. 3. Postural alignment in standing

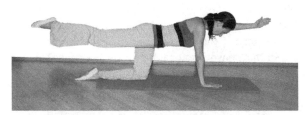

Fig. 4. Stability and endurance training: core muscle activation with limbs exercises

4. Body-mind exercise system

The purpose of the system of fitness exercises developed by Pilates is to develop harmony of body, mind and spirit by improving muscle strength and increasing the elasticity of active movement structures. The movements are carried out slowly and fluently with focused attention. These exercises are referred to as a "body-mind exercise system". Other such systems include also Yoga, Tai Chi and Feldenkreis' method.

"Body-mind exercises" is not the name of the exercise, but rather a description of how an exercise should be performed. Their common features are: mind control during exercises, relaxation of muscles and joints not involved in exercise movement, and maintaining muscles' physiological elasticity, with movement starting from body centre.

Understanding one's individual optimal postural alignment (neutral posture) will allow economy of movement, a natural flow of compensatory patterns, so that no muscle is overworked or misused, without aiming for perfect symmetry. Pilates explained the balance of body and mind as the conscious control of all muscular movements of the body. It is the correct utilisation and application of the leverage principles afforded by the bones comprising the skeletal framework of the body, a complete knowledge of the mechanism of the body, and a full understanding of the principles of equilibrium and gravity as applied to the movements of the body in motion, at rest and sleep. Concentration and awareness is one of the fundamental principles of Pilates' system. It determines movement in a particular muscle group. It is very important, especially when other sectors of locomotors apparatus do not act properly or are not in natural alignment because of trauma or sport injury. That is why Pilates' system is nowadays recognized as a relatively safe alternative for intensive aerobic or weight bearing exercises. (Latey, 2001, as cited in Latey, 2002).

Awareness of the performed movement improves its efficiency and quality of movements. According to the original assumptions of the Pilates' system it requires at least an elementary knowledge of biomechanics and functional anatomy by the practitioner. It facilitates the process of learning new movement patterns, especially those to be transferred into functional tasks such as walking, reaching, lifting and other daily living or sport activities (Lange et al., 2000).

Focusing on the therapeutic movement, particularly in the case of sport injuries helps to avoid errors in repeating the exercises without therapeutic supervision. Proper learning of movement can be also achieved with the help of hands-on guiding, assisting correct movement (touch can improve muscle engagement and relaxation). Verbal cues also play a very important role in increasing awareness of the therapeutic movement being performed and learnt. This applies particularly in the case of a limited amount of information such as typically used with elderly or stroke patients (Lange et al., 2000; Latey, 2000). Verbal cues of the Pilates based exercise instructor as well as his tactile stimulation (hands-on) aim to motivate the exercisers to increase the focus on how to perform movement and maintain the desired body position, so that sensorimotor integration is stimulated. Moreover, connecting the mind and body requires the exercising person to tune into their bodily sensory systems.

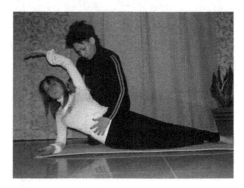

Fig. 5. "Hands on" for body alignment execution

Touch can improve muscle recruitment, a client's awareness and also introduce better body biomechanics and relaxation. Awareness of the sensations, touching the muscles and joints helps to focus concentration. Awareness of the body also assists in reducing overwork, strain and tension. Sportsmen particularly need awareness of their body, particularly the muscular sensations, so as to direct mental and physical efforts efficiently. Attending to the feedback from the proprioceptor system makes the individual aware of what is being done. Precision assists coordination; this is the practical application of focused awareness.

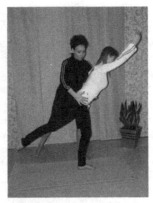

Fig. 6. Manual stimulus for increasing body awareness and desired muscle recruitment

5. "Powerhouse" – The strong core

Popular weight lifting in a gym studio typically focuses on improving muscle strength by shortening the muscles; the complex role of the supporting muscles is ignored. However, as the body lengthens, the diagonally opposed supporting muscles also have to work well. Stretching the muscles is an important part of sport training and in order to regain muscle balance, with the muscles lengthening and working at the same time, eccentric muscle contractures with proper support from stabilizing deep muscles and the body centre is needed.

Major emphasis in the Pilates concept should be placed upon the muscles forming 'powerhouse'- the body centre. Joseph Pilates himself never set down in writing what the exact parameters of the powerhouse were and there does not seem to be exact agreement amongst the master teachers of Pilates today. In a recent legal decision, the ability to trademark the name Pilates, and consequently the sole right of certification of Pilates instructors was lost. This means that there is no longer one certifying or governing body that determines exactly what the Pilates method is or is not. As a result, the Pilates based exercise, along with the underlying biomechanical basis, has been diverging greatly in recent years. There are now many techniques within the Pilates world, some adhering strictly to the system of exercises developed by Joseph Pilates, and others that are incorporating changes into this system.

The powerhouse is the core centre of the body from which peripheral muscle actions are carried out. The idea of centring is to create not only a strong structural powerhouse, but also a flexible one. Indeed, Joseph Pilates had the following maxim on his business card: "A man is only as old as his spine is inflexible". Profound muscle strengthening is a very important supplementation for training in various sports disciplines where big, superficial muscle groups are mainly reinforced. Skipping profound muscles in strength training leads to imbalance, which increases the risk of trauma, and often is the reason for serious sport injury. It is suggested that treatment of muscle imbalances should start with exercises that isolate specific core muscles and then progress into functional activities or complex sports movements where these muscle should act in synergy to stabilize the lumbo-pelvic region. Pilates method of body conditioning may be generalized to have three major effects upon the powerhouse. First, Pilates affects the posture of the pelvis, which results in postural changes to the lumbar spine. Second, it works directly upon the musculoskeletal structure of the spine (the lumbar spine in particular) by strengthening, stretching, and lengthening the spine. Third, Pilates affects the structural integrity or tone of the abdomino-pelvic cavity as a whole. The posture of the pelvis largely determines the posture of the spine. The spine sits upon the base of the sacrum; therefore, any change in the sagittal posture of the pelvis will change the level of the base of the sacrum. The level of the base of the sacrum will in turn affect the curve of the lumbar spine. However, once the base of the sacrum is uneven to any degree, the spine must have a curve in it to compensate. This curve is necessary to eventually create a level base for the head to sit upon. This righting mechanism to create a level base for the head is necessary to place the eyes and the labyrinthine receptors of the inner ear on a level plane, this being necessary for proper static and dynamic proprioception of our body.

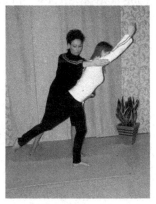

Fig. 7. Execution of strong core with body alignment before and during movement

One of the major emphases of Pilates is to address the posture of the pelvis by addressing the musculature of the pelvis. Pilates further corrects this imbalance by placing a strong emphasis on stretching the low back musculature. In this manner, Pilates aims to create a neutral pelvis, and thereby create a healthy lumbar lordosis. (Muscolino& Cipriani, 2004 as cited in Selby, 2002; Siler, 2000; Winsor, 1999).

6. Breathing in Pilates

Body posture has an impact on the functioning of the entire human organism. There are reasons to believe that correct posture is a prerequisite for correct breathing patterns (Fiz & Gnitecki, 2008). Deficient respiratory capacity reduces the amount of oxygen delivered to body cells, which hampers both physical and intellectual performance. Symptoms of oxygen deficiency include headache, vertigo, lack of appetite as well as concentration and memory malfunctions. Lower oxygen levels have a negative impact on muscles, which are likely to work deficiently under such circumstances and tire faster, which can lead to general fatigue and listlessness. The body tries to compensate for the oxygen loss, involving additional breathing muscles in the respiratory process, which then requires higher energy consumption and reduces its efficiency. The entire body is involved in breathing. During respiration, the functioning of the breathing muscles changes the dimensions of the chest. Shoulders and particular backbone sections are also part of the breathing cycle. Any immobilization, disfigurement, pain, lesions or developmental defects of the chest, as well as breathing muscles palsy can have important consequences for mobility and thus reduce the lungs' ventilation range. It needs to be stressed that most pathological processes, not only such severe ones as pneumonia, bronchitis, chronic obstructive pulmonary disease and heart failure, but also those of lesser clinical importance, including meteorism, intercostal nerve pains, or shoulder neuralgia clearly change the breathing mechanics (Dyszkiewicz et al., 2003). Changes in posture and its incorrect models related to the synchronized functioning of the muscles of the neck, upper body, abdomen, shoulders and pelvis are crucial for breathing (and in consequence for chest mobility). Other remote factors, seemingly unrelated to chest biomechanics, include the impairment of the motoric function of the lower extremities and the backbone, with a modification of the movement patterns. Research carried out by Szczygieł (Szczygieł et al., 2010) on healthy people indicated that even momentary slightly forced posture distortions can have a strong impact on breathing parameters. The research was an attempt to specify the plane in which posture distortions most severely influence the functioning of the respiratory system. Results show that the body arrangement most likely to lead to a reduction of the VC is posture with counter-lateral head, shoulder and hip rotation. The position responsible for the greatest reduction of other factors (VC- Vital Capacity, FEV1- Forced Expiratory Volume in One Second, MEF75- Maximal Expiratory Flow at 75% of Force Vital Capacity, MEF50- Maximal Expiratory Flow at 50% of Force Vital Capacity, MEF25- Maximal Expiratory Flow at 25% of Force Vital Capacity and PEF- Peak Expiratory Flow) was frontal stooping. Positions with sagittal plane changes had the smallest effect on breathing mechanics. Therefore, optimum conditions for breathing require an axial arrangement of particular body segments.

According to Joseph Pilates "breathing is the principal art of life. Our life depends on it. Millions have never learned the art of correct breathing." From the day we were born, we have been breathing unconsciously, without worrying if our breathing is correct.

Correct coordination of breathing with a particular exercise is the rule of thumb applied while teaching the Pilates method. Correct breathing improves blood oxidation, brain function and movement control.

In Pilates, costal-diaphragmatic breathing is used, accentuating protracted exhalation with simultaneous drawing of the navel closer to the spine. While inhaling, the chest expands in three planes, and while exhaling, abdominal oblique muscles become involved. This is called "lateral breathing". Lateral breathing causes the chest to expand, and the air penetrates the back and lateral parts of the chest. This stimulates intercostal muscles, allowing them to expand and making the upper body more agile.

Normally, our breath is too shallow, and stress compounds the problem, making our breathing faster and even shallower (Rakowska, 1990). Women tend to breathe with the tip or the upper part of the lungs, raising their shoulders and the upper body. Men are more likely to breathe using their diaphragm, making their abdomen expand with every breath.

An important element of the Pilates method is being able to expand the ribs laterally, which helps you to draw in your abdomen, at the same time relaxing the upper body. While accentuating the axial arrangement of the body, the method ensures the optimum conditions for the respiratory system and helps to stabilize the backbone. This is of crucial importance for people practicing sports, who are likely to adopt forced body posture. This increases the risk of overload changes in the body, and hampers the functioning of the respiratory system (Bliss et al., 2005). Unlike other exercises based on passive breathing, the Pilates breathing method involves active respiration. It activates outer intercostal muscles and abdominal muscles. The most efficient muscle participating in breathing out, and thus in increasing the pressure in the abdominal cavity is the transverse abdominal muscle (Zocchi et al., 1993).

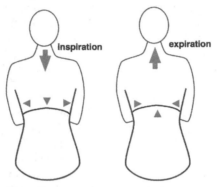

Fig. 8. Pilates method breathing

Deep breathing is an important element of exercise optimisation. The fact that the basic movements in the exercise are made while breathing out, sets the method apart from others. In addition, prolonging exhalation helps to counteract the occurrence of undesirable tension (protracted additional respiratory muscle cramps) and ensures greater stabilization in the most difficult phases of the exercise. While considering reports on the effectiveness of the method, an issue that must be mentioned is the case of diaphragm rupture while breathing deeply using the Pilates method (Yang et al., 2010). Cases of such spontaneous diaphragm rupture, without prior antecedents in patients, are extremely rare. They may occur e.g. with abrupt coughing. They account for ca. 1% of similar diaphragm problems (Gupta et al., 2005). The causes are related to a rapid increase in abdominal pressure. Weighted against the benefits of the method, such cases seem to be of marginal importance.

Meanwhile, both scientific magazines and popular science publications frequently look at bronchial asthma in athletes. Statistics regarding asthma indicate that it occurs more frequently in athletes than in the general population (Weiler et al., 1998). This topic is quite controversial. On the one hand, it is suggested that prolonged intensive training may lead to the development of bronchial asthma (Weiler et al., 1998) and (Helenius et al., 1998). At the same time, the issue of the use of medicines by asthmatic athletes in the context of pharmacological doping is raised. In light of the above, the Pilates breathing method may be a valuable element of physical training. There is no doubt that optimum breathing allows for longer and more intensive training without running the risk of excess fatigue. The asthma debate is exhaustively discussed in an article by Wroński. The author believes that Pilates breathing exercises can be used to complement drug therapy in children and young people with bronchial asthma (Wroński& Nowak ,2008).

7. Muscle imbalances and Pilates practising by sportsman

The muscle balance in any joint is determined by the ratio of torques between agonist and antagonist muscle groups. The coordination of movements depends on the coordinated actions of muscles on the opposite sides of a joint. This prevents injuries of muscles, tendons, and joint elements during fast movements. The deficiency of strength in one muscle or muscle group can lead to imbalance in the joint actions, which in turn can cause traumas of muscles and joints due to the anomalous distribution of mechanical stresses and strains.(Pontaga, 2003) The terms muscle balance or imbalance do not refer to equal or unequal torque values, but to the balance between the torque ratios of agonistic and antagonistic muscle groups (Gioftsidou et al., 2008). There is a failure of the agonist-antagonist relationship and to their balance between the torque ratios. Muscle imbalances resulting in overloaded movement apparatus can result from frequent repetition of movement patterns specific to the sport's discipline. Static overload refers to the maintenance of posture of the body for a longer period of time such as the trunk flexion in cycling, downhill, speed skating, alpine skiing. Dynamic overload can result from forced movement which is typical of the discipline, leading to the development of muscle imbalances. Because the human physiological motor activities take place in the area of the force of gravity to align the existing muscle imbalances Pilates method offers exercises in various starting positions with multidimensional movements in which skeletal muscle are activated in a manner conducive not only to development of their strength but also endurance, flexibility and neuromuscular coordination. Therefore, this system, with appropriate supervision and adjustment of the degree of difficulty of the exercises to be performed without losing the flow of movement and dynamic stabilization of the deep muscle system appears to be appropriate in the eradication of unwanted muscle imbalances. Recent studies hypothesized a common muscle imbalance pattern of weakness in gluteus medius and tightness of the iliotibial band in chronic musculoskeletal pain syndromes in the lumbar-pelvic-hip area such as chronic low back pain. Investigators categorized muscles, based on their primary functions, as "phasic" or "postural", and indicated that in response to dysfunction or overuse, the phasic muscles tend to be inhibited or weakened; while the postural muscles tend to develop higher tone and ultimately shorten. [Jull&Janda, 1987, Janda 1992,1993 as cited in Arab&Nourbakhsh, 2010] Tight muscles are activated more readily during movement patterns and become overactive. Once the phasic and postural muscles are no longer activated in balance, they are unable to protect the body's joints from the effects of gravity.(Page, 2005)

In this classification, the gluteus medius; primary muscle for hip abduction, is categorized as phasic and the tensor fasciae latae and iliotibial band the synergist muscle, is categorized as postural muscle. It is speculated that the iliotibial band shortness in patients with low back pain is a compensatory mechanism following hip abductor weakness. (Jull&Janda, 1987 as cited in Arab&Nourbakhsh, 2010). Controversial results have been reported in the studies which examined the relationship between hip abductor strength and the iliotibial band syndrome in runners. Some researchers concluded after conducting a study with runners with the iliotibial band problems that strengthening of the hip abductors has been recommended for symptom improvement in subjects with the iliotibial band dysfunction (Fredericson&Weir, 2006, MacMahon et al. 2000 as cited in Arab&Nourbakhsh, 2010) while others in contrast (Grau et al., 2008 as cited in Arab&Nourbakhsh, 2010) concluded that weakness of hip abductors does not seem to play a role in the etiology of the iliotibial band syndrome in runners. Some reports have also demonstrated an association between LBP and hip abductor muscle weakness.

Considering the above reports and the promising results of research on the effects of Pilates exercises to reduce chronic low back pain seems to be a reasonable recommendation to use Pilates techniques for athletes with low back pain. Note, however, that the scientific evidence demonstrating the efficacy of this method in the treatment of back pain are incomplete. Modern group sports such as soccer is marked by a faster speed of play than in the past, and this inevitably translates into an increase in the intensity of practice sessions. This may justify an increase in the percentage of muscle strains occurring during practice.

We suggest an assessment whether it is observed that a player's muscle imbalances is only an adaptive response to the athlete's body to the demands of the discipline and is tolerated by him, or results of biomechanical changes in articular' trajectory caused by the development of the areas in the body with reduced resistance to overload (locus minores resistanci). It is worth to check if after previous trauma protective mechanisms of the damaged area have extinguished and not result in persistently maintaining the stiffness and the development of undesirable tissue compensation. Because such mechanism may change a whole myofascial chain and neuromuscular coordination it is possible that pain may also occurs in a place located far away from the primary pathology. Also, persistent pain or fear of its occurrence may lead to changes in motor programs resulting in the development of muscle imbalance syndromes, particularly in muscle tone and their flexibility. For example, examining the strength and elasticity of muscles of lower limbs, often stated gluteal muscles weakness and their function of the hip' extension is overtaken by hamstring muscles which results in excessive tension and shortening. In turn, the weakening of the abductors and external hips' rotators, usually cause the hypertone in the area of iliotibial band. Certain muscles in the human body are especially subjected to strain traumas, for example, the posterior muscle group of thigh. The simultaneous extension of the hip joint and flexion of the knee stretch the posterior muscle group of thigh and, if the movements are very fast and forceful (sprinting, bobsledding, jumping, and other athletic sports), these muscles can be injured.(Pontaga, 2003). In the study analysing muscle injuries suffered in Italian major-league soccer team during the period 1995–2000 it was found that among the overall injuries, muscle accidents were the most frequent, representing 30% (103 cases), followed by contusions (28%), sprains (17%) and tendinopathies (9%). Proposed causes of muscle strains were: lack of training, insufficient warming up, excessive fatigue, strength imbalances, flexibility deficiencies, muscle weakness and insufficient rehabilitation. (Volpi et al., 2004)

A study of the role of eccentric muscular work in the development of muscle strains found a residual eccentric-strength deficit in sprinters with a history of hamstring injury compared to runners with no injuries. (Jonhagen et al. 1994 as cited in Volpi et al., 2004)

Factors increasing the risk of developing acute muscle injuries, include decreased muscle strength, mainly eccentric muscle strength and muscle imbalance (decreased eccentric work of antagonist to concentric work of agonist (Schwellnus, 2004 as cited in Gioftsidou et al., 2008). In running and kicking there is an important eccentric activation of thigh muscles. When decelerating in running, the hamstrings act eccentrically to slow extension at the knee, and the quadriceps act eccentrically to control the lowering of body weight when athletes approach a stop. In kicking muscles, activation follows "the soccer paradox" meaning that flexor activity is dominant during extension and extensor activity dominates during flexion. Quadriceps activity is greatest during the loading phase when it is antagonistic to the movement and hamstrings are most active during the forward swing when they are antagonistic to the movement (Volpi et al., 2004).

There is no knee extensor activity immediately prior to ball contact. The eccentric activation of knee flexors reduces the angular velocity at the knee. Such a mechanism protects the knee from hyperextension, but it is extremely stressful for hamstrings. (Robertson&Moshe,1985 as cited in Volpi et al., 2004). Electromyography studies have confirmed hamstring peak activity near the time of ball contact. (Wahrenberg et al., 1978 as cited in Volpi et al., 2004)

Recuperation of flexibility (Kujala et al., 1997 as cited in Volpi et al., 2004), amelioration of muscle strength (Worrell, 1994 as cited in Volpi et al., 2004) and correction of muscle imbalances (Welsch, 1988 as cited in Volpi et al., 2004) represented the primary goals in muscle-strain rehabilitation. It is important to underline that prevention of recurrences, not speed of recovery, is the primary goal in muscle- strain rehabilitation. It is suggested that athletes who have suffered a muscle injury must never give up eccentric work for the rest of their careers (Volpi et al., 2004).

As Pilates method offers different eccentric exercises for trunk and leg muscle e.g. rolling the spine in different position with or without using the equipment or tools (Swiss ball, Thera-band) in our opinion this method can be suggested as a complementary sport training. Elasticity of the leg muscles, especially hamstrings, iliopsoas, quadriceps, hip rotators, plays very important role in maintaining the proper body posture both in rest and in motion. Weakness and contractions of this muscles lead to improper pelvic alignment in standing position, and consequently in spine and total body. In athletes practicing e.g. cycling, leg muscles work intensively in contracting position, while complementary Pilates training provides the eccentric exercises.

It is indicated that fatigue of the shoulder complex muscles, which may occur in overhead athletes or workers with regular exposure to overhead work, is proposed to be a neuromuscular alteration that contributes to shoulder pathology. Acute muscle fatigue may create short-term muscle force imbalances and disrupt normal synergistic activation of the muscles at the shoulder region. These activation imbalances may in turn result in the scapulothoracic kinematic alterations. Acute fatigue of the serratus anterior may be particularly problematic as this muscle has been noted to be the primary contributor to both normal three-dimensional scapula rotations and scapulothoracic stability. In addition, the serratus anterior is considered to be one component of several muscle synergies at the shoulder complex and its fatigue may alter the balance of these synergies. (Szucs et al., 2009)

Precise control of movement at the shoulder complex during upper extremity use is considered critical to the health of the shoulder region. In Pilates based exercise it is strongly recommended to keep scapulas in position of "soft V" at starting positions so the intention is to voluntarily "fix" the scapula in the position of posterial depression. It is generally accepted that serratus anterior and the trapezius (upper and lower) should work with proper timing to provide normal, three-phases humero-scapular rhythm. In first phase upper trapezius should be relaxed and scapula fixation should be provide by lower trapezius. In second phase scapula external rotation is achieved by the activation of serratus anterior and at last upper trapezius with other scapula's elevators need to fire to lift the scapula up. (Horst, 2010)

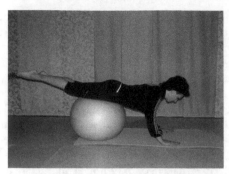

Fig. 9. Push-up exercise on Swiss ball, starting position without "locked elbows"

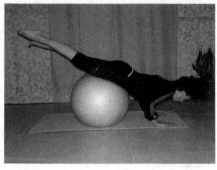

Fig. 10. Push-up exercise on Swiss ball , movement with activation of strong core

It was found that the upper trapezius and serratus anterior are under differing cortical control mechanisms, with trapezius but not serratus demonstrating both contralateral and ipsilateral responses to cortical magnetic stimulation. Increased upper trapezius tone and constant readiness to activate disturbs the humero-scapular rhythm and is also an indication of fatigue or compensation of serratus anterior. As muscle fatigue can be a central phenomenon as well as a peripheral phenomenon, the upper trapezius may have been recruited differently during or after the task. (Alexander et al., 2007, Hunter et al., 2006 as cited in Szucs et al., 2009) It is ball, important that performing Pilates Push-up, which is an exercise in close kinematic chain, serratus anterior muscle should be activated rather than a dominant role of upper trapezius muscle which can be achieved by the alignment of spine, unlocked elbow joints, lower – costal breathing and touching stimulus of an instructor during execution of an exercise.

The Push-up exercise has been recommended as a rehabilitative exercise for individuals with shoulder pathology because it strongly activates serratus anterior while minimizing upper trapezius co-activation (Ekstrom et al., 2005, Lear&Gross 1998, Ludewig et al., 2004 as cited in Szucs et al., 2009). Using this task as a rehabilitative exercise may be too strenuous for most patients, but it may have potential as an assessment tool to help determine the success of serratus anterior strengthening and endurance training or the readiness for return to high demand overhead work. (Szucs et al., 2009)

The results of the controlled study with 19 participants show that a 12-week long Pilates training program was effective in improving core strength and posture (exercising subjects showed smaller static thoracic kyphosis during quiet standing) as well as certain aspects of scapula and upper trunk displacement during a shoulder flexion task. As deficits in neck–shoulder biomechanics have previously been associated with symptoms in the neck–shoulder region, these results could support the use of the Pilates method in the prevention of neck–shoulder disorders.(Emery K., 2010)

In our opinion Pilates can be recommened as a complementary exercising method for many sports discipline to reduce muscle imbalances, increase body awareness, sensomotoric coordination, economical breathing, body aligment, precision and fluency in movement however deep understanding and proper implementation in the practise the main Pilates principles under close supervision of certified and experienced Pilates instructor is needed.

8. Pilates method in evidence based medicine

Current state of neurophysiological and biomechanical knowledge has caused that classical Pilates technique evaluated into Pilates based exercises which are recommended for use by people of varying age and physical proficiency. We conducted database searches (SPRINGER LINK, SCIENCE DIRECT, EBSCO HEALTH SOURCE, MEDLINE, PUBMED, COCHRANE, EMBASE) up to the June 2011 to investigate the application and effectiveness of this method using the key word "Pilates".

8.1 Pilates based exercise programs effects in different age population

Rogers and Gibson explains that studies concerning Pilates method primary concentrated on its effects in rehabilitation or to increase specific component of movement – such as tennis serve velocity (Sewright, 2004 as cited in Rogers&Gibson, 2009), leaping ability (Hutchinson 1998 as cited in Rogers&Gibson, 2009) or muscular strength and endurance in specific population.

In a controlled experiment of Rogers and Gibson with healthy, young objects (n=28) in which novice practitioners (n=9) participated 3–times a week, 1-hour session in 8-week traditional mat Pilates program, it was concluded that in experimental group body composition, muscle endurance and flexibility improved compared to participants of university wellness centre forming the control group. (Rogers&Gibson, 2009)

In the controlled study of Siqueira Rodriges with 52 elderly females, 27 persons formed the Pilates group participating in Pilates exercises twice a week for eight weeks. The researchers concluded that the practice of the Pilates method can improve the functional autonomy and static balance of elderly individuals (Siqueira Rodrigues et al., 2010)

In pilot study with 7 older adults who participated in a novel Pilates inspired exercise program specifically designed to improve balance in an upright position, referred to as postural stability it was indicated that the effect in relation to static balance can be a consequence of postural stability, reached by the harmony of opposing muscle groups. (Kaesler et al., 2007)

Siqueira Rodrigues introduce Pilates as a method consisting of a physical exercise that uses resources such as gravity and the resistance of springs, either to resist or assist movement execution (Gagnon, 2005 as cited Siqueira Rodrigues et al., 2010). It aims to prevent automatic movements, which are responsible for unwanted muscle activity that can cause injuries (Petrofsky et al., 2005 as cited in Siqueira Rodrigues et al., 2010). Siqueira Rodrigues also indicates that Pilates method has been studied in relation to its positive effects on posture (Blum, 2002 as cited in Siqueira Rodrigues et al., 2010), pain control (Gladwell et al.,

2006 as cited in Siqueira Rodrigues et al., 2010), improved muscle strength (Schroeder et al., 2002 as cited in Siqueira Rodrigues et al., 2010), flexibility (Segal et al., 2004 as cited in Siqueira Rodrigues et al., 2010), and motor skills (Lange et al., 2000 as cited in Siqueira Rodrigues et al., 2010).

The positive influence of Pilates exercise on dynamic balance and personal autonomy in healthy adults was assessed in the controlled study with the 17 participants of 10 Pilates-based exercise sessions performed on a Reformer and including a tall arm series, open leg rocker, leg press series and tall kneel arm series. After the Pilates training significant change in dynamic balance was found in the Functional Reach Test, while control, non-exercising group (n=17) demonstrated no significant change. These findings suggest that Pilates-based exercise may be a useful tool for clinicians and trainers to incorporate with their patients and clients who are looking to improve their dynamic balance and also benefit athletes who are seeking small gains to improve performance through precise, controlled movements. (Johnson et al., 2007)

Some authors indicates that Pilates encouraged the importance of proprioceptive stimulation for motor learning improvement using the powerhouse exercise (transversus abdominus, obliques, and multifidi muscles) and repetition of correct movement to achieve the training standard, leading to a better motor performance and less risk of injuries. (Anderson & Spector, 2000 as cited in Siqueira Rodrigues et al., 2010)

An observational study was conducted to assess and compare the contraction of the transversus abdominis muscle among 36 healthy females (mean age 36.2) trained in Pilates, traditional abdominal curls and a control group. To indirectly measure contraction of the transversus abdominis muscle and to monitor lumbar–pelvic stability, a stabilizer pressure biofeedback unit (Chattanooga Group Inc.) was employed and a tester, blinded to group category, conducted the measurements. For the lumbar–pelvic stability test, only 5 (42%) Pilates group subjects passed this test, with all others failing this test, leaving 14% overall who were able to stabilize the lumbar–pelvic area. The authors concluded that females who train in Pilates may be better able to recruit and utilize their deep abdominal muscles and stabilize the pelvic area compared to those not trained in Pilates. (Herrington & Davies, 2005)

In the controlled, experiment with 34 pain-free health club members with no Pilates experience who were randomly assigned to an unsupervised twice weekly of eight weeks Pilates mat exercises or strength training it was concluded that transversus abdominis activation increased following a programme of unsupervised Pilates mat exercises that is practical and requires no special equipment, however, there was no change in abdominal muscle activation during functional postures. The researchers suggested that supervision of exercises and progression to more functional exercises may be required to increase functional abdominal activation. (Critchley et al., 2011)

Performing Pilates exercise might prove to be a useful means of increasing activity and thereby curbing the obesity epidemic of female teenagers. It was proven in a randomised, controlled study that 4 weeks long physical training with the Pilates technique lowered the BMI percentile of 10- to 12-year-old girls. (Jago et al., 2006)

8.2 Pilates method and low back pain

Two systematic reviews of all controlled clinical trials of Pilates to treat low back pain were recently conducted. In the most recent review the search strategy was filled up to May 2010 and generated a total of 199 references, of which 51 were considered potentially relevant. Study quality was assessed using the Oxford scale. Four eligible randomized controlled clinical trials (n ¼ 4) involving Pilates for the management of low back pain were included. They originated from the United Kingdom (Gladwell et al., 2006 as cited in Posadzki et al., 2010), the United States (Head et al., 2006 as cited in Posadzki et al., 2010), Italy (Rydeard et al., 2006 as cited in Posadzki et al., 2010) and Canada (Vad et al., 2007 as cited in Posadzki et al., 2010). Although some of the authors of the reviewed studies conclude that Pilates yielded better therapeutic results than usual or standard care, the findings of this review suggest that the evidence available for its clinical effectiveness is inconclusive. (Posadzki et al., 2011)

The second systematic review published this year with meta-analysis aimed to compare pain and disability in individuals with persistent nonspecific low back pain who were treated with Pilates exercises compared to minimal or other interventions based on 7 randomized controlled trials. In conclusion they stated that Pilates-based exercises are superior to minimal intervention for reduction of pain in individuals with nonspecific low back pain. However, Pilates-based exercises are no more effective than other forms of exercise to reduce pain. In addition, Pilates exercises are no more effective than minimal intervention or other exercise interventions to reduce disability related to chronic low back pain. (Lim at al., 2011)

These two systematic reviews show that the evidence base for Pilates method effectiveness in treatment of chronic low back pain remains scarce and therefore larger and better-designed clinical trials are needed.

8.3 Pilates based exercise in post-surgery rehabilitation

Pilates practice applied in post-surgery rehabilitation were found in conference review, preliminary report and case study article.

It possible to use different tools and special equipment when incorporating Pilates based exercise into treatment process. In the review which aims was to establish an evidence-based approach to the postoperative rehabilitation of the knee following anterior cruciate ligament reconstruction, arthroscopic meniscectomy and meniscal repair surgery exercises performed with the use of Pilates Reformer machine were investigated.

The authors emphasized that there has been a gradual move away from traditional methods towards accelerated rehabilitation programs for anterior cruciate ligament reconstruction following the observation that patients who had been noncompliant with traditional rehabilitation progressed more rapidly. (Decarlo et al., 1992, Shelbourne et al., 1990 as cited in Atkinson et al., 2010) They claim that accelerated rehabilitation programs, which aim to overcome the common post-surgical problems of prolonged knee stiffness, anterior knee pain, difficulty gaining full extension and delays in the strength recovery, maintaining knee stability may include following types of exercise: closed and open kinetic chain, eccentric, concentric, isometric, isokinetic, plyometric, sport-specific and Pilates method. The Pilates Reformer machine exercises allowing the patient to be positioned in such way as to help to remove gravity from the equation and other equipment exercise for core stability strength and co-ordination are included after the 4-week in post-operative anterior cruciate ligament reconstruction protocol. The author indicates that additional use of Pilates Reformer machines according to the principles of the Australian Physiotherapy and Pilates Institute may allow for earlier progressive load bearing and introducing squatting or lunging activities in treatment process. The theory behind this approach is to introduce consistent motion and defined joint ranges early in the rehabilitation period, using zero-gravity spring-based resistance. This allows for exact functional patterns and muscle memory to be retrained and thus, when the patient is ready to weight bear into a squat or lunge, the motion has already been learned. Though there is currently little scientific data to support this new approach, it may shorten rehabilitation by as much as 4 weeks, with the largest effect seen within the first 2 months. The authors of the survey proposed at the 3-month post-operative review functional exercise for neuromuscular coordination and also Pilates exercises for core stability and strength with the application of all equipment. (Atkinson et al., 2010)

In a preliminary report with 38 participants Pilates method was introduced into modified exercises programme developed to account for the postoperative precautions and needs of total hip and knee arthroplasty. At 1 year follow up, review of patient charts and follow up telephone calls revealed; 25 patients were extremely satisfied and 13 were satisfied with their outcome and use of Pilates in their rehabilitation. From these observations of a small number of patients it was concluded that this technique can be utilized without early complications, however, further studies are necessary to confirm its utility and safety. (Levine et al., 2009)

Other report which documented the use of the Pilates method in medical rehabilitating of postsurgical patients and for recuperation of musculoskeletal condition was case study concerning treatment of scoliosis of adult woman who had progressive severe low back pain. She had worsened over the years after her surgery and had prevented her from activities such as carrying her son or equipment necessary for her job as a photographer. The patient was provided a series of Pilates exercises used to overcome her chronic habituation and muscle weakness. It was concluded that addition of Pilates based exercise to therapy can be useful to care for patients with chronic low back pain and deconditioning (Blum, 2002).

8.4 Pilates based exercise in specific disorder treatment

In a randomized clinical trial comparing pelvic floor muscle training to a Pilates exercise program for improving pelvic muscle strength 62 women with little or no pelvic floor dysfunction were randomized to Pilates or a pelvic floor muscle-training. The results of the study demonstrated only the feasibility of a Pilates exercise program for strengthening the pelvic floor muscles with the important note that these findings are only relevant to those women who can "find" their pelvic floor muscles however are encouraging and may eventually lead to widespread use of Pilates-based exercise programs to treat and prevent pelvic floor dysfunction. (Culligan et al., 2010)

In a randomised, controlled trail with 52 breast cancer patients and also in one pilot study of with 4 women who had undergone axillary dissection and radiation therapy for breast cancer it was concluded that Pilates exercises are safe and efficient for women with breast cancer but there is a need for further studies to confirm these statements. (Eyigor et al., 2010, Keays at al., 2008)

In a randomized, prospective, controlled, and single-blind trial with 55 participants the effects of Pilates on pain, functional status, and quality of life in patients with ankylosing spondylitis were investigated. Pilates exercise program of 1 h was given by a certified trainer to 30 participants of experimental group 3 times a week for 12 weeks. It was the first clinical study designed to investigate the role of Pilates method in ankylosing spondylitis treatment with a conclusion that this exercise technique is as an effective and safe method to improve physical capacity in ankylosing spondylitis patients. (Altan et al., 2011)

9. Conclusion

Studies concerning effects of performing Pilates based exercise suggest its beneficial influence on body posture, pain control, muscle strength, endurance, flexibility, body composition, static balance, functional autonomy, motor skills and specific component of sport activities. There is an increasing number of scientific reports suggesting application of Pilates method into modern, mind-body post-operation rehabilitation treatment. Despite a lack of convincing evidence to date to prove its medical effectiveness, the results of reports are promising and we suggest further studies to be carried out using a more representative sample and a longer period of intervention, to more precisely evaluate the results of practising Pilates based exercises.

10. Acknowledgment

We would like to thank:
Anna Schabowska, an International Certified Coach of Pilates Method for providing the photos used in the chapter; Jagiellonian University Medical College in Krakow, Andrzej Frycz Modrzewski Krakow University, and the University School of Physical Education in Krakow for support to cover the cost of publication process.

11. References

Altan, L.; Korkmaz, N. ; Dizdar, M.&Yurtkuran, M. (2011). Effect of Pilates training on people with ankylosing spondylitis. *Rheumatol Int.* Apr 17. [Epub ahead of print]

Arab, AM. & Nourbakhsh, MR. (2010). The relationship between hip abductor muscle strength and iliotibial band tightness in individuals with low back pain. *Chiropractic & Osteopathy*, 18, pp. 1-5

Atkinson,DE.; Laver, JM. & Sharpvi, E. (2010). Physiotherapy and rehabilitation following soft-tissue surgery of the knee. *Mini-symposium: soft tissue surgery in the knee. Elsevier Ltd. Orthopaedics and Trauma.* Vol. 24, No.2, pp. 129-138

Bliss, L. & Teeple, P. (2005). Core stability: the centerpiece of any training program. *Current Sports Med. Reports*, Vol 4, pp. 179-183

Blum, CL. (May 2002). Chiropractic and pilates therapy for the treatment of adult scoliosis. *J Manipulative Physiol Ther.*Vol.m 25, No. 4, pp E3

Critchley, DJ.; Pierson, Z.& Battersby, G. (2011). Effect of Pilates mat exercises and conventional exercise programmes on transversus abdominis and obliquus internus abdominis activity: pilot randomised trial. *Man Ther.*Vol.16, No. 2, pp. 183-9

Culligan, PJ, ;Scherer, J. ; Dyer, K. ; Priestley, JL. ;Guingon-White, G. ;Delvecchio,D.& Vangeli, M. (2010). A randomized clinical trial comparing pelvic floor muscle training to a Pilates exercise program for improving pelvic muscle strength. *Int Urogynecol J Pelvic Floor Dysfunct*. Vol. 21, No 4,pp. 401-8

Dyszkiewicz, A.; Wróbel, Z. & Rumanowski, M. (2003). The 3-D system of breathing track analysis in selected clinical cases. *Physiotherapy*. Vol. 11,pp. 13-20

Emery, K.; De Serres, SJ.; McMillan, A & Côté, JN. (2010). The effects of a Pilates training program on arm–trunk posture and movement. *Clin Biomech*. 25, pp. 124–130

Eyigor, S.; Karapolat, H.; Yesil, H.; Uslu, R.& Durmaz, B. (2010). Effects of Pilates exercises on functional capacity, flexibility, fatigue, depression and quality of life in female breast cancer patients: a randomized controlled study. *Eur J Phys Rehabil Med*. Vol. 46, No. 4, pp. 481-7

Fiz, J. & Gnitecki, J. (2008). Effect of body possition on lung sounds in healthy young man. *Chest,* 133:729- 736

Gioftsidou, A.; Ispirlidis, I.; Pafis, G., Malliou, P., Bikos, C.& Godolias, G.(2008) Isokinetic strength training program for muscular imbalances in professional soccer players. 2, pp 101–105

Gupta, V.; Singhal, R.& Ansari, M. (2005). Spontaneous rupture of the diaphragm. *Eur. Emerge*. Med. Vol. 12, pp. 43-44

Helenius, I.; Tikkanen, H. & Haahtela, T. (1998). Occurence of exercise induced bronchospasm in elite runners. Dependence on atopy and exposure to cold air and pollen. *Br. J. Sports Med*. Vol. 32, pp. 125 – 129

Herrington, L. &Davies, R. (2005).The influence of Pilates training on the ability to contract the Transversus Abdominis muscle in asymptomatic individuals. *J Bodyw Mov Ther*. 9, pp. 52–57

Horst, R. (2010). Trening strategii motorycznych i PNF. Motor strategy training and PNF.*Top School*. ISBN: 9788392984207

Jago, R.; Jonker, ML.; Missaghian, M. & Baranowski, T. (2006). Effect of 4 weeks of Pilates on the body composition of young girls. *Prev Med*. Vol. 42, No.3, pp. 177-80

Johnson, EG.; Larsen, A.; Ozawa, H.; Wilson, CH.& Kennedy, K. (2007). The effects of Pilates-based exercise on dynamic balance in healthy adults. *J Bodyw Mov Ther*. 11, pp. 238–242

Kaesler, DS.; Mellifont, RB,; Swete Kelly, P.& Taaffe, P. (2007). A novel balance exercise program for postural stability in older adults: A pilot study. *J Bodyw Mov Ther*. 11,pp. 37–43

Keays, KS.; Harris, SR.; Lucyshyn, JM.& MacIntyre, DL. (2008). Effects of Pilates Exercises on Shoulder Range of Motion, Pain, Mood, and Upper-Extremity Function in Women Living With Breast Cancer: A Pilot Study. *Phys Ther,* Vol. 88, No.4, pp. 494-510

Lange, C.; Unnithan, V.; Larkam, E.& Latta, PM. (2000). Maximizing the benefits of Pilates-inspired exercise for learning functional motor skills. *J Bodyw Mov Ther*, Vol. 4, No. 2.pp 99-108

Latey, P. (2001).The Pilates method: history and philosophy. *J Bodyw Mov Ther*, Vol. 5, No.4, pp. 275-282

Latey, P. (2002). Upadating the principles of the Pilates method – Part 2. *J Bodyw Mov Ther*, Vol. 6, No. 2, pp. 94-101

Levine, B.; Kaplanek, B. & Jaffe, WL. (2009). Pilates Training for Use in Rehabilitation after Total Hip and Knee Arthroplasty. *Clin Orthop Relat Res*. Vol. 467, No. 6, pp. 1468–1475 Symposium: advanced techniques for rehabilitation after total hip and knee arthroplasty.

Lim, EC.; Poh, RL.; Low, AY.&Wong, WP. (2011). Effects of Pilates-based exercises on pain and disability in individuals with persistent nonspecific low back pain: a systematic review with meta-analysis. *J Orthop Sports Phys Ther*. Vol. 41, No.2,pp. 70-80

McNeill, W. (2011) Decision making in Pilates. *J Bodyw Mov Ther*. 15,pp. 103-107

Mętel, S. & Milert A. (2007) Metoda Josepha Pilatesa oraz możliwości jej zastosowania w fizjoterapii (Joseph Pilates' method and its application in physiotherapy). *Reh Med* 11 (2): 27-36

Muscolino, JE. & Cipriani, S. (2004). Pilates and the "powerhouse". *J Bodyw Mov Ther*. 8, pp.15–24

Page, P. (2005). Muscle Imbalances in Older Adults. *Journal of Active Aging* 4(2):30-39

Pontaga.(2003). Muscle strength imbalance in the hip joint caused by fast movements Mechanics of Composite Materials, 39:4,365-368 *Latvian Academy of Sports Education*, Riga, LV-1006, Latvia. Translated from Mekhanika Kompozitnykh Materialov, Vol. 39, No. 4, pp. 549-554

Rakowska, J. (1990). Breathing in the diagnosis tootsy resistance. *Psychotherapy*, 4; pp. 75-82

Rogers, K. & Gibson, AL. (2009). *Eight-week traditional mat Pilates training-program effects on adult fitness characteristics*. Res Q Exerc Sport. 2009. Vo. 80, No.3:pp.569-74

Siqueira Rodrigues, BG.; Ali Cader, S.; Bento Torres, NV.; Oliveira, EM. & Martin Dantas, EH. (2010). Pilates method in personal autonomy, static balance and quality of life of elderly females. *J Bodyw Mov Ther*. Vol.14, No.2 :pp. 195-202

Szczygieł, E.; Rojek, M. & Golec, J. (2010). Forced postural distortions and the level of spirometric values. *Orthop. Quart.*, Vol. 3; pp. 439-451

Szucs, K.; Navalgund, A.& Borstad, JD. (2009). Scapular muscle activation and co-activation following a fatigue task. *Med Biol Eng Comput*. 47:pp. 487-495

Weiler, J.; Layton, T.& Hunt, M. (1998). Asthma in United States Olympic athletes who participated in the 1996 Summer Games. *J. Allergy Clin. Immunol*. Vol. 102, pp. 722 – 726

Wroński, W.; Nowak, M. (2008). Pilates breathing exercise method as a form of pneumological rehabilitation in children and youths with bronchiale asthma. *Przegląd Lekarski*. Vol. 65, Suppl 2, pp. 9-11

Volpi, P.; Melegati, G.; Tornese, D.& Bandi ,M. (2004). Muscle strains in soccer: a five-year survey of an Italian major league team. *Knee Surg Sports Traumatol Arthrosc*. 12 : pp. 482–485

Yang, Y.; Park, J. & Kim, J. (2010). Spontaneous diaphragmatic rupture complicated with perforation of the stomach during Pilates. *Am. J. Emerg. Medic.*, Vol. 28, pp. 259.e1-259.e3

Zocchi, L.; Fitting, W. & Majani, U. (1993). Effect of pressure and timing of contraction on human rib cage muscle fatigue. *Am Rev Respir Dis*, Vol 147, pp. 857- 864

7

Syndesmotic Injuries in Athletes

Jeffrey R. Thormeyer, James P. Leonard
and Mark Hutchinson
*Department of Orthopaedic Surgery, University of Illinois, Chicago,
USA*

1. Introduction

Ankle injuries are the most common presenting injury in the athletic population, with the ankle sprain accounting for 10% to 30% of all single-sport injuries [1-4]. Lateral ankle sprains make up a majority of these injuries, and the literature describes a high degree of success with quick return to play afterward. Injuries to the syndesmotic ligaments occur far less frequently, with reported values between 1% and 18% of all ankle sprains [5-8]. However, the incidence of these "high ankle sprains" has been increasing recently due to an increase in the knowledge and understanding of the clinical diagnosis, biomechanics, and cause of syndesmotic injuries. More recent reports have the incidence ranging from 17% to 74% of all ankle injuries in young athletes [9-11]. Despite the improved awareness for this injury, there still exists a paucity of information on optimal conservative and operative management. In a recent survey, health care providers caring for professional athletes identified syndesmotic injuries as the most difficult foot and ankle injury to treat [12]. Athletes have shown a delayed return to play, higher incidence of chronic pain, and significant long-term disability compared to lateral ankle sprains [8, 13, 14]. A study from the United States Military Academy found that involvement of the syndesmosis was the most predictive factor of chronic ankle dysfunction six months after an injury [14]. This review will describe the anatomy of the biomechanics of the distal tibiofibular ligament, followed by an assessment of the clinical evaluation and diagnosis of syndesmotic ligament injuries. Finally, the indications and treatment options for both nonoperative and operative intervention will be discussed and evaluated with a current review of the literature.

2. Anatomy

A syndesmosis is defined as a fibrous joint in which two adjacent bones are linked by a strong membrane or ligaments [15]. The distal tibiofibular joint is a syndesmotic joint between the tibia and fibula, linked by four ligaments: the anterior inferior tibiofibular ligament (AITFL), the interosseous ligament (IOL), the posterior inferior tibiofibular ligament (PITFL), and the inferior transverse ligament (ITL). The distal tibiofibular joint employs both its bony and ligamentous structure for stability (FIGURE 1).
The architecture of the bony components of the syndesmosis provide significant stability to this joint. The fibula sits in a groove created by bifurcation of the lateral ridge of the tibia into the anterior and posterior margins of the tibia, approximately 6-8cm above the level of

the talocrural joint [16]. The anterior margin ends in the anterolateral aspect of the tibial plafond called the anterior tubercle, or Chaput's tubercle. The posterior margin ends in the posterolateral aspect of the tibial plafond called the posterior tubercle, or Volkmann's tubercle. The apex of this fibular notch is the incisura tibialis, which has a depth that varies from concave (60-75%) to shallow (25-40%) [17, 18]. Its depth varies from 1.0 to 7.5mm [19, 20] and is a little less in women than in men [21]. A shallow notch may predispose to recurrent ankle sprains or syndesmotic injury with fracture-dislocation [15]

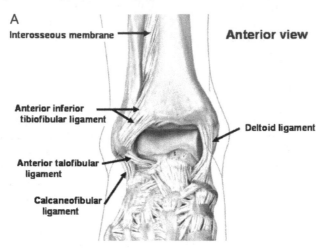

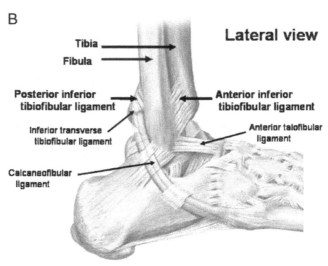

Fig. 1. Anatomy of syndesmosis, A) anterior; B) lateral. AITFL = anterior tibiofibular ligament; IOL = interosseous ligament; PITFL = posterior tibiofibular ligament; ITL = inferior tibiofibular ligament. (Reprinted from Browner B, Jupiter J, Levine A, Trafton P. Skeletal Trauma: Fractures, Dislocations, Ligamentous Injuries, 3rd edition. Philadelphia: Saunders, 2002; p. 2307Y74. Copyright * 2002 Saunders.

The bony architecture of the fibula mirrors that of the fibular notch. The medial aspect of the fibula forms a convex structure that complements that of the tibia, with an anterior and posterior margin, as well as a ridge that bifurcates that margins and aligns itself with the incisura tibialis.

The AITFL originates from the anterior tibial tubercle and runs distally and laterally in an oblique fashion to insert onto the anteromedial distal fibula. This ligament has a width of approximately 18mm, length between 20 and 30mm, and a thickness of 2 to 4 mm. It is the most commonly sprained ligament in syndesmotic injuries and is always disrupted with joint space widening or frank diastasis [15]. It is often multifascicular, and its most inferior fascicle has been described as a discrete structure called the accessory AITF ligament. The fibers can be seen during ankle arthroscopy and have been reported to be a source of impingement [22]. The PITFL originates on the posterior aspect of the fibula and runs horizontally to Volkmann's tubercle (FIGURE 5). This ligament has an approximate width of 18mm and a thickness of 6mm and is the strongest component of the syndesmosis. Because of its extensive breadth of attachment coupled with elasticity, the PITFL is able to withstand greater forces without failure than the AITFL and reaches maximal tension during dorsiflexion [23, 24]. The inferior transverse ligament is deep and inferior to the PITFL, extending over to the posterior aspect of the medial malleolus. The inferior transverse ligament is often difficult to distinguish from the PITFL as it runs just distally in the same plane. It forms the most distal aspect of the articulation. A portion of this ligament lies below the posterior tibial margin preventing posterior translation of the talus and deepening the ankle mortise to increase joint stability by functioning as a labrum. The interosseous ligament spans the space between the lateral tibia and medial fibula and is confluent with the proximal interosseous membrane. It is the main restraint to proximal migration of the talus between the tibia and the fibula [25] (FIGURES 2 and 3).

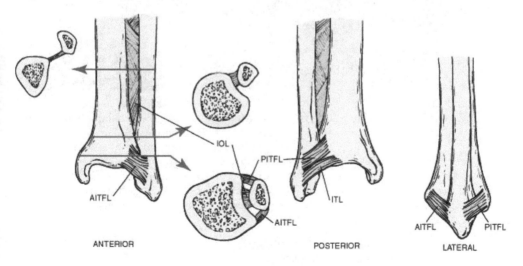

Fig. 2. The anatomy of the ankle syndesmosis in anterior, posterior, lateral positions; anterior inferior tibiofibular ligament (AITFL), interosseous ligament (IOL), posterior inferior tibiofibular ligament (PITFL), inferior transverse ligament (ITL). Copyright: Mark Hutchinson, University of Illinois

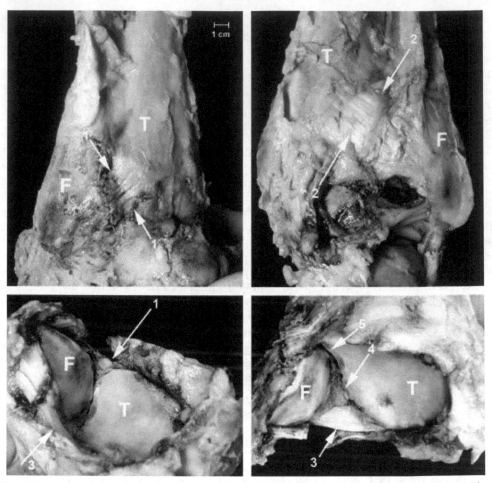

Fig. 3. Exposure of syndesmotic ligaments ina dissected right ankle (male, 92 years). (A) The trapezoid multifascicular anterior tibiofibular ligament (AITFL) (1) runs obliquely upwards from the anterior fibular tubercle towards the anterior tibial tubercle. (B) The band-like posterior tibiofibular ligament (PITFL) (2) runs obliquely upwards from the posterior fibular tubercle towards the posterior tibial tubercle. (C) View from below after removal of the talus shows the curved and horizontally running transverse ligament (3) and the inferior margin of the AITFL. In (D) fat (4) from the synovial fold is visible in the tibial incisure between the transverse ligament and the small contact area between the tibia and fibula (5). F, fibula; T, tibia. Picture courtesy of:

Title: Anatomy of the distal tibiofibular syndesmosis in adults: a pictorial essay with a multimodality approach
Author: John J. Hermans,Annechien Beumer,Ton A. W. De Jong,Gert-Jan Kleinrensink
Publication: Journal of Anatomy
Publisher: John Wiley and Sons
Date: Dec 1, 2010

3. Biomechanics

The ankle joint undergoes extreme loading which places stresses upon the bones, ligaments and dynamic stabilizers. Failure or injury to any of these components can lead to instability and pain. As a weight-bearing joint, the ankle can experience a multitude of different forces, reaching up to 6 times body weight at times [23]. The syndesmotic ligamentous complex maintains the integrity of the ankle mortise necessary to perform its hinge and glide movements. In simple terms, the ligaments stabilize the syndesmosis by preventing lateral displacement of the fibula. If any or all of the structures fail and the lateral malleolus displaces laterally, the talus usually follows. When the syndesmosis is disrupted, the normal gliding and rotational motion of the talar dome within the distal part of the tibia is altered. In addition to maintaining the integrity between the tibia and fibula, the syndesmosis complex resists axial, rotational, and translational forces. The deep portion of the deltoid ligament also contributes to the stability of the syndesmosis and must be evaluated after injury [26].

Normal motion exists between the distal fibula and tibia. The fibula can move medially, laterally, proximally, and distally in small increments. It also has a rotational component in relation to the tibia. The ankle joint undergoes triplanar motion from plantarflexion to dorsiflexion [27]. The movements require the talus and malleoli to remain in intimate contact. The superior portion of the talus is wider anterior vs. posterior, often described as a trapezoid. In dorsiflexion, the wider portion of the talus is set between both malleoli, providing maximum stability. The reverse process happens with plantarflexion. The syndesmotic ligaments provide such strong stabilization to the articulation that the fibula only rotates externally about 2 degrees, and the intermalleolar distance widens only about 1mm when the ankle joint is brought from full plantar flexion to full dorsiflexion [28]. The talus rotates an average of 5 degrees with dorsiflexion. The fibula moves approximately 2-4 mm distally with weight bearing. Mechanical disruption of the syndesmosis may result in increased compressive stresses seen by the tibia, increased likelihood of lateral subluxation of the distal fibula, and incongruence of the ankle joint articulation [29]. The relative joint position of the talus under the tibial plafond and dynamic joint motion would be altered with resulting abnormalities in contact pressures and a medium for development of degenerative joint disease.

Radiostereometric analysis of normal ankles by Beumer et al [30] showed that with an external rotation moment of 7.5N-m applied to the foot, the fibula externally rotated between 2-5 degrees, translated medially between 0 and 2.5mm, and moved posterior between 1 and 3.1mm. The extremes of motion are seen in the stance phase of gait. Oglivie-Harris et al. performed a biomechanical study to determine the relative contribution of each of these ligaments during 2 mm of lateral displacement of the fibula [31]. Their results showed the AITFL contributed 35% of the restraining force, the inferior transverse ligament contributed 33%, the intraosseous ligament contributed 22%, and the PITFL contributed 9%. They proposed that injury to two of the ligaments may lead to instability. Another study used cadaver specimens to determine the effects of sequential sectioning of the syndesmotic ligaments to resistance of an external rotation force. The distal tibiofibular diastasis was 2.3mm after sectioning of AITFL, 5.5mm with the additional sectioning of distal 8cm of the intraosseous ligament, and 7.3mm after division of the PITFL [29]). Sectioning of all 3 ligaments allowed for close to 5 degrees of pathologic external rotation at ankle joint. The AITFL has been found to prevent excess fibular movement and rotation of the talus and maximum tension is achieved in plantar flexion. The posterior ligaments are able to withstand greater forces without failure than the AITFL and reach maximum tension during dorsiflexion [23]. The posterior structures combination of strength and elasticity make them the last structures to tear in an injury [24]. The IOL is the shortest but primary bond between tibia and fibula [32]. The IOL restrains posterolateral bowing of the fibula and transmits a small portion of the weight bearing load to the fibula [33]. It is thought to behave as a spring, allowing for slight separation of tibia and fibula during dorsiflexion [34]. Normal axial loading within the leg segment during walking involves a transfer of between 6% to 15% of the compressive axial load from the tibia to the fibula through the distal interosseous ligament and membrane [27].

4. Mechanism of injury

Athletes may present with a variety of mechanisms for injury. The exact mechanisms are not known for certain and despite the fact that researchers have been unable to duplicate the lesions of a syndesmotic sprain, most syndesmotic injuries are caused by external rotation [29, 35, 36]. Any measure that widens the mortise may damage the syndesmosis. Most proposed mechanisms of injury were based on the observations of clinicians who have interviewed patients with these injuries. The mechanism of external rotation is supported by multiple biomechanical studies that demonstrate increased external rotation of the talus and fibula upon sequential sectioning of the ligaments involved [37]. With this external rotation moment, the fibula separates from the tibia, causing initially a disruption of the AITFL. Commonly, the medial deltoid ligament is also injured. Nussbaum produced a study of 60 athletes with syndesmotic sprains without diastasis [38]. 55% of the injuries occurred when an athlete collided with another with a planted foot in external rotation; after the contact, the player fell forward, dorsiflexing the ankle and further externally rotating the foot. 37% caught their toe and twisted their ankle without receiving contact. No significant correlation existed between the mechanism of injury and the severity of injury. External rotation of the talus also occurs, with possible injury to the deltoid ligament medially. The severity of the force and the duration are determining factors on how far the injury extends; sometimes the proximal extent of the fibular injury component results in a fracture.

Clinicians should be aware of other possible mechanisms of injury. Others have reported on syndesmotic injuries that were due to hyperdorsiflexion, inversion, and plantarflexion [39-42]. Brosky reported that when maximal tension is achieved with external rotation, either dorsiflexion or plantarflexion may result in damage [43]. Other more recent cadaveric studies have looked at whether syndesmotic injuries can cause result from and cause multidirectional instability [44].

Mechanisms during individual sporting activities have been described. Fritschy noted that despite the protection offered by the rigid ski boot, syndesmotic injuries were common among elite skiers because of extremely rapid turns and sudden forceful external rotation of the foot. The external rotation forces acting on the individual ski are caused by a relatively long moment arm [45]. Skiers typically catch the inner edge of the ski which causes forceful external rotation of the foot. Football players often encounter 2 possible scenarios involving contact for high ankle sprains. One involves a direct blow to the lateral leg with a planted foot causing interal rotation of the leg relative to the foot. The other scenario involves a blow to the lateral knee with the foot planted in external rotation relative to the body being internally rotated [9]. (FIGURE 4) Other injuries include falls, twisting weight-bearing injuries, and motor vehicle accidents. Athletes often are incapable of providing an exact mechanism; but they often recognize that the injury is not consistent with a typical ankle sprain.

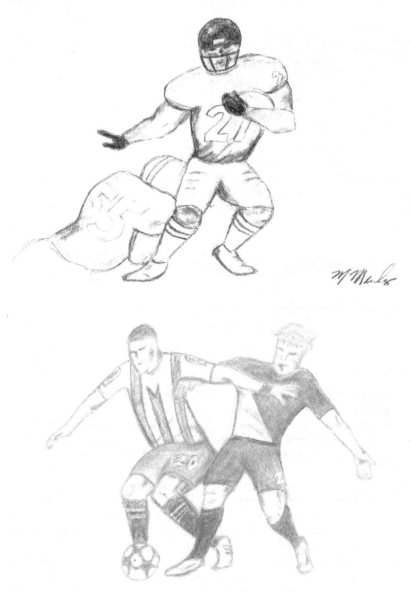

Fig. 4. The mechanism of syndesmotic injury typically seen in sports such as (a) soccer and (b) football is a direct or indirect external rotation force placed on the foot relative to leg and trunk. Figures copyright is owned by Jeffrey R. Thormeyer. Artist: Matthew Mendoza

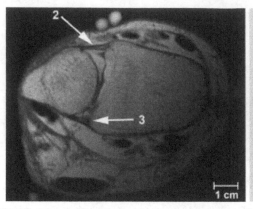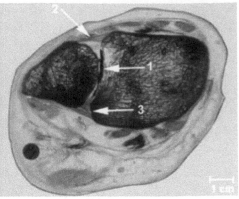

Fig. 5. Correlation between MR image (left) and plastinated slice (right) at the same level through the tibiofibular syndesmosis (female, 84 years). The intra-articularly injected green dye is visible in the tibiofibular recess (1), which extends between the anterior (2) and posterior (3) tibiofibular ligament. As the MR image is obtained without intra-articular contrast, the recess is not visible here. The incisura fibularis is shallow with an irregular contour.

Picture courtesy of :

Title: Anatomy of the distal tibiofibular syndesmosis in adults: a pictorial essay with a
             multimodality approach
Author: John J. Hermans,Annechien Beumer,Ton A. W. De Jong,Gert-Jan Kleinrensink
Publication:Journal of Anatomy
Publisher: John Wiley and Sons
Date: Dec 1, 2010

5. Epidemiology

Isolated ankle syndesmosis injuries are not very common disruptions. They are seen more often in conjunction with deltoid ligament injury and fractures in the malleoli. The real prevalence of ankle syndesmosis injuries is likely underestimated because many are missed or are not treated in a timely fashion. Hopkinson and colleagues suggested that ankle syndesmosis injuries account for 1% of all ankle injuries in the United States military. This was a study of cadets at West Point, who must participate in a contact sport, and showed 15 syndesmotic injuries out of a total of 1344 total ankle sprains [39]. Fallat and colleagues followed all ankle injuries that presented at a local emergency department and a primary care clinic prospectively for 33 months. The diagnosis of a high ankle sprain was made on physical examination alone. Of 639 patients who had 547 soft tissue injuries and 92 ankle fractures, the prevalence of syndesmosis injuries was 5% [46].
In populations of high-level sports participation or high impact activities, the incidence has shown to be higher [10, 47]. In ice hockey and skiing syndesmotic sprains are occurring more frequently than lateral ankle sprains most likely due to the rigid nature of the footwear as observed by Fritschy in world class skiers [45]. Boytim and colleagues reported a prevalence of 18% for syndesmosis injuries in a prospective study of 98 ankle injuries, and close to 40% of ankle sprains in an American professional football team [9]. Vincellete and

colleagues showed that close to a 1/3 of Canadian football players had calcification of the syndesmosis, documenting evidence of old, chronic, syndesmotic injuries [48]. A retrospective study by Wright et al showed syndesmotic sprains accounting for 74% of ankle sprains in two professional hockey teams over 10 years [11]. A study using arthography demonstrated high incidences (50% direct and 36% indirect signs of syndesmotic injury) [49]. In a retrospective study using MR to assess injuries to the ankle in 90 severe sprains, Brown et al. found a syndesmotic injury in almost 2/3 (24% acute; 38% chronic) [50].

Syndesmosis injuries are increasing in incidence in the athletic population, and in collision sports such as football, hockey, and rugby. They account for an increasingly significant proportion of ankle sprains. For athletes, the increase in risk stems from the intensity of play, twisting and cutting demands, as well as risk of contact and collision. Risk factors were identified in a study performed with data over 4 years looking at injuries sustained by cadets at the United States Military Academy. Syndesmotic and medial ankle sprains accounted for about 12% of ankle sprains in this young, athletic population. Important risk factors noted included male sex, higher level of competition, and exposure to selected sports such as football, team handball, basketball and soccer [51]. Using all available data, the incidence of high ankle sprains in the general athletic population is increasing as a percentage of all ankle sprains and is higher with more intense sporting activities.

Despite syndesmotic injuries being less common, they are often more difficult to diagnose than lateral or medial ankle sprains and recovery from the injury can be very protracted. Common complications of syndesmotic sprains are heterotopic ossification or frank synostosis, prolonged dysfunction of the ankle, and diastasis. Taylor and colleagues reported the findings on 50 syndesmosis injuries in 44 football players [52]. Reported that Hopkinson [39] reported that 90% of syndesmotic injuries showed HO (although asymptomatic), while Boytim [9]demonstrated a 75% rate. McMaster and Scranton found radiographic evidence of synostosis in seven patients who had persistent pain 3 to 11 months after a high ankle sprain [53]. Veltri et al. reported 2 cases of symptomatic synostosis in 2 football players [54]. A different study conducted by Bassett et al [52] reported that 50% of players who sustained syndesmotic injuries had evidence of HO and that their recovery period was on average 11 additional days as compared to those without HO. In a survey of NFL head athletic trainers, the mean return to play time was 30 days with a range of 5-56 days [55]. Boytim et al reported that football players with a high ankle sprain averaged 6.3 missed or limited practices (range 2-21) and averaged 1.4 missed games (range 0-5) as compared to 1.1 missed or limited practices and 0.04 games missed for lateral ankle sprains [9]. Difficulties in ankle function become apparent as soon as the athlete returns to high demand activities such as cutting, twisting, turning, jumping or pushing off. A study revealed that an ankle syndesmotic sprain requires a recovery period almost twice as long as that of a severe lateral ankle sprain [39]. Furthermore, residual chronic pain is more common than in an isolated lateral ankle sprain [38, 56]. Failure to reduce or stabilize a syndesmotic injury and the associated lateral talar translation may cause abnormal joint mechanics, diastasis, and degenerative changes. Accordingly, early recognition and treatment of high ankle sprains is paramount for a normal non-antalgic gait and return to sport.

6. Clinical evaluation

As with all injuries, a thorough history and physical exam are mandatory. Paramount within the history is relevant information concerning mechanism of injury and prior ankle injuries or instability. It is important to detail the time interval between injury and evaluation. A simple classification system into acute (<3 weeks), subacute (3 weeks to 3 months), or chronic (> 3 months) is useful. Because many ankle injuries can appear similar on initial presentation, an understanding of the mechanism of injury is crucial. A grade III lateral ankle sprain (non-surgical) from an inversion type injury can look similar to an unstable syndesmotic injury (surgical). Differential diagnoses begins with mechanism of action, location of injury, type of sport, position of limb, direction of forces, and magnitude and velocity of injury. Elapsed time from injury allows correlation with amount and timing of swelling. Severity of injury can be correlated with ability to bear weight. Athletes complain of generalized pain with weight-bearing or push off during gait if they are able to bear weight. A heel-raise gait pattern may be observed to avoid excessive ankle dorsiflexion and to avoid pain during pushoff [43]. In chronic situations, the athlete may complain of stiffness and feelings of instability, especially on rough or uneven terrain [57] Patients with chronic injuries may show prolonged recovery as compared to those with ordinary lateral ankle sprains [56].

Inspection may reveal edema and ecchymoses about the lateral aspect of the ankle. Palpation is necessary for differentiation. Palpation is necessary as the patient will often have well-localized anterolateral pain located over the anterior syndesmosis of the ankle. The pain and swelling in acute syndesmotic injuries are often more precisely localized than in patients with the common inversion lateral ankle sprain. Careful palpation over the anterior talofibular and calcaneofibular ligaments should reveal minimal if any tenderness. The degree of swelling tends not to be as substantial as with lateral inversion injuries. Note any tenderness along the interosseous membrane and the length of the tenderness. Nussbaum et al found that days lost from competition could be predicted by measuring the distance over which the interosseous membrane was tender to palpation [38] There may be tenderness about the medial aspect of the ankle if they injury involved an abduction component. Fites et al. recommend that if swelling about the joint between tibia and fibula occurs less than 24 hours after injury, consider it a syndesmotic injury until proven otherwise [58]. The deep deltoid ligament and posterior syndesmotic ligaments are structures deep within the ankle and difficult to palpate independently. Each may be ruptured without isolated palpable tenderness. Because of the uncertainty with presentation, repeat clinical exams are often necessary to delineate between stable and occult unstable injuries. A missed, unstable injury that is undertreated can lead to a poor result. Range of motion is often limited in both directions of sagittal plane motion with an empty or painful end feel at terminal dorsiflexion [55] If the athlete is unable to bear weight, the Ottawa fracture rules should be applied to determine the need for radiographs before provocative stress tests are performed [59].

To evaluate syndesmotic injuries, numerous clinical exam tests have been described. However, the accuracy, prognostic potential, ability to detect severity of injury, or capability to correlate with the degree of instability present have not been well established [55]. A number of exam tests have been developed that include the external rotation test, the Cotton test, the fibular-translation test, the squeeze test, and the crossed-leg test [60].

The squeeze test is performed by compressing the tibia and fibula at midcalf level [61]. Pain in the area of AITFL is a positive test and may herald a syndesmotic injury (FIGURE 6). Teitz et al confirmed that compression of the two bones proximal to the midpoint of the calf caused separation at the origin and insertion of the AITFL [62]. Reliability remains in question with reported low positive predictive value as well as poor intra-examiner reliability [63, 64]. Studies have indicated that a positive test is correlated with a prolonged recovery time or presence of heterotopic ossification [39, 52].

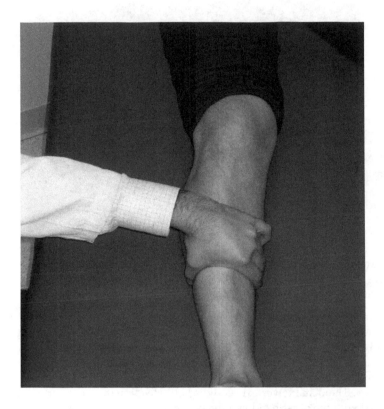

Fig. 6. The squeeze test. The tibia and fibula are compressed at the level of the mid-calf. Pain at the ankle joint indicates a positive test. The examiner should palpate the fibula along its entire length. Copyright: Mark Hutchinson, University of Illinois

The external rotation test is performed with the patient sitting facing the examiner with hips and knees at 90 degrees. The leg is stabilized and an external rotation force is applied to the ankle with the foot in dorsiflexion (FIGURE 7). The largest displacement of the syndesmosis and creation of tension within the ligamentous structures occurs here as the broadest portion of the talus is present in this position. Reproduction of pain in the syndesmotic area is a positive test. Medial sided pain points toward a deltoid ligament injury. Alonso [63] reported a high degree of inter-tester agreement, low rate of false positives and a protracted recovery if coupled with palpatory tenderness and a positive squeeze test.

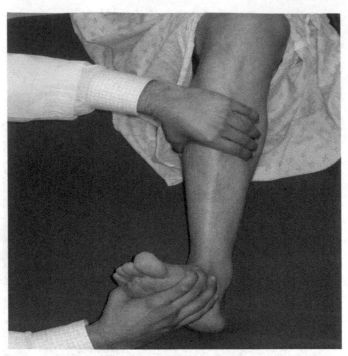

Fig. 7. The external rotation test. With the knee bent to 90- and keeping the leg steady, an external force is applied to the ankle. Pain at the ankle indicates a positive test. Copyright: Mark Hutchinson, University of Illinois

The fibular-translation test is performed by applying an anterior and posterior drawer force to the fibula with the tibia stabilized. Increased translation as compared to contralateral side accompanied by pain defines the test as positive. This test has shown poor correlation to syndesmotic injury both in cadaveric sectioning studies as well as clinically [55].

The Cotton or shuck test is done by attempted translation of the talus within the mortise in a lateral direction. The distal lower extremity is held steady with one hand while the plantar heel is grasped with the other hand and the heel is moved side to side. Increased translation or pain may be indicative of a syndesmotic injury along with a concomitant deltoid injury. A high degree of false positives secondary to subjective interpretation has been shown. Excessive translation is more often seen with the most severe injuries [65, 66].

The crossed-leg test is a more recently described test. The patient rests the midtibia of his affected extremity on the knee of the other extremity, in a figure 4 type position. The patient then applies a downward force on the medial side of the knee. The test is positive if pain is felt in the syndesmotic region. The authors reported 7 of 9 patients with radiographic abnormalities tested positive with this maneuver [67].

The heel thump test was described as a test to target ligamentous injury in the absence of a fracture. The patient rests with leg dangling over edge of table or chair with the foot in gravity induced equinus. The examiner delivers a firm thump to the heel in line with the long axis of tibia with the intention of delivering talus into the mortise. A positive test is aggravation of pain above the ankle briefly. The utility of this test may lie in the ability to examine the structures when swelling precludes palpation or ligamentous stressing [68]. However, the test is not specific as it has been described as a method for identifying tibial stress fractures also [69].

Stability of the ankle joint may be further examined by asking the patient to perform some active maneuvers including performing a toe raise, walking and jumping. Spaulding found in gait analysis that syndesmotic injury decreased the ability to effectively push off the toes while walking [70]. The above mentioned actions should be painful or prevent normal motion if a syndesmotic injury is present. Improvement with these measures by tightly taping the ankle just above joint is an adjunctive test described by Williams and Amendola [71] to further confirm suspicion. Additionally, functional ability may be assessed by having the athlete perform a single leg hop. Disability was defined by Nussbaum as an inability to hop 10 times without significant pain [38] Nussbaum concluded that 4 parameters may help determine severity of the syndesmosis injury: AITFL tenderness, the length of tenderness along the interosseous membrane, a positive external rotation test, and functional disability. This study reported 55 out of 60 patients had a positive external rotation test which also required longer rehab and return to play time. They also found that return to play time could be correlated directly with the tenderness length with a 95% confidence interval.

Although the presence of positives with any of these tests should generate suspicion to a syndesmotic injury, there are no good studies demonstrating that one test is reliably predictable as to the severity of the injury. Beumer and colleagues al performed a biomechanical evaluation of 5 special tests (squeeze, fibula translation, Cotton, external rotation, and anterior drawer) to determine the degree of distal tibiofibular displacement induced by each test in intact cadaveric ankles and after sectioning of the anterior talofibular ligament, the posterior talofibular ligament, and the deltoid ligament [60]. The average increase in displacement after sectioning of all ligaments was only approximately 1 mm. This study showed that the degree of distal displacement between tibia and fibula exhibited with specific exam maneuvers combined with creation of syndesmotic specific ligament injuries failed to show that any of the tests can be used to predict extent of injury.

7. Imaging

Evaluation of the syndesmosis should include three views (AP, lateral, mortise) of the ankle as well as orthogonal views of the entire tibia and fibula especially if any tenderness along the proximal leg exists. A mortise view taken with the patient positioned in unilateral weight bearing is the most accurate way to assess instability radiographically but many patients with mortise instability may not be able to tolerate unilateral standing due to pain [72]. Bilateral weight-bearing or non-weight bearing radiographs can be considered instead. Weight bearing films provide physiologic stress to unveil occult unstable injuries. CT scans and MRI scans may be of value in more subtle cases. Radiographs are evaluated for the relationship of the tibia and fibula as well as for fractures along the entire lengths of the bones. Disruption of the normal relationship between distal tibia and fibula is often representative of a syndesmotic injury. Radiographic evaluation with full length views of the leg is needed to evaluate pronation or external rotation injuries resulting in a Maisonneuve type fracture. The more proximal the fibular fracture, the greater risk for syndesmotic injury and resulting instability. Beumer et al [30] studied motion of the distal fibular before and after syndesmotic injuries on cadavers. The fibula tended to externally rotate after disruption but this was difficult to see on plain radiographs. Posterior translation on the lateral view was described as a secondary pathology. Radiographic parameters have been developed to help identify syndesmotic injuries: increased tibiofibular clear space decreased tibiofibular overlap, and medial clear space widening.

Tibiofibular clear space is defined as the distance between the medial border of the fibula and the lateral border of the posterior tibia as it extends into the incisura fibularis. This distance is measured at 1 cm proximal to the tibial plafond and should be less than 6mm in both the AP and mortise projections. This measurement provides the most reliable indicator of injury to syndesmosis [73]. Tibiofibular overlap is the overlap of the lateral malleolus and the anterior tibial tubercle. This is also measured 1 cm above the plafond. The overlap should be greater than 6mm in the AP view, and greater than 1 mm in the mortise view. Medial clear space is defined by the distance between the lateral border of the medial malleolus and the medial talus at the level of the talar dome (FIGURE 8). With the ankle in neutral, the clear space should be less than or equal to the space between talar dome and tibial plafond. A widening of the medial clear space correlates with a concomitant deltoid ligament injury [61]. Avulsion fractures may occur and aid in identification; calcification above syndesmosis or at tibial attachment of PITFL may also aid in diagnosis.

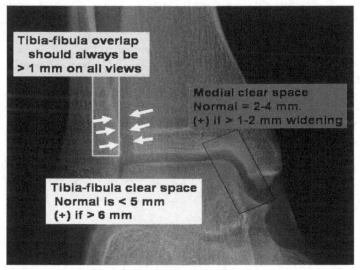

Fig. 8. Diastasis of the tibiofibular clear space greater than 6 mm is considered one of the most reliable indicators of syndesmotic injury. There should be at least 1 mm of tibiofibular overlap on all views. The medial clear space of greater than 4 mm or greater than 2 mm difference compared with the opposite side is indicative of instability. Copyright: Mark Hutchinson, University of Illinois

Reliability of evaluation of syndesmotic injuries by measuring diastasis of the tibia-fibula interval and tibia-fibula overlap on standard radiographs has been questioned. There is considerable variation in the size and depth of the notch which can make radiographic interpretation of separation difficult [74]. Absolute values of distances do not take into account anatomic differences in size or with gender. To account for these, Ostrum et al. introduced the concepts of measurements based on ratios [75]. They concluded that there was an injury to the syndesmosis if the ratio of the tibiofibular overlap: fibular width was greater than 24%; ratio of tibiofibular clear space: total fibular width less than 44%. In addition to gender differences, rotation effects measurement of tibiofibular overlap. Pneumaticos et al [76] demonstrated that overlap changed with rotation but the clear space remained same during rotation from degrees of external rotation to 25 degrees of internal rotation. They concluded that the tibiofibular clear space is the most reliable parameter for measuring widening on plain radiographs. Takao et al. published results of ankle arthroscopy in tibiofibular syndesmotic rupture [77]. Evaluating 38 patients who had Weber B ankle fractures, they identified disruption on AP and mortise radiography in 42% and 55% respectively. During arthroscopy, the diagnosis actually increased to 87% [78]

Some authors have suggested stress radiographs to aid in identification; stress radiography with an external rotation force placed on the foot is a useful imaging approach (FIGURE 10). It may require local anesthesia to obtain these views. Alternatively, a gravity stress view may be obtained by performing an AP radiograph with the leg horizontal and without support under the foot/ankle. The resultant displacements are then compared to the uninjured side. Lateral views may allow for easier interpretation to assess possible posterior and lateral displacement of the fibula [29] . However, studies evaluating translation after rotation forces applied show that after sectioning of ligaments, distance is negligible and stress views cannot be reliable used for predictive purposes because of the high false negative rate.

CT scans are more sensitive than plain radiography in detecting syndesmotic injuries based on diastasis. Ebrahiem et al noted that CT is more effective at picking out 2-mm and 3-mm diastasis[79]. Avulsion fracture may occur on either the anterior or posterior aspect of the tibia and have been noted to occur in up to 50% of syndesmotic injuries. CT imaging utilized in this case can pick up avulsion fractures without evidence of diastasis [80].

MRI can be used for diagnosis and has shown to effectively display the components of the syndesmotic complex with high interobserver agreement [81]. A study by Takao et al. revealed 100% specificity and 93% sensitivity of injury of AITFL and 100% specificity and sensitivity for PITFL as compared to arthroscopy in acute studies [82]. While useful for confirmation, it is unclear if MRI imaging has shown to alter treatment plans or prognosis. MRI allows for the grading of ligamentous injuries. Grade 1 injuries represent stretching of the ligament without fiber disruption. The ligament is intact on MR imaging but often has edema present adjacent to the ligament and within overlying soft tissues. Grade II injuries represent partial tearing of the ligament. MR images demonstrate thickening of the ligament with partial fiber disruption and associated edema within the ligament and overlying soft tissues. Grade III injuries represent discontinuity of the ligament. MR images demonstrate this along with extensive edema. The normal AITFL is dark on all MR sequences and has an oblique course. This structure may have normal fenestrations and accessory fascicles[83]. MR imaging findings of acute injuries include abnormal T2 signal with thickening, waviness, or disruption of the AITFL and interosseous membrane, usually with fluid extending superiorly within the distal tibiofibular joint. MR imaging findings of more chronic injuries include thickening, attenuation or disruption without associated edema. Associated injuries also are common with these injuries and are picked up by MR imaging. Brown et al looked at associated injuries in 59 patients with acute and chronic injuries. AITFL injuries were present in 74%; bone contusions in 24%, osteochondral lesions in 28%, joint incongruence in 33%, and osteoarthritis in 10% [50].

Recent interest has been garnered for the use of ultrasound with its inherent advantages as a method of diagnosis. Ultrasound can be performed in the office setup in both real time and dynamic modes. It is inexpensive, fast and does not have radiation exposure (FIGURE 9). Mei-Dan et al conducted ultrasound evaluations on athletes with syndesmotic injuries and compared them to athletes who sustained lateral ankle sprains as well as a control group without injury. The results were encouraging for accurately diagnosing a syndesmotic injury in cases of latent high grade syndesmotic sprains. Exams within two weeks of injury increased the ability of ultrasound to detect injury [84]. Milz et al compared US examination and MRI studies for lateral ligament injuries and syndesmotic injuries. The study showed a sensitivity of 66% and specificity for AITFL of 91% [85].

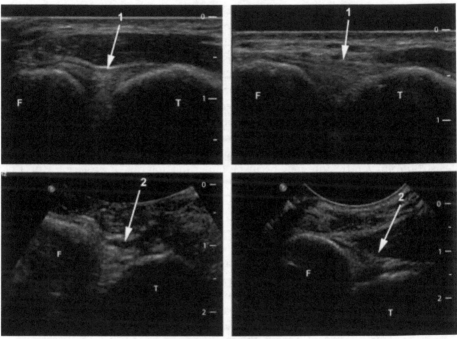

Fig. 9. Ultrasound images of anterior (1) (A,B) and posterior (2) (C,D) tibiofibular ligament (female, 20 years). F, fibula; T, tibia. In plantar flexion the ATIFL is slack (A). In dorsiflexion the talus pushes the tibia and fibula outwards, with stretching of the anterior tibiofibular ligament as a result (B). The same mechanism applies for the PTIFL. In plantar flexion the ligament is slack with a resulting increase in echogenicity (C). In dorsiflexion the fibres are stretched and are more longitudinally aligned (D). F, fibula; T, tibia

Title: Anatomy of the distal tibiofibular syndesmosis in adults: a pictorial essay with a
              multimodality approach
Author: John J. Hermans,Annechien Beumer,Ton A. W. De Jong,Gert-Jan Kleinrensink
Publication:Journal of Anatomy
Publisher: John Wiley and Sons
Date: Dec 1, 2010

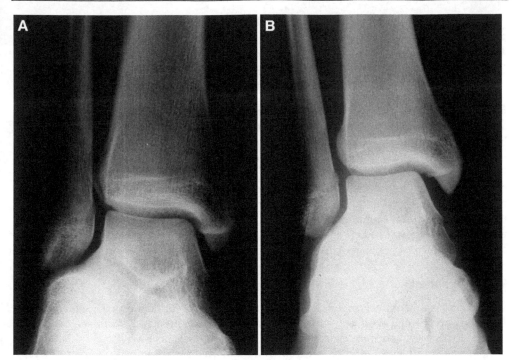

Fig. 10. Mortise radiographs of subject 1, 1 day after injury. (A), at rest, there is a suggestion of widening of the syndesmosis without widening of the medial clear space. (B), with external rotation stress, there is obvious widening of the medial clear space and distal syndesmosis

Source: American Journal of Sports Medicine
Aggressive Surgical Treatment and Early Return to Sports in Athletes With Grade III Syndesmosis Sprains
1. Dean C. Taylor, MD, COL (Ret)†,*,
2. Joachim J. Tenuta, MD, MC, COL‡,
3. John M. Uhorchak, MD, COL (Ret)§, and
4. Robert A. Arciero, MD, COL (Ret) | |
5. Am J Sports Med November 2007 vol. 35 no. 11 1833-1838

8. Classification

There are two classification systems for syndesmotic injuries. The West Point Ankle Grading system provided by Gerber and colleagues is more applicable to athletes [10] and is based on amount of edema, tenderness, ability to bear weight, stress testing, and abnormal radiographic parameters. It distinguishes the following categories of pure ligamentous syndesmotic injuries: grade I—no evidence of instability (partial tear of the AITFL; grade II—no or slight evidence of instability (tear of the AITFL, partial tear of the IOL); and grade III—definite instability (complete tear of the syndesmotic ligaments). A grade II injury poses a particular diagnostic challenge because the extent of injury and its occult instability often requires provocative measures to recognize. Underestimating or undertreating the injury can have devastating consequences.

The other classification system is based on whether diastasis is acute or latent. Based on radiographic findings, Edwards and DeLee [86] classified traumatic syndesmotic sprains into latent diastasis (seen on stress radiographs only) and frank diastasis, which is obvious on plain radiographs.

Because the existing classification systems do not offer a clear therapeutic algorithm, clinical and radiographic examination should focus on detecting and documenting the amount of latent and frank diastasis, as well as documenting the time course of injury. Traumatic injuries can be catergorized into acute, subacute, and chronic. Acute injuries, identified within three weeks of injury, are divided into sprains without diastasis, sprains with latent diastasis, and sprains with frank diastasis based on clinical examination, routine radiographs, stress radiographs, and futher imaging studies. Injuries to the syndesmosis of longer than 3 weeks' duration are considered subacute. Syndesmotic injuries more than 3 months old are considered chronic. The latter two entities can be further subdivided based on variables such as presence of arthritic changes, and presence or absence of a synostosis.

9. Management

(TABLE 1) Treatment intervention is based on the severity of the syndesmotic injury. Grade 1 injuries are treated with non-surgical management. Symptomatic treatment includes a period of rest, ice, and immobilization for comfort and assistance with rehabilitation. For mild injuries in athletes, casting is generally not required and may impede course of therapy because of risk of disuse atrophy and stiffness. Patients often utilize crutches only 1 to 2 weeks for comfort in a controlled ankle motion walker boot. This immobilization allows

	Grade I	Grade II	Grade III
Clinical	Stable exam	Mid laxity	Unstable exam
	Good end point	Soft but positive end point	No end point
			Gross instability
X-rays	Stable on stress radiographs	0-1 mm laxity on stress x-rays	Unstable stress radiographs
Treatment	Rest, ice		
		Consider surgery; Cast immobilization may be 6-8 wk	
	Bracing and crutches for comfort	Return to play may be delayed for 6-8 wk until able to pass functional testing	Followed by functional bracing
	Functional brace at 2-4 wk	Take another x-ray at 2-3 wk to ensure no displacement	After surgery, follow same return to play as Grade II
	Return to play when no symptoms appear on functional testing	Then treat the same as Grade I injury	

Table 1.

athlete early mobilization but protects against external rotation. The athlete is then switched to a functional brace usually between weeks 2 and 4. Exercises are initiated during this transition. They include gradual increases in range of motion and stretching with eventual balance and bicycle program additions. Of note, patients need repeat examinations and radiographs every 1 to 2 weeks during this initial period to determine continued stability [87].

Nussbaum et al[38] and Williams et al [71] have described a 3-phase approach to rehabilitation. The acute phase aims at protecting the joint and decrease pain and swelling through immobilization and pain control. The subacute phase includes an increase in exercise intensity with goals of restoration of strength and basic functional motion. This includes cardiovascular conditioning. The final stage has its goal of returning the patient back to sport participation with strengthening, neuromuscular training, and sport-specific exercises. Determining the timing of return to sports is difficult and is based on examination as well as ability to perform sport specific tasks.

Grade II and III injuries are inherently unstable. The consensus concerning Grade III injuries is that operative fixation is necessary to maintain anatomic reduction of the mortise. The optimum treatment plan for Grade II injuries is less clear [88]. Nonoperative treatment for this injury includes initial splinting and protection from rotation as well as strict non-weight bearing status. Once swelling has retreated and the syndesmosis remains reduced on exam, the patient is transitioned to a short leg cast for 6 to 8 weeks. The athlete is then transitioned to progressive weight bearing in a walking cast, and then eventually to a soft ankle brace. If conservative approach is undertaken, again, serial evaluations are needed to ensure maintenance of reduction. Rehabilitation should focus on range of motion, balance, proprioception, strength, and return to play exercises specific to his/her sport [32]. Some investigators have suggested more aggressive treatment in athletes, including arthroscopic debridement and percutaneous screw fixation; however, this approach has not yet been substantiated by biomechanical or clinical data ([89] Early anatomic reduction and fixation ensures that the ligaments are in an optimal position for healing. Early fixation avoids the potential of a subtle missed diagnosis or for a delayed slip while attempting cast immobilization.

10. Operative treatment

10.1 Indications

The goal of surgical stabilization is to restore and maintain the normal tibiofibular relationship to allow appropriate healing of the ligamentous structures of the syndesmosis. Therefore, any sign of instability, either frank diastasis on radiograph or diastasis on stress radiographs, direct treatment towards syndesmotic fixation. However, these clear indications for surgical intervention represent a small percentage of the population. Taylor et al [90] noted that only 0.25% of ankle injuries and 1.7% of syndesmotic sprains are Grade III injuries with unstable radiographs. In addition, stress radiographs have been shown to be unreliable [91, 92] on biomechanical studies with a high false negative rate [32].

Chronic sprains with recalcitrant pain and functional instability are another indication for surgical fixation of the syndesmosis. Often times, these patients present with chronic ankle pain of an unknown etiology requiring an ankle arthroscopy to make the appropriate diagnosis [93, 94]. Thus, arthroscopic evidence of syndesmotic instability is another indication for surgical intervention. However, this modality is mostly used for chronic ankle pain, as it is unrealistic to perform an ankle arthroscopy on every ankle injury without radiographic signs of instability.

The challenge becomes identifying those patients with injuries that will result in prolonged recovery, recurrent symptoms, or chronic pain and instability despite normal radiographs. Amendola et al[95] performed a systematic review of syndesmotic sprains, and was only able to find six prospective studies investigating isolated syndesmotic sprains without radiographic widening or associated fracture in athletes. The average amount of time lost due to injury between studies was from 10 days to 52 days, but the range of missed time was from 0 days to 137 days. Surgical intervention was required in only two of these studies, with Wright et al [13] reporteding 1 out of 14 cases and Hopkinson et al [5] reporting 1 out of 15 cases. Recurrent or prolonged symptoms were not recorded in all the studies, but Hopkinson et al [5] noted no recurrences, Nussbaum et al [96] documented a 6% recurrence and Taylor et al [97] a 43% recurrence of ankle instability. Because of the small size, varied follow-up and heterogeneous outcome measures of these studies no conclusion could be made regarding risk factors or prognostic signs regarding prolonged symptoms, recurrent symptoms, or surgical intervention.

11. Surgical implants

There are a multitude of different implants employed for syndesmotic fixation. Metal screws are the most common hardware utilized, however recently the development of bioabsorbable screws and suture-button fixation has been analyzed as alternatives. Each mode of fixation has its own advantages and disadvantages, and several biomechanical studies are available in the literature evaluating each implant, as well as comparing different methods of fixation.

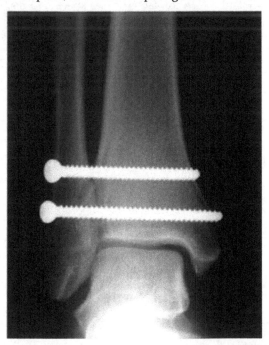

Fig. 11. Proper orientation of syndesmotic screws. Copyright: Mark Hutchinson, University of Illinois

There are multiple different methods to choose from when using a metal syndesmotic screw, such as composition of the screw, size of the screw and number of cortices of fixation (FIGURE 11). Several biomechanical studies have evaluated these parameters, and for the most part no difference in strength of fixation was found. Beumer et al[98] evaluated the difference between stainless steel and titanium screws, and found no difference in strength of fixation. The same study also noted no difference between three and four cortical fixation. No biomechanical advantage was found using a 4.5-mm screw over a 3.5-mm screw in tricortical fixation of the syndesmosis [99]. However, with quadricortical fixation the 4.5-mm screw did show improved resistance to shear stresses during axially loading compared to a 3.5-mm screw [100].

Syndesmotic fixation of the tibiofibular joint prevents its normal physiologic movement that occurs during normal weight bearing and ankle range of motion. Needleman et al [101] demonstrated that quadricortical fixation with a 4.5-mm screw decreases tibiotalar external rotation, and may result in fatigue fracture of the screw [102]. Three cortical fixation may decrease the rigidity of fixation and increase physiologic motion, but may also lead to hardware loosening [103]. Other complications associated with the metal screw include inferior tibiofibular synostosis [104] and osteolysis around the implant [102].

To avoid the hardware complications associated with metal screws, bioabsorbable screws have been proposed as an alternative mode of fixation. The goal of the bioabsorbable implant is to temporarily hold the tibiofibular joint in place while the syndesmosis heals, but over time hydrolyze and degrade to the point of failure after weight bearing as started to allow for normal physiologic motion of the ankle. Two cadaveric, biomechanical studies compared the load to failure and stiffness of fixation between a stainless steel screw and a polylactide bioabsorbable screw of the same size [105, 106]. Both studies found no difference in syndesmotic fixation between the metal and bioabsorbable screw group. Two randomized, clinic trials evaluating bioabsorbable and metallic screws found no loss of reduction in either group, with no different in subjective and objective outcomes between the two groups [107, 108]. In fact, patients were more likely to return to their previous level of activity when treated with a bioabsorbable screw rather than a metal screw [108].

The material of these bioabsorbable screws has caused concern regarding possible biologic reactions with the body. Several studies have reported osteolysis [109], foreign-body reaction [110, 111], late inflammatory reaction [112] and osteoarthritis due to polymer debris entering the joint [113] with use of bioabsorbable screws. However, these studies were either case reports, or involved treatment of ankle fractures or talar neck fractures. In the previous four studies comparing metal and bioabsorbable screws, there was no osteolysis or inflammatory reaction recorded.

Another alternative to screw fixation is the suture button. This method resists tibiofibular diastasis while allowing for some movement at the distal tibiofibular joint (FIGURE 12). Proponents of this technique believe that it is simple, safe and effective when compared to the syndesmotic screw [114, 115]. Several biomechanical studies have been published recently comparing this technique to metal syndesmotic screws. These studies were in agreement that the metal screw has on average increase strength to failure compared to the suture button, but that the suture button has more consistent strength [114, 116, 117]. Failure of the suture button occurs through the button, whereas failure of the screw is relative to cortical thickness. Forsythe et al [118] found the suture-button was not as strong, with increased diastasis compared to a metal screw.

However, the studies did not agree on the amount of motion that suture-button allowed. Klitzman et al [119] noted in their biomechanical analysis that suture-button fixation allowed more physiologic motion of the fibula in the sagittal plane when compared to tricortical screw fixation. On the other hand, Soin et al [117] denied observing a difference in fibular motion during cyclic loading for the suture-button and syndesmotic screw. They described ankle motion for both constructs as being similar, and stated that neither was normal.

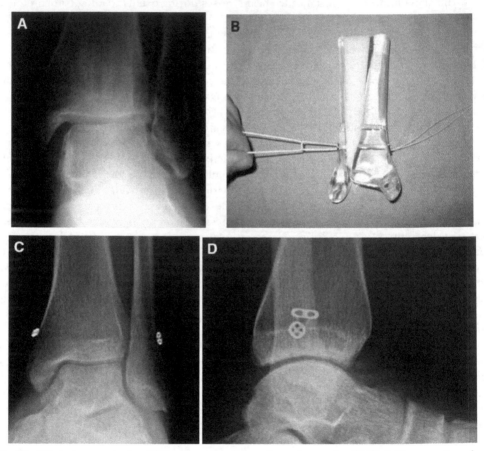

Fig. 12. (A) Anteroposterior (AP) view of a widened syndesmosis. (B) TightRope system for syndesmosis fixation.(C, D) AP and lateral weight-bearing radiographs 6 months after a TightRope fixation of a syndesmosis disruption

Title: Ankle Syndesmosis Injuries
Author: Fernando A. Peña,J. Chris Coetzee
Publication: Foot and Ankle Clinics
Publisher: Elsevier
Date: March 2006

12. Surgical intervention

The AO technique for syndesmotic fixation recommends that diastasis screws be placed parallel and 2cm to 3cm above the ankle joint angled 20° to 30° anteromedially to match the anatomic relationship of fibula and tibia axially [120] (Figure 14). Two different cadaveric studies evaluated the level of placement of fixation, yielding conflicting data. McBryde et al examined syndesmotic fixation at 2 cm and 3.5 cm above the tibial plafond, and found 2cm above the tibial plafond gave improved syndesmotic fixation. Miller et al [121] found improved holding strength and decreased displaced with fixation at 5cm above the tibial plafond compared to 2cm regardless of using tricortical metal screws or suture button. The AO technique also warns about placing screws within 2cm of the tibial plafond for fear of inferior tibiofibular synostosis, although Kukreti et al [104] did not find a significant difference in synostosis when placed within 2cm of the ankle joint and between 2 – 5cm from the joint. Therefore, no conclusions can be made regarding the appropriate height of diastasis fixation.

No recommendations have been made between tricortical and quadricortical fixation. As previously discussed, there is no biomechanical difference between three cortical and four cortical fixation [98]. A prospective, randomized trial comparing two tricortical screws with one quadricortical screw showed improved subjective outcomes at three months for tricortical fixation [122]. By one year, the outcomes were not statistically different. Ankle motion between the two groups was equivalent at all time periods. All quadricortical screws were routinely removed at two months, while tricortical screws were removed in two patients because of discomfort.

The AO technique recommends one screw for syndesmotic fixation, with an additional screw being used with concurrent multiple fractures of the fibula [120]. Biomechanical studies have shown two screws increase the fixation strength of the tibiofibular joint [123], but there are no clinical studies comparing one-screw versus two-screw fixation. Another biomechanical study evaluated single versus double suture-button fixations[124]. The second suture-button added very little strength to the construct, which was still significantly less than an intact syndesmosis. However, this study did show that an "anatomic" suture-button fixation provided significantly improved strength compared to the original technique that was equivalent to the intact syndesmosis. This technique provides fixation at the posterior cortex of the fibula to the anterolateral edge of the tibia (FIGURE 13).

Traditional, syndesmotic fixation has been performed with the ankle in maximum dorsiflexion [101, 125]. This maneuver accounts for the narrower posterior talus engaging in the mortise during plantarflexion, which theoretically could cause overtightening of the mortise and prevent dorsiflexion when the wider anterior talus attempt to engage into the mortise. Lately, recent studies have shown that fixation in any amount of ankle flexion results in equivalent range of motion [126, 127].

13. Postoperative management

Most biomechanical studies evaluated in this review report fixation of the tibiofibular syndesmosis does not restore the strength or diastasis of the normal syndesmosis during normal weight bearing conditions. The only study that published data suggesting full strength and resistance to diastasis with loading is Teramoto et al [124] with use of their "anatomic suture-button" technique. However, their study also showed metal screw fixation that was stronger than the intact syndesmosis, which is contradictory to every other study regarding syndesmotic metal screw fixation. Because normal weight bearing results in

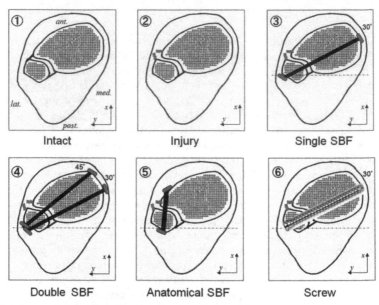

Fig. 13. Axial View of Different Fixation Devices for Ankle Syndesmosis. (1) Intact syndesmosis (2) Injured syndesmosis (3) Single Suture Button Fixation (4) Double Suture Button Fixation (5) Anatomic Suture Button Fixation (6) Screw Fixation
Reference: Figure 13 is from Teramoto A et al. Comparison of Different Fixation Methods of the Suture-Button Implant for Tibiofibular Syndesmosis Injuries. AJSM October 2011.

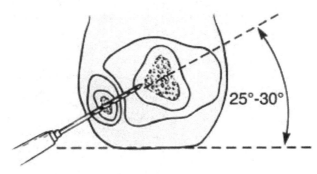

Fig. 14. Is from Browner BD, Jupiter JB, Levine AM, Trafton PG (eds). Skeletal Trauma ed 3. Philadelphia PA, WB Sauders, 2003, vol 2, p 2309.

increased diastasis regardless of surgical technique or implant, non-weight bearing is recommended for the first six weeks to allow the syndesmotic ligaments to heal. Weight bearing is then slowly progressed as tolerated.

Another controversy specific to metal screws is their removal postoperatively. As described previously, metal screws are at risk to loosen with tricortical fixation or break with quadricortical fixation. Other complications, such as symptomatic hardware, osteolysis and synostosis, are also possible postoperatively. Bell et al [102] retrospectively reviewed patients with syndesmotic screws, and compared those that had the screw removed versus those in which the screw was maintained. There was no statistical significance between the two groups in ankle scores, range of motion or functional outcome. The only difference was a higher incidence of osteolysis and screw breakage in the retained screw group. Manjoo et al retrospectively divided patients into two groups: patients with intact screws and patients with fractured, loosened or removed screws. An intact syndesmotic screw was associated with worse function scores compared to loose, fractured or removed screws. No difference was noted in functional outcomes between patients with loose, fractured or removed screws. Intact syndesmotic metal screws are routinely removed as early as 8-12 weeks postoperatively [25, 128], but should not postpone weight bearing or limit rehabilitation. De Souza et al[129] did not show any adverse clinical outcomes to patients that began weight bearing prior to screw removal.

Rehabilitation can progress to functional activities when the patient demonstrates the ability to perform activities of daily living, ambulate on uneven/soft surfaces, and ascend/descend stairs without difficulty. Patients may return to sports participation when they demonstrate the ability to perform aggressive sports-specific tasks like running, jumping, kicking, and cutting/pivoting at competition/practice speed without noteworthy symptoms during or after participation. The expected time frame to return is around 12 to 14 weeks.

14. Outcomes

The literature has many outcome studies evaluating syndesmosis fixation in patients with concurrent ankle fractures. Most of these studies are retrospective case series. They show the most important predictor of functional outcome is accurate reduction of the syndesmosis [130-132]. A cadaveric study showed that 1mm of lateral talar displacement is associated with a 42% decrease in tibiotalar contact area [133].

Fewer studies have evaluated surgical fixation of pure syndesmotic injuries, and most of these studies are retrospective case series. There is a paucity of published data comparing the clinical results of different methods of surgical fixation. Edwards and DeLee[134] and Taylor et al[90] both published their case series of six patients with isolated, unstable ankle syndesmotic injuries that were treated with syndesmotic screw fixation. Edwards and DeLee reported 4 excellent and 2 good results, but no other information regarding functional outcome and return to sports. Taylor et al treated six intercollegiate athletes, and using aggressive rehabilitation was able to get the athletes to return to full activity in 41 days on average.

Degroot et al[135] followed 24 patients with suture button repair for syndesmotic injuries for an average of 20 months. Syndesmotic parameters returned to normal after surgery and remained normal throughout the followup period. However, one in four patients required removal of the suture endobutton device due to local irritation or lack of motion. Osteolysis of bone with subsidence of the device was noted in four patients, and three patients developed heterotopic ossification. This is somewhat surprising as the main advantage of suture button devices was the lack of hardware problems seen with metal screws. This study illustrates the point that clinical studies need to be performed to fully investigate outcomes of these devices. Although there is a significant amount of biomechanical data available, without good clinical evidence true recommendations regarding the best implant and technique for syndesmotic fixation will remain in question

15. Conclusion

Controversy surrounds almost every aspect of syndesmosis injuries from diagnosis to treatment to return of play. More research will help in defining these areas more clearly as the awareness has increased recently. Isolated injury to the syndesmosis is associated with chronic pain, prolonged recovery, recurrent sprains, and the heterotopic ossification. The delay in fixation that can occur with either a delayed or missed diagnosis with resultant instability takes the athlete out of the crucial period of ligamentous healing where the response to surgery is often decreased. Optimizing outcomes from these complex injuries requires early recognition through awaremess of mechanism of injury, a detailed physical exam, and appropriate imaging to assess for subtle changes. Successful treatment depends on early identification and timely intervention; anatomic reduction is required of any treatment modality. While the injury is difficult one, appropriate management can return the athlete to preinjury levels of participation, although their return will likely be delayed compared to lateral ankle sprains.

16. Acknowledgment

The authors would like to recognize the participation and dedication of Dr. Brandon Hill, Madigan Army Medical Center, to this project.

17. References

[1] Waterman, B.R., et al., *Epidemiology of ankle sprain at the United States Military Academy.* The American journal of sports medicine, 2010. 38(4): p. 797-803.

[2] Waterman, B.R., et al., *The epidemiology of ankle sprains in the United States.* The Journal of bone and joint surgery. American volume, 2010. 92(13): p. 2279-84.

[3] Hootman, J.M., R. Dick, and J. Agel, Epidemiology of collegiate injuries for 15 sports: summary and recommendations for injury prevention initiatives. Journal of athletic training, 2007. 42(2): p. 311-9.

[4] Fong, D.T., et al., A systematic review on ankle injury and ankle sprain in sports. Sports Med, 2007. 37(1): p. 73-94.

[5] Hopkinson, W.J., et al., *Syndesmosis sprains of the ankle.* Foot & ankle, 1990. 10(6): p. 325-30.

[6] Cedell, C.A., *Ankle lesions.* Acta orthopaedica Scandinavica, 1975. 46(3): p. 425-45.

[7] Fallat, L., D.J. Grimm, and J.A. Saracco, *Sprained ankle syndrome: prevalence and analysis of 639 acute injuries.* The Journal of foot and ankle surgery : official publication of the American College of Foot and Ankle Surgeons, 1998. 37(4): p. 280-5.

[8] Boytim, M.J., D.A. Fischer, and L. Neumann, *Syndesmotic ankle sprains.* The American journal of sports medicine, 1991. 19(3): p. 294-8.

[9] Boytim, M.J., D.A. Fischer, and L. Neumann, *Syndesmotic ankle sprains.* Am J Sports Med, 1991. 19(3): p. 294-8.

[10] Gerber, J.P., et al., Persistent disability associated with ankle sprains: a prospective examination of an athletic population. Foot Ankle Int, 1998. 19(10): p. 653-60.

[11] Wright, R.W., et al., *Ankle syndesmosis sprains in national hockey league players*. Am J Sports Med, 2004. 32(8): p. 1941-5.

[12] Clanton, T.O. and P. Paul, *Syndesmosis injuries in athletes*. Foot Ankle Clin, 2002. 7(3): p. 529-49.

[13] Wright, R.W., et al., *Ankle syndesmosis sprains in national hockey league players*. The American journal of sports medicine, 2004. 32(8): p. 1941-5.

[14] Gerber, J.P., et al., *Persistent disability associated with ankle sprains: a prospective examination of an athletic population*. Foot & ankle international / American Orthopaedic Foot and Ankle Society [and] Swiss Foot and Ankle Society, 1998. 19(10): p. 653-60.

[15] Hermans, J.J., et al., Anatomy of the distal tibiofibular syndesmosis in adults: a pictorial essay with a multimodality approach. J Anat, 2010. 217(6): p. 633-45.

[16] Kelikian, H. and A.S. Kelikian, *Disorders of the Ankle*. 1985: Saunders. 893.

[17] Elgafy, H., et al., Computed tomography of normal distal tibiofibular syndesmosis. Skeletal Radiol, 2010. 39(6): p. 559-64.

[18] Hocker, K. and A. Pachucki, [The fibular incisure of the tibia. The cross-sectional position of the fibula in distal syndesmosis]. Der Unfallchirurg, 1989. 92(8): p. 401-6.

[19] Sora, M.C., et al., Evaluation of the ankle syndesmosis: a plastination slices study. Clin Anat, 2004. 17(6): p. 513-7.

[20] Grass, R., *[Injuries of the inferior tibiofibular syndesmosis]*. Der Unfallchirurg, 2000. 103(7): p. 519.

[21] Yildirim, H., et al., *Evaluation of the fibular incisura of the tibia with magnetic resonance imaging*. Foot & ankle international / American Orthopaedic Foot and Ankle Society [and] Swiss Foot and Ankle Society, 2003. 24(5): p. 387-91.

[22] Bassett, F.H., 3rd, et al., Talar impingement by the anteroinferior tibiofibular ligament. A cause of chronic pain in the ankle after inversion sprain. J Bone Joint Surg Am, 1990. 72(1): p. 55-9.

[23] Rammelt, S., H. Zwipp, and R. Grass, Injuries to the distal tibiofibular syndesmosis: an evidence-based approach to acute and chronic lesions. Foot Ankle Clin, 2008. 13(4): p. 611-33, vii-viii.

[24] Kelikian, H. and A.S. Kelikian, *Disorders of the ankle*. 1985, Philadelphia: Saunders. vi, 893 p.

[25] Williams, G.N., M.H. Jones, and A. Amendola, *Syndesmotic ankle sprains in athletes*. The American journal of sports medicine, 2007. 35(7): p. 1197-207.

[26] Jones, M.H. and A. Amendola, *Syndesmosis Sprains of the Ankle: A Systematic Review*. Clinical Orthopaedics and Related Research, 2007. 455: p. 173-175 10.1097/BLO.0b013e31802eb471.

[27] Espinosa, N., J.P. Smerek, and M.S. Myerson, *Acute and chronic syndesmosis injuries: pathomechanisms, diagnosis and management*. Foot Ankle Clin, 2006. 11(3): p. 639-57.

[28] Sarsam, I.M. and S.P. Hughes, The role of the anterior tibio-fibular ligament in talar rotation: an anatomical study. Injury, 1988. 19(2): p. 62-4.

[29] Xenos, J.S., et al., The tibiofibular syndesmosis. Evaluation of the ligamentous structures, methods of fixation, and radiographic assessment. J Bone Joint Surg Am, 1995. 77(6): p. 847-56.

[30] Beumer, A., et al., Kinematics of the distal tibiofibular syndesmosis: radiostereometry in 11 normal ankles. Acta Orthop Scand, 2003. 74(3): p. 337-43.

[31] Ogilvie-Harris, D.J., S.C. Reed, and T.P. Hedman, *Disruption of the ankle syndesmosis: biomechanical study of the ligamentous restraints.* Arthroscopy, 1994. 10(5): p. 558-60.

[32] Press, C.M., A. Gupta, and M.R. Hutchinson, *Management of ankle syndesmosis injuries in the athlete.* Curr Sports Med Rep, 2009. 8(5): p. 228-33.

[33] Evans, J.M. and W.G. Schucany, *Radiological evaluation of a high ankle sprain.* Proc (Bayl Univ Med Cent), 2006. 19(4): p. 402-5.

[34] Norkus, S.A. and R.T. Floyd, *The anatomy and mechanisms of syndesmotic ankle sprains.* J Athl Train, 2001. 36(1): p. 68-73.

[35] Amendola, A., Controversies in diagnosis and management of syndesmosis injuries of the ankle. Foot Ankle, 1992. 13(1): p. 44-50.

[36] Lin, C.F., M.L. Gross, and P. Weinhold, Ankle syndesmosis injuries: anatomy, biomechanics, mechanism of injury, and clinical guidelines for diagnosis and intervention. J Orthop Sports Phys Ther, 2006. 36(6): p. 372-84.

[37] Close, J.R., Some applications of the functional anatomy of the ankle joint. J Bone Joint Surg Am, 1956. 38-A(4): p. 761-81.

[38] Nussbaum, E.D., et al., Prospective evaluation of syndesmotic ankle sprains without diastasis. Am J Sports Med, 2001. 29(1): p. 31-5.

[39] Hopkinson, W.J., et al., *Syndesmosis sprains of the ankle.* Foot Ankle, 1990. 10(6): p. 325-30.

[40] Orthner, E., R. Weinstabl, and R. Schabus, [Experimental study for clarification of the pathogenic mechanism in traumatic peroneal tendon dislocation]. Unfallchirurg, 1989. 92(11): p. 547-53.

[41] Pankovich, A.M., Fractures of the fibula at the distal tibiofibular syndesmosis. Clin Orthop Relat Res, 1979(143): p. 138-47.

[42] Frick, H., [The isolated tear of the tibio-fibular syndesmosis-mechanism, clinical observations, diagnosis and therapy (author's transl)]. Unfallheilkunde, 1978. 81(8): p. 542-5.

[43] Brosky, T., et al., The ankle ligaments: consideration of syndesmotic injury and implications for rehabilitation. J Orthop Sports Phys Ther, 1995. 21(4): p. 197-205.

[44] Teramoto, A., et al., Three-dimensional analysis of ankle instability after tibiofibular syndesmosis injuries: a biomechanical experimental study. Am J Sports Med, 2008. 36(2): p. 348-52.

[45] Fritschy, D., *An unusual ankle injury in top skiers.* Am J Sports Med, 1989. 17(2): p. 282-5; discussion 285-6.

[46] Fallat, L., D.J. Grimm, and J.A. Saracco, *Sprained ankle syndrome: prevalence and analysis of 639 acute injuries.* J Foot Ankle Surg, 1998. 37(4): p. 280-5.

[47] Crim, J.R., Winter sports injuries. The 2002 Winter Olympics experience and a review of the literature. Magn Reson Imaging Clin N Am, 2003. 11(2): p. 311-21.

[48] Vincelette, P., C.A. Laurin, and H.P. Levesque, *The footballer's ankle and foot.* Can Med Assoc J, 1972. 107(9): p. 872-4 passim.

[49] Weissman, J.A. and A.K. Lazis, [The radiological features of the distal tibio-fibular syndesmosis (author's transl)]. Rofo, 1980. 133(1): p. 46-51.

[50] Brown, K.W., et al., MRI findings associated with distal tibiofibular syndesmosis injury. AJR Am J Roentgenol, 2004. 182(1): p. 131-6.

[51] Waterman, B.R., et al., *The epidemiology of ankle sprains in the United States.* J Bone Joint Surg Am, 2010. 92(13): p. 2279-84.

[52] Taylor, D.C., D.L. Englehardt, and F.H. Bassett, 3rd, *Syndesmosis sprains of the ankle. The influence of heterotopic ossification.* Am J Sports Med, 1992. 20(2): p. 146-50.

[53] McMaster, J.H. and P.E. Scranton, Jr., *Tibiofibular synostosis: a cause of ankle disability.* Clin Orthop Relat Res, 1975(111): p. 172-4.

[54] Veltri, D.M., et al., Symptomatic ossification of the tibiofibular syndesmosis in professional football players: a sequela of the syndesmotic ankle sprain. Foot Ankle Int, 1995. 16(5): p. 285-90.

[55] Mulligan, E.P., *Evaluation and management of ankle syndesmosis injuries.* Phys Ther Sport, 2011. 12(2): p. 57-69.

[56] Katznelson, A., E. Lin, and J. Militiano, *Ruptures of the ligaments about the tibio-fibular syndesmosis.* Injury, 1983. 15(3): p. 170-2.

[57] Grass, R., et al., *[Injuries of the inferior tibiofibular syndesmosis].* Unfallchirurg, 2000. 103(7): p. 520-32.

[58] Fites, B., et al., *Latent syndesmosis injuries in athletes.* Orthopedics, 2006. 29(2): p. 124-7.

[59] Stiell, I.G., et al., *Implementation of the Ottawa ankle rules.* JAMA, 1994. 271(11): p. 827-32.

[60] Beumer, A., et al., A biomechanical evaluation of clinical stress tests for syndesmotic ankle instability. Foot Ankle Int, 2003. 24(4): p. 358-63.

[61] Zalavras, C. and D. Thordarson, *Ankle syndesmotic injury.* J Am Acad Orthop Surg, 2007. 15(6): p. 330-9.

[62] Teitz, C.C. and R.M. Harrington, A biochemical analysis of the squeeze test for sprains of the syndesmotic ligaments of the ankle. Foot Ankle Int, 1998. 19(7): p. 489-92.

[63] Alonso, A., L. Khoury, and R. Adams, Clinical tests for ankle syndesmosis injury: reliability and prediction of return to function. J Orthop Sports Phys Ther, 1998. 27(4): p. 276-84.

[64] Beumer, A., et al., Radiographic measurement of the distal tibiofibular syndesmosis has limited use. Clin Orthop Relat Res, 2004(423): p. 227-34.

[65] Beumer, A., et al., A biomechanical evaluation of the tibiofibular and tibiotalar ligaments of the ankle. Foot Ankle Int, 2003. 24(5): p. 426-9.

[66] Beumer, A., B.A. Swierstra, and P.G. Mulder, Clinical diagnosis of syndesmotic ankle instability: evaluation of stress tests behind the curtains. Acta Orthop Scand, 2002. 73(6): p. 667-9.

[67] Kiter, E. and M. Bozkurt, The crossed-leg test for examination of ankle syndesmosis injuries. Foot Ankle Int, 2005. 26(2): p. 187-8.

[68] Lindenfeld, T. and S. Parikh, *Clinical tip: heel-thump test for syndesmotic ankle sprain.* Foot Ankle Int, 2005. 26(5): p. 406-8.

[69] Starkey, C., Injuries and Illnesses in the National Basketball Association: A 10-Year Perspective. J Athl Train, 2000. 35(2): p. 161-167.

[70] Spaulding, S.J., Monitoring recovery following syndesmosis sprain: a case report. Foot Ankle Int, 1995. 16(10): p. 655-60.

[71] Williams, G.N., M.H. Jones, and A. Amendola, *Syndesmotic ankle sprains in athletes.* Am J Sports Med, 2007. 35(7): p. 1197-207.

[72] Smith, A.H. and B.R. Bach, Jr., *High ankle sprains: minimizing the frustration of a prolonged recovery.* Phys Sportsmed, 2004. 32(12): p. 39-43.

[73] Harper, M.C., An anatomic and radiographic investigation of the tibiofibular clear space. Foot Ankle, 1993. 14(8): p. 455-8.

[74] Bonnin, J.G., *Injuries to the ankle.* 1970, Darien, Conn.,: Hafner Pub. Co. xvi, 412 p.

[75] Ostrum, R.F., P. De Meo, and R. Subramanian, A critical analysis of the anterior-posterior radiographic anatomy of the ankle syndesmosis. Foot Ankle Int, 1995. 16(3): p. 128-31.

[76] Pneumaticos, S.G., et al., The effects of rotation on radiographic evaluation of the tibiofibular syndesmosis. Foot Ankle Int, 2002. 23(2): p. 107-11.

[77] Takao, M., et al., Arthroscopic and magnetic resonance image appearance and reconstruction of the anterior talofibular ligament in cases of apparent functional ankle instability. Am J Sports Med, 2008. 36(8): p. 1542-7.

[78] Takao, M., et al., Arthroscopic diagnosis of tibiofibular syndesmosis disruption. Arthroscopy, 2001. 17(8): p. 836-43.

[79] Ebraheim, N.A., et al., Anatomical evaluation and clinical importance of the tibiofibular syndesmosis ligaments. Surg Radiol Anat, 2006. 28(2): p. 142-9.

[80] Sclafani, S.J., Ligamentous injury of the lower tibiofibular syndesmosis: radiographic evidence. Radiology, 1985. 156(1): p. 21-7.

[81] Jones, M.H. and A. Amendola, *Syndesmosis sprains of the ankle: a systematic review.* Clin Orthop Relat Res, 2007. 455: p. 173-5.

[82] Takao, M., et al., Diagnosis of a tear of the tibiofibular syndesmosis. The role of arthroscopy of the ankle. J Bone Joint Surg Br, 2003. 85(3): p. 324-9.

[83] DeLee, J., D. Drez, and M.D. Miller, *DeLee & Drez's orthopaedic sports medicine : principles and practice.* 3rd ed. 2010, Philadelphia: Saunders/Elsevier. 2 v. (xxv, 2219, lv p.).

[84] Mei-Dan, O., et al., A dynamic ultrasound examination for the diagnosis of ankle syndesmotic injury in professional athletes: a preliminary study. Am J Sports Med, 2009. 37(5): p. 1009-16.

[85] Milz, P., et al., Lateral ankle ligaments and tibiofibular syndesmosis. 13-MHz high-frequency sonography and MRI compared in 20 patients. Acta Orthop Scand, 1998. 69(1): p. 51-5.

[86] Edwards, G.S., Jr. and J.C. DeLee, *Ankle diastasis without fracture.* Foot Ankle, 1984. 4(6): p. 305-12.

[87] Porter, D.A., Evaluation and treatment of ankle syndesmosis injuries. Instr Course Lect, 2009. 58: p. 575-81.

[88] Jenkinson, R.J., et al., Intraoperative diagnosis of syndesmosis injuries in external rotation ankle fractures. J Orthop Trauma, 2005. 19(9): p. 604-9.

[89] Jelinek, J.A. and D.A. Porter, Management of unstable ankle fractures and syndesmosis injuries in athletes. Foot Ankle Clin, 2009. 14(2): p. 277-98.

[90] Taylor, D.C., et al., Aggressive surgical treatment and early return to sports in athletes with grade III syndesmosis sprains. The American journal of sports medicine, 2007. 35(11): p. 1833-8.

[91] Beumer, A., et al., Kinematics of the distal tibiofibular syndesmosis: radiostereometry in 11 normal ankles. Acta orthopaedica Scandinavica, 2003. 74(3): p. 337-43.

[92] Beumer, A., et al., External rotation stress imaging in syndesmotic injuries of the ankle: comparison of lateral radiography and radiostereometry in a cadaveric model. Acta orthopaedica Scandinavica, 2003. 74(2): p. 201-5.

[93] Schafer, D. and B. Hintermann, Arthroscopic assessment of the chronic unstable ankle joint. Knee Surg Sports Traumatol Arthrosc, 1996. 4(1): p. 48-52.

[94] Takao, M., et al., Arthroscopic diagnosis of tibiofibular syndesmosis disruption. Arthroscopy : the journal of arthroscopic & related surgery : official publication of the Arthroscopy Association of North America and the International Arthroscopy Association, 2001. 17(8): p. 836-43.

[95] Amendola, A., G. Williams, and D. Foster, Evidence-based approach to treatment of acute traumatic syndesmosis (high ankle) sprains. Sports Med Arthrosc, 2006. 14(4): p. 232-6.

[96] Nussbaum, E.D., et al., Prospective evaluation of syndesmotic ankle sprains without diastasis. The American journal of sports medicine, 2001. 29(1): p. 31-5.

[97] Taylor, D.C., D.L. Englehardt, and F.H. Bassett, 3rd, Syndesmosis sprains of the ankle. The influence of heterotopic ossification. The American journal of sports medicine, 1992. 20(2): p. 146-50.

[98] Beumer, A., et al., Screw fixation of the syndesmosis: a cadaver model comparing stainless steel and titanium screws and three and four cortical fixation. Injury, 2005. 36(1): p. 60-4.

[99] Thompson, M.C. and D.S. Gesink, Biomechanical comparison of syndesmosis fixation with 3.5- and 4.5-millimeter stainless steel screws. Foot & ankle international / American Orthopaedic Foot and Ankle Society [and] Swiss Foot and Ankle Society, 2000. 21(9): p. 736-41.

[100] Hansen, M., et al., Syndesmosis fixation: analysis of shear stress via axial load on 3.5-mm and 4.5-mm quadricortical syndesmotic screws. The Journal of foot and ankle surgery : official publication of the American College of Foot and Ankle Surgeons, 2006. 45(2): p. 65-9.

[101] Needleman, R.L., D.A. Skrade, and J.B. Stiehl, Effect of the syndesmotic screw on ankle motion. Foot & ankle, 1989. 10(1): p. 17-24.

[102] Bell, D.P. and M.K. Wong, Syndesmotic screw fixation in Weber C ankle injuries--should the screw be removed before weight bearing? Injury, 2006. 37(9): p. 891-8.

[103] Heim, D., U. Heim, and P. Regazzoni, [Malleolar fractures with ankle joint instability--experience with the positioning screw]. Unfallchirurgie, 1993. 19(5): p. 307-12.

[104] Kukreti, S., A. Faraj, and J.N. Miles, Does position of syndesmotic screw affect functional and radiological outcome in ankle fractures? Injury, 2005. 36(9): p. 1121-4.

[105] Thordarson, D.B., et al., Biomechanical evaluation of polylactide absorbable screws used for syndesmosis injury repair. Foot & ankle international / American Orthopaedic Foot and Ankle Society [and] Swiss Foot and Ankle Society, 1997. 18(10): p. 622-7.

[106] Cox, S., et al., Distal tibiofibular syndesmosis fixation: a cadaveric, simulated fracture stabilization study comparing bioabsorbable and metallic single screw fixation. The Journal of foot and ankle surgery : official publication of the American College of Foot and Ankle Surgeons, 2005. 44(2): p. 144-51.

[107] Thordarson, D.B., et al., Bioabsorbable versus stainless steel screw fixation of the syndesmosis in pronation-lateral rotation ankle fractures: a prospective randomized trial. Foot & ankle international / American Orthopaedic Foot and Ankle Society [and] Swiss Foot and Ankle Society, 2001. 22(4): p. 335-8.

[108] Kaukonen, J.P., et al., Fixation of syndesmotic ruptures in 38 patients with a malleolar fracture: a randomized study comparing a metallic and a bioabsorbable screw. Journal of orthopaedic trauma, 2005. 19(6): p. 392-5.

[109] Bostman, O.M. and H.K. Pihlajamaki, Late foreign-body reaction to an intraosseous bioabsorbable polylactic acid screw. A case report. The Journal of bone and joint surgery. American volume, 1998. 80(12): p. 1791-4.

[110] Hovis, W.D. and R.W. Bucholz, Polyglycolide bioabsorbable screws in the treatment of ankle fractures. Foot & ankle international / American Orthopaedic Foot and Ankle Society [and] Swiss Foot and Ankle Society, 1997. 18(3): p. 128-31.

[111] Partio, E.K., et al., Self-reinforced absorbable screws in the fixation of displaced ankle fractures: a prospective clinical study of 152 patients. Journal of orthopaedic trauma, 1992. 6(2): p. 209-15.

[112] Yoshino, N., et al., Delayed aseptic swelling after fixation of talar neck fracture with a biodegradable poly-L-lactide rod: case reports. Foot & ankle international / American Orthopaedic Foot and Ankle Society [and] Swiss Foot and Ankle Society, 1998. 19(9): p. 634-7.

[113] Bostman, O.M., Osteoarthritis of the ankle after foreign-body reaction to absorbable pins and screws: a three- to nine-year follow-up study. J Bone Joint Surg Br, 1998. 80(2): p. 333-8.

[114] Thornes, B., et al., Suture-endobutton fixation of ankle tibio-fibular diastasis: a cadaver study. Foot & ankle international / American Orthopaedic Foot and Ankle Society [and] Swiss Foot and Ankle Society, 2003. 24(2): p. 142-6.

[115] Thornes, B., et al., Suture-button syndesmosis fixation: accelerated rehabilitation and improved outcomes. Clinical orthopaedics and related research, 2005(431): p. 207-12.

[116] Seitz, W.H., Jr., et al., Repair of the tibiofibular syndesmosis with a flexible implant. Journal of orthopaedic trauma, 1991. 5(1): p. 78-82.

[117] Soin, S.P., et al., *Suture-button versus screw fixation in a syndesmosis rupture model: a biomechanical comparison*. Foot & ankle international / American Orthopaedic Foot and Ankle Society [and] Swiss Foot and Ankle Society, 2009. 30(4): p. 346-52.

[118] Forsythe, K., et al., *Comparison of a novel FiberWire-button construct versus metallic screw fixation in a syndesmotic injury model*. Foot & ankle international / American Orthopaedic Foot and Ankle Society [and] Swiss Foot and Ankle Society, 2008. 29(1): p. 49-54.

[119] Klitzman, R., et al., *Suture-button versus screw fixation of the syndesmosis: a biomechanical analysis*. Foot & ankle international / American Orthopaedic Foot and Ankle Society [and] Swiss Foot and Ankle Society, 2010. 31(1): p. 69-75.

[120] Hahn, D. and C. Colton, *Malleolar Fractures*. AO Principles of Fracture Management, ed. T. Ruedi and W. Murphy. Vol. 2. 2000, New York: Thieme.

[121] Miller, R.S., P.S. Weinhold, and L.E. Dahners, Comparison of tricortical screw fixation versus a modified suture construct for fixation of ankle syndesmosis injury: a biomechanical study. Journal of orthopaedic trauma, 1999. 13(1): p. 39-42.

[122] Hoiness, P. and K. Stromsoe, Tricortical versus quadricortical syndesmosis fixation in ankle fractures: a prospective, randomized study comparing two methods of syndesmosis fixation. Journal of orthopaedic trauma, 2004. 18(6): p. 331-7.

[123] Xenos, J.S., et al., The tibiofibular syndesmosis. Evaluation of the ligamentous structures, methods of fixation, and radiographic assessment. The Journal of bone and joint surgery. American volume, 1995. 77(6): p. 847-56.

[124] Teramoto, A., et al., Comparison of Different Fixation Methods of the Suture-Button Implant for Tibiofibular Syndesmosis Injuries. The American journal of sports medicine, 2011.

[125] Barnett, C.H. and J.R. Napier, The axis of rotation at the ankle joint in man; its influence upon the form of the talus and the mobility of the fibula. J Anat, 1952. 86(1): p. 1-9.

[126] Tornetta, P., 3rd, et al., *Overtightening of the ankle syndesmosis: is it really possible?* The Journal of bone and joint surgery. American volume, 2001. 83-A(4): p. 489-92.

[127] Bragonzoni, L., et al., The distal tibiofibular syndesmosis during passive foot flexion. RSA-based study on intact, ligament injured and screw fixed cadaver specimens. Archives of orthopaedic and trauma surgery, 2006. 126(5): p. 304-8.

[128] Zalavras, C. and D. Thordarson, *Ankle syndesmotic injury*. The Journal of the American Academy of Orthopaedic Surgeons, 2007. 15(6): p. 330-9.

[129] de Souza, L.J., R.B. Gustilo, and T.J. Meyer, *Results of operative treatment of displaced external rotation-abduction fractures of the ankle*. The Journal of bone and joint surgery. American volume, 1985. 67(7): p. 1066-74.

[130] Chissell, H.R. and J. Jones, The influence of a diastasis screw on the outcome of Weber type-C ankle fractures. J Bone Joint Surg Br, 1995. 77(3): p. 435-8.

[131] Leeds, H.C. and M.G. Ehrlich, *Instability of the distal tibiofibular syndesmosis after bimalleolar and trimalleolar ankle fractures*. The Journal of bone and joint surgery. American volume, 1984. 66(4): p. 490-503.

[132] Weening, B. and M. Bhandari, Predictors of functional outcome following transsyndesmotic screw fixation of ankle fractures. Journal of orthopaedic trauma, 2005. 19(2): p. 102-8.

[133] Ramsey, P.L. and W. Hamilton, *Changes in tibiotalar area of contact caused by lateral talar shift.* The Journal of bone and joint surgery. American volume, 1976. 58(3): p. 356-7.

[134] Edwards, G.S., Jr. and J.C. DeLee, *Ankle diastasis without fracture.* Foot & ankle, 1984. 4(6): p. 305-12.

[135] Degroot, H., A.A. Al-Omari, and S.A. El Ghazaly, *Outcomes of suture button repair of the distal tibiofibular syndesmosis.* Foot & ankle international / American Orthopaedic Foot and Ankle Society [and] Swiss Foot and Ankle Society, 2011. 32(3): p. 250-6.

8

Better Association Between Q Angle and Patellar Alignment Among Less Displaced Patellae in Females with Patellofemoral Pain Syndrome: A Correlation Study with Axial Computed Tomography

Da-Hon Lin[1], Chien-Ho Janice Lin[2],
Jiu-Jenq Lin[3], Mei-Hwa Jan[3,4],
Cheng-Kung Cheng[5] and Yeong-Fwu Lin[4,5]
[1]Department of Orthopedic Surgery, En Chu Kong Hospital, Taipei,
[2]Department of Neurology, University of California Los Angels, CA,
[3]School and Graduate Institute of Physical Therapy,
National Taiwan University, Taipei,
[4]Yeong-An Clinic, Orthopedics & Rehabilitation, Taipei,
[5]Graduate Institute of Biomedical Engineering,
National Yang-Ming University, Taipei
[1,3,4,5]Taiwan
[2]USA

1. Introduction

Q angle, as an isolated clinical tool, is of uncertain and limited clinical value. [1] The Q angle, defined as the angle between the lines joining the anterior superior iliac spine, the center of the patella, and the center of the tibial tubercle, has been studied widely [2,3]. As a routine assessment tool in physical examination for clinical knee problems, with great inherent diversity in serving as a relevant clinical tool, the Q angle has long met debates in day to day orthopaedic practice. An increase in Q angle has long been looked as a pathologic factor in PFPS [4, 5]. Presumably the larger the Q angle, the larger the lateral pulling force on the patella [2], but reportedly Q angle rarely correlated with patellofemoral pain syndrome(PFPS)[6, 7]. Livingston and Mandigo [7] reported that no correlations between the Q angle measures and the magnitude of discomfort experienced in unilateral knee pain sufferers; while these relationships were weak yet significant in bilateral knee pain sufferers.

Since last decade, computer tomography (CT) has become an important diagnostic tool for better assessment of patellofemoral disorders [8, 9, 10]. Biedert and Warnke [6] have carried out a correlation study between the Q angle and the patella position by axial CT evaluation in patients with PFPS, but failed to establish the diagnostic relevance of the Q angle in the related patellofemoral disorders [6]. Other studies have revealed no significant correlation between Q angle and the position of patella in patients with PFPS. It has been stated that the patella may be translated laterally in patients with patellofemoral malalignment and thereby articially affect the measurement.[1] Reider has found a decrease in Q angle in chronic recurrent dislocation of patella, an increase in Q angle in the classic patellar pain pattern, often called "chondromalacia patella, and a normal mean Q angle in subluxated patellae.[11] Lin et al had a disclosure of a more apparent statistic trait via a deep exploration into the patellar alignment subtypes in a study of PFPS.[12] Given this; we speculated that patellar displacement exerts an effect on the Q angle to some extent. Since lateral displacement of the patella was found in most patients with PFPS, the Q-angle might be undervalued over the already laterally displaced patellae in patients with PFPS[13]. A deep exploration into the effect of lateral patellar displacement on Q angle measures might render a better disclosure of how the measure of Q angle and related clinical implication were affected by patellar displacement. The current study is thus aimed to execute a deeper prospective study of the correlation between Q angle and patellar alignments by treating the more displaced patellae and less displaced patellae separately to see whether Q angle might be varied with difference in patellar displacement. The hypothesis of this study was that the interaction dynamics between Q angle and patellar alignment may be varied with various status of patellar displacement.

Clinical Relevance: To endorse Q angle with a certain clinical value is important to clinical assessment of PFPS that prevails among females.

2. Materials and methods

2.1 Subjects

Among 50 female PFPS patients enrolled in the current study, there were 28 patients with PFPS over their both knees and 22 patients with PFPS unilaterally. All patients were examined with axial computed tomography for all knees. All PFPS knees came into the current study to explore the probable correlation between the Q angle and the patellar position. The inclusion criteria of PFPS were patients who were suffering from pain with more than three kinds of knee-flexing activities as sitting, getting up from sitting, walking upstairs or downstairs, squatting, getting up from squatting, running, kneeling, or jumping. The exclusion criteria included the presence of any major medical disease, rheumatoid arthritis, or gouty arthritis; past history of previous knee surgery, image findings of osteoarthritis, or any deformity of lower limbs. All were measured for body weight, body height, BMI, and Q angle. The Q angle was measured, with the patient lying supine, as the angle between the lines joining the anterior superior iliac spine, the center of the patella, and the tibia tubercle [2, 3]. The same goniometer was used for every patient and the same senior doctor taking all of the measurements. All patients underwent CT imaging of the knees in the same way as Gigante's methods [9].

2.2 CT imaging

Computed tomography was performed with a Pace General Electric machine (GE Medical Systems). The patient was in the supine position and the scans were obtained in knee extension with the quadriceps relaxed. The ankles were restrained with felt strips to prevent external rotation of the foot. An axial image was obtained through the widest diameter of the patella, which allows the best view of the patellofemoral joint for the related measurement of patellar alignment [9].

2.3 CT measurements of patellar displacement

Lateral patella shift of Sasaki (LS)[14], used to represent patellar positions, is the ratio of the lateral portion of transverse patellar line relative to the medial one (AC /BC). "C" is the point on the transverse patellar line (AB) intersected by a line that is drawn from the most convex point of the lateral femoral condyle and perpendicular to the line (Line D) along the anterior border of femoral condyles.. (Figure 1) The interrelation between the Q angles and CT measurements were investigated.

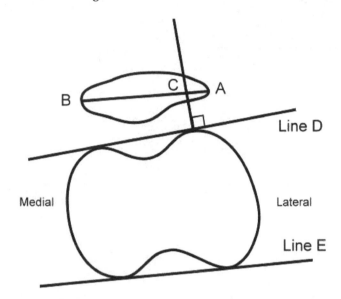

Lateral Shift of Sasaki (LS): AC/BC*100%

Fig. 1. Measurement made from CT images for lateral patella shift of Sasaki (LS). "LS" is the ratio of the lateral portion of transverse patellar line relative to the medial one (AC /BC). "C" is the point on the transverse patellar line (AB) intersected by a line that is drawn from the most convex point of the lateral femoral condyle and perpendicular to the line (Line D) along the anterior border of femoral condyles.

2.4 Statistical analysis

SPSS (version 11.5, SPSS Inc, Chicago, IL) statistical soft ware was used to execute all statistical analyses. The statistic tool used includes t test for the difference in measurement between study groups. The Pearson's correlation was used to investigate the relation between the Q angle and the measurement for patellar displacement, LS. For all statistical tests, the significance level was set at $p< .05$. To further examine the relationship between the Q angle and the measurements for patellar positions, the whole sample was grouped as: group 1 that was divided into those knees whose mean LS were below 20 percentiles of the whole sample and those knees whose mean were over 20 percentiles, group 2 that was divided into those knees whose mean LS were below 30 percentiles of the whole sample and those knees whose mean were over 30 percentiles, and group 3 that was divided into those knees whose mean LS were below 40 percentiles of the whole sample and those knees whose mean were over 40 percentiles. And a test with ROC curve was done for the specificity and sensitivity of the presence of patellar pain relative to Q angle. The area under the ROC curve was used to anticipate the pathognomonic potential of the Q angle. (Figure 2)

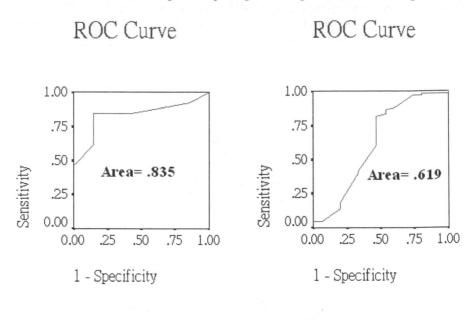

Fig. 2. Test with ROC curve for the specificity and sensitivity of the presence of patellar pain relative to Q angle.

3. Results

Q angle was significantly correlated to the measure of patellar displacement, LS, in the less displaced half of LS measures of each group. And an area of .730 to .835 was revealed by the test with ROC curve in the subgroups of less displaced patellae.

In total, the subjects aged 40.14±9.99 years, and their the basic demographics was: body weight, 57.18±8.55 kg, body height, 158.48±5.48 cm, and BMI, 22.75±3.09. The Q angle was 23.98±7.61 degrees, and LS, 35.99±14.03 in %. The Q angle and LS measures in each group and subgroup were shown in Table 1. There was no significant difference in Q angle between the subgroups in each group. ($p < 0.05$) (Table 1)

Statistic correlation was undertaken to explore the probable correlation between Q angle and patellar position, measured in LS. There was no correlation between Q angle and LS when the whole sample of 100 knees was calculated as a whole. After analysis into subgroups of different cutoff, a significant correlation was disclosed between Q angle and LS in the subgroup of knees with less displaced patellae in each group of respective way of cutoff. ($p < 0.05$) (Table 2)

	Group 1 Cutoff 20%: 24.00mm		Group 2 Cutoff 30%: 27.87mm		Group 3 Cutoff 40%: 32.16mm	
	Lower 20 percentiles (n= 20)	Upper 80 percentiles (n= 80)	Lower 30 percentiles (n= 30)	Upper 70 percentiles (n= 70)	Lower 40 percentiles (n= 40)	Upper 60 percentiles (n= 60)
Q angle (deg)	21.45±6.08	24.61±7.85	23.37±7.09	24.24±7.86	24.35±7.83	23.72±7.52
LS (%)	18.60±4.28**	40.33±12.10	21.11±5.06**	42.36±11.58	23.34±5.90**	44.42±11.24

There was significant difference in LS between any two subgroups within any group ($p< 0.01$).
There was no significant difference in Q angle between the subgroups within any group. ($p< 0.05$)

Table 1. Measurements of Q angles and patellar position (LS) in study groups

Via the test with ROC curve for the specificity and sensitivity of the presence of patellar pain relative to Q angle, an area of .730 to .835 was revealed in the less displaced half of LS measures of each group, indicating that Q angle would be more pathognomonic of PFPS among patients or knees of less displaced patellae. (Figure 2, Table 2)

	Group 1 Cutoff 20%: 24.00mm		Group 2 Cutoff 30%: 27.87mm		Group 3 Cutoff 40%: 32.16mm	
	Lower 20 percentiles (n= 20)	Upper 80 percentiles (n= 80)	Lower 30 percentiles (n= 30)	Upper 70 percentiles (n= 70)	Lower 40 percentiles (n= 40)	Upper 60 percentiles (n= 60)
Correlation coefficient[a]	0.481*	-0.175	0.502**	-0.142	0.453**	-0.096
Area under ROC curve[b]	0.835	0.619	0.780	0.634	0.730	0.657

[a]: Correlation coefficient between Q angle and lateral shift of patella (LS)
[b]: Diagnostic tests: probability of correctly distinguishing between painful and non-painful knees
*: p <0.05; **: p<0.01

Table 2. Correlation coefficient between Q angle and lateral shift of patella (LS). And diagnostic tests between subjects with and without painful knees.

4. Discussion

We have hypothesized that the interaction dynamics between Q angle and patellar alignment may be varied with various status of patellar displacement. After deep exploration into the subgroups of LS, the current study has demonstrated that Q angle was significantly correlated to the measure of patellar alignment, LS, in the less displaced half of LS measures of each group of respective cutoff point for LS. And via the test with ROC curve for the specificity and sensitivity of the presence of patellar pain relative to Q angle, an area of .730 to .835 was observed to be under the ROC curve in the less displaced half of LS measures of each group, indicating that Q angle would be more pathognomonic of PFPS among patients or knees of less displaced patellae.

Reportedly, a decrease in Q angle has been observed in chronic recurrent dislocation of patella, an increase in Q angle in the classic patellar pain pattern, often called "chondromalacia patella, and a normal mean Q angle in subluxated patellae.[11] While, Biedert and Warnke's reported failure to conclude any correlation between the Q angle and the patellar displacement in their experiment[6]. Quite similar to Biedert and Warnke's work [6]. Our current study also showed no correlation between the Q angle and the patellar displacement when analyzing all the subject knees of PFPS as a whole. When the more displaced patellae and the less displaced half were evaluated separately, a significant correlation was observed between the Q angle and the patellar displacement among those with less displaced patellae in our study.

The concept of the "larger the Q angle, the larger the lateral pulling force on the patella" has been challenged, one after another, in the literature. Dandy has reported that an unstable, subluxated patella lies more laterally than normal, thereby decreasing the Q angle[15]. By statistically treating the more displaced patellae and the less displaced ones separately in the 3 ways of cutting off for the LS measures, the current study has revealed a positive correlation between Q angle and patellar displacement among those with less displaced patellae. The Q angle has been presumed to be responsible for the bowstring effect [3], whereby the patella tends to move laterally as the quadriceps contracts. Actually it is the underlying valgus vector force of the Q angle, rather than the Q angle per se, that dominates the way that the instantaneous bowstring assumes. As thus the Q angle and the instantaneous center of the patella landmarks the way the instantaneous bowstring assumes. Apparently Q angle failed to mean a comparable degree of the valgus vector across the knee of PFPS. As revealed in the current study, Q angle was equivocally obscured by patellar displacement that was the presumed result of the valgus across the knee. As thus the degree of valgus across the knee could be better represented by Q angle together with patellar displacement. In the current study there was no significant difference in Q angle between the subgroups in each group. We failed to observe Q angle as being undervalued by patellar displacement even if a consistent trait of negative association between Q angle and patellar displacement (LS) has been demonstrated in each subgroup of more displaced patellae in each group. (Table 2) We failed to verify Post's concept that the patella may be translated laterally in patients with severe patellofemoral malalignment and thereby artificially decrease the measurement of the Q angle[1, 2].

The natural valgus of the lower limb and the lateral pulling vector of the quadriceps migrates the patella laterally.[15, 16] An abnormal or increased Q angle is considered a relevant pathologic factor in patellofemoral disorder [6]. When the Q angle exceeds 15-20° it is thought to contribute to knee extensor mechanism dysfunction by increasing the tendency for lateral patella malpositioning [17]. Previous investigations of the quadriceps angle (or Q angle) and its relationship to knee disorders have yielded equivocal results.[6, 9, 10, 18] Reportedly Q angle failed to dictate the PFPS symptom and the presumed patellar malalignment leading to PFPS. Previous studies from various investigators have failed to correlate Q angle measurements with patient complaints. Fairbank et al have demonstrated no significant difference between painful and pain free knees [19]. There is no specific correlation between patellar symptomatology and an increased Q angle, as thus the clinical value of measuring the Q angle has been much controversial [20]. In the current study, via the test with ROC curve for the specificity and sensitivity of the presence of patellar pain relative to Q angle, an area of .730 to .835 was observed under the ROC curve in the less displaced half of LS measures of each group of respective cutoff point, indicating that Q angle would be more pathognomonic of PFPS among patients or knees of less displaced patellae. Likewise, the current study has endorsed Q angle with a certain clinical value among people who are with less displaced patellae. The result will be important to clinical assessment of PFPS that prevails among females and athletes[20].

For the time being, the diagnostic relevance of the Q angle is highly equivocal. The Q angle has been subjected to a radical modification in order to play a positive clinical tool and provide a certain clinical value. Fithian et al has proposed a modified Q angle by measuring it in 30° of knee flexion with the patella manually reduced into the trochlea [21]. By analyzing all subject knees into different subtypes of patellar displacement to reveal an association between Q angle and patellar alignment and to endorse the Q angle with a promising pathognomonic value among PFPS patients or knees of less displaced patellae, the current study would help motivate further revision and endorsement of the Q angle in regard.

Reportedly a significant difference in Q angle between sides has led to a statement that symmetry in right versus left lower limb Q angle measures may be erroneous. And this is why both knees of PFPS patients with bilateral knee pain were enrolled into the current study instead of one person one knee [7, 22] Additionally, in our series, there was a significant difference in Q angle between sexes in our unopened observations ($p < 0.01$) This is why the male were excluded from the current study. As thus the current design merely focused on female population. Women have been stated to have higher Q angles than men, on the basis of a wider pelvis [23, 24]. Some has reported minimal difference in the Q angle measure between men and women [3]; while some has reported higher Q angle in men [19, 25].

The limitation of this study is failure to execute the interaction dynamics between Q angle and patellar position under weight bearing condition. A further study with open MR would make possible the related study under weight bearing condition.

In conclusion, Q angle was significantly correlated to patellar alignment among people with less displaced patellae. Q angle was more pathognomonic of patellar pain in those people with less displaced patellae.

5. Acknowledgements

The authors thank Dr. Ming-Chang Chiang of UCLA for the critical review of the study design and the logics that goes through the article.

6. References

[1] Post WR, Teitge R, Amis A., Fimech E: Patellofemoral malalignment: looking beyond the viewbox. Clin Sports Med 2002; 21:521-546.

[2] Caylor D, Fites R, Worrel TW: The relationship between quadriceps angle and anterior knee pain syndrome. J Orthop Sports Phys Ther 1993; 17: 11-15.

[3] Grelsamer RP, Dubey A, and Weinstein CH: Men and women have similar Q angles. A clinical and trigonometric evaluation. J Bone Joint Surg Br 2005; 87:1498-501.

[4] Ford DH, Post WR: Open or arthroscopic lateral release, indication, techniques, and rehabilitation. Clin Sports Med 1997; 16: 29-49.

[5] Rillmann P, Dutly A, Kieser C, Berbig R: Modified Elmslie-Trillat procedure for instability of the patella. Knee Surg Sports Traumatol Arthrosc 1997; 6:31-35.

[6] Biedert RM, Warnke K: Correlation between the Q angle and the patella position: a clinical and computed tomography evaluation. Arch Orthop Trauma Surg 2001; 121:346-349.

[7] Livingston LA, Mandigo JL: Bilateral Q angle asymmetry and anterior knee pain syndrome. Clin Biomech 1999; 14:7-13.

[8] Biedert RM, Gruhl C: Axial computed tomography of the patellofemoral joint with and without quadriceps contraction. Arch Orthop Trauma Surg. 1997; 116: 77-82.

[9] Gigante A, Pasquinelli FM, Paladini P, Ulisse S, and Greco F: The effects of patellar taping on patellofemoral incongruence: A computed tomography study. Am J Sports Med. 2001; 29:88-92.

[10] Guzzanti V, Gigante A, Di Lazzaro A, Fabbriciani C: Patellofemoral malalignment in adolescents: Computerized tomographic assessment with or without quadriceps contraction. Am J Sports Med 1994; 22: 55-60.

[11] Reider B, Marshall JL, Warren RF. Clinical characteristics of patellar disorders in young athletes. Am J Sports Med 1981; 9:270-274.

[12] Lin YF, Lin JJ, Jan MH, Wei TC, Shih HY, and Cheng CK. Role of vastus medialis obliquus in repositioning the patella: A dynamic computed tomography study. Am J Sports Med. 2008; 36:741-746.

[13] Herrington L, Nester C: Q-angle undervalued? The relationship between Q-angle and medio-lateral position of the patella. Clin Biomech 2004; 19:1070-1073.

[14] Sasaki T, Yagi T. Subluxation of the patella: Investigation by computerized tomography. Int Orthop. 1986; 10:115-120.

[15] Dandy DJ: Chronic patellofemoral instability. J Bone Joint Surg Br 1995; 78: 328-335.

[16] Goh JC, Lee PY, Bose K. A Cadaver Study of the Function of the Oblique Part of Vastus Medialis. J Bone Joint Surg 1995; 77:225-231.

[17] Byl T, Cole J, and Livingston L: What determines the magnitude of the Q-angle? A preliminary study of selected skeletal and muscular measures. J Sports Rehab 2000; 9: 26-34.

[18] Kujala UM, Kormano M, Osterman K, et al: Magnetic resonance imaging analysis of patellofemoral congruity in females. Clin J Sport Med. 1992; 2:21-26.

[19] Fairbank JC, Pynsent PB, Van Poortvliet JA, Phillips H: Mechanical factors in the incidence of knee pain in adolescents and young adults. J Bone Joint Surg Br 1984; 66: 685-93.

[20] Hughston JC. Subluxation of the Patella. J Bone Joint Surg 1968; 50A:1003-1026.

[21] Fithian DC, Mishra DK, Balen PF, Stone ML, and Daniel DM: Instrumented measurement of patellar mobility. Am J Sports Med 1995; 23: 607-15.

[22] Livingston LA, Mandigo JL: Bilateral within-subject Q angle asymmetry in young adult females and males. Biomed Sci Instrum. 1997; 33:112-7.

[23] Frey C: Foot health and shoe wear for women. Clin Orthop Relat Res 2000; 372:32-44.

[24] Fulkerson JP, Arendt EA: Anterior knee pain in females. Clin Orthop Relat Res 2000; 372: 69-73.

[25] Aglietti P, Insall JN, CerulliG: Patellar pain and incongruence. I: Measurement of incongruence. Clin Orthop Relat Res 1983; 176:217-24.

9

Consequences of Ankle Inversion Trauma: A Novel Recognition and Treatment Paradigm

Patrick O. McKeon[1], Tricia J. Hubbard[2] and Erik A. Wikstrom[2]
[1]University of Kentucky,
[2]University of North Carolina at Charlotte
USA

1. Introduction

Diseases associated with physical inactivity (i.e. hypokinetic diseases) include, but are not limited to: cardiopulmonary disease, hypertension, obesity, metabolic disorders, non-smoking related cancers, and osteoporosis.(Admirall et al., 2011; CDC, 2009; Liu et al., 2008; Sesso, Paffenbarger, & Lee, 2000; Steanovv, Vekova, Kurktschiev, & Temelkova-Kurktschiev, 2011; Weiderpass, 2010) Physical inactivity remains one of the most important public health concerns as objective measures demonstrate that less than 5% of Americans participate in the recommended amount of physical activity necessary for health benefits.(Troiano et al., 2008) Additionally, physical inactivity is currently identified as the second leading actual cause of death, implicated in more deaths than the next seven causes of death combined.(Mokdad, Marks, Stroup, & Gerberding, 2004) Further, injury associated with sport, exercise, and recreation is a leading cause for the cessation of regular physical activity.(Koplan, Powell, Sikes, & Campbell, 1982; Pate, Pratt, Blair, & al., 1995) With lateral ankle sprains (LAS) being the most commonly occurring orthopedic pathology (Fernandez, Yard, & Comstock.R.D., 2007; Hootman, Dick, & Agel, 2007), and with such a high percentage of disability occurring after the initial injury(McKay, 2001; Verhagen, de Keizer, & Van Dijk, 1995) its role in potentially limiting physical activity is significant.(Verhagen et al., 1995) Despite the obvious public health problem that ankle sprains represent, no significant inroads have been made at preventing the injury and/or treating the associated sequelae using traditional treatment paradigms. Thus the evidence regarding the presentation and treatment of the consequences associated with LAS will be described within the context of a new recognition and treatment paradigm known as the PCL(McKeon PO, Medina McKeon JM, Mattacola CG, Lattermann C. Finding, 2011) (patient-, clinician-, laboratory-oriented) model which addresses the sequelae of lateral ankle sprains from a holistic perspective. Further, this model will be situated within the dynamic systems theory to provide the framework for understanding how all of the individual post-injury adaptations create a singular pathology that predisposed an individual to fall into a continuum of disability that will affect them for the remainder of their lives.

2. Ankle sprain epidemiology

2.1 Observation and description of the clinical phenomenon

Lateral ankle sprains are the most common injuries associated with physical activity and athletic participation. (Fernandez et al., 2007; Hootman et al., 2007) Forceful plantar flexion and inversion is the most common mechanism of injury causing damage to the passive lateral ligamentous structures of the ankle.(Baumhauer, Alosa, Renstrom, Trevino, & Beynnon, 1995) Specifically, the anterior talofibular ligament (ATFL), reported to be the weakest, is the first ligament injured.(Brostrom, 1964) Rupture to the ATFL is followed by damage to the calcaneofibular ligament (CFL) and finally to the posterior talofibular ligament (PTFL).(Brostrom, 1964) Isolated injury to the ATFL occurs in 66% of LAS while ATFL and CFL ruptures occur concurrently in another 20%.(Brostrom, 1964) The PTFL is not commonly injured because of the large amount of dorsiflexion needed to strain the ligament places the ankle in a closed packed and thus more stable position. The current literature suggests it takes over 6 weeks for ligament damage to heal, (Avci & Sayh, 1998; Brostrom, 1966; Cetti, Christensen, & Corfitzen, 1984; Freeman, 1965b; Konradsen, Holmer, & Sondergaard, 1991; Munk, Holm-Christensen, & Lind, 1995) however, studies have also documented joint laxity 6 months after injury.(Brostrom, 1966; Cetti et al., 1984) In addition to the lateral ligamentous structures of the talocrural joint, the subtalar ligaments can also be injured. However, injury to the subtalar joint often occurs in combination with injury to the lateral ankle ligaments as evidenced by the estimated 75 to 80% incidence of subtalar instability in those with CAI.(Hertel, Denegar, Monroe, & Stokes, 1999; Meyer, Garcia, Hoffmeyer, & Fritschy, 1986) Damage to the ligaments of the ankle can lead to the development of an unstable or hypermoble ankle joint which ultimately leads to an increase in the accessory motion available at a joint. Increased accessory motion places further strain on the injured ligaments and it is hypothesized that increased mobility of the talus, due to hypermobility, may lead to the axis of rotation becoming more anterior or posterior in the frontal plane.

With injury to ligaments, mechanoreceptors may also be damaged. If damaged, the afferent (i.e. sensory) input from ligamentous mechanoreceptors may be altered and further disrupt the axis of joint rotation causing the injured individual to compensate in an effort to maintain proper function.(Konradsen & Magnusson, 2000) However, there is a lack of consistent empirical data to confirm that alterations in function are due to the loss and/or disruption of afferent input from ligament mechanoreceptors.(Hubbard & Hertel, 2006a) Despite the inconsistency of the literature, evidence does exist to suggest that a loss of afferent information from the lateral ligaments can have both local and global consequences on sensorimotor function in both asymptomatic individuals (Myers, Riemann, Hwang, Fu, & Lephart, 2003; McKeon, Booi, Branam, Johnson, & Mattacola, 2010) and those with CAI.

In addition to ligamentous mechanoreceptors, musculotendinous mechanoreceptors may also become altered with ankle instability.(Freeman, 1965a) Increased mobility of the talus stresses the joint capsule (Wilkerson & Nitz, 1994) which then negatively affects (via the gamma motorneurons) the activation threshold of the muscle spindles in muscles and tendons that cross the ankle joint. Further, the gamma motor neurons may also increase co-contraction levels (Wilkerson et al., 1994) resulting in altered afferent signals being sent to the central nervous system. Evidence of these altered afferent signals are the early recruitment of proximal muscles such as the gluteals to help provide stability (i.e. the development of a hip strategy).(Beckman & Buchanan, 1995; Bullock-Saxton, janda, &

Bullock, 1994) A vicious and continuous cycle is thus put into motion when proper healing and joint alignment are not restored due to inappropriate treatment.(Hubbard et al., 2006a) Unfortunately, inappropriate or totally absent treatment occurs far too often for lateral ankle sprains. Indeed, LAS are often erroneously considered to be an inconsequential injury with no lasting consequences. However, LAS account for approximately 60% of all injuries during interscholastic and intercollegiate sports in the United States.(Fernandez, Yard, & Comstock, 2007; Hootman et al., 2007) Further, more than 23,000 LAS are estimated to occur per day in the United States which equates to approximately one sprain per 10,000 people daily.(Kannus & Renstrom, 1991) In addition, health care costs for acute LAS have been estimated to be over $4 billion dollars annually in the United States alone when accounting for inflation in 2011.(Soboroff, Pappius, & Komaroff, 1984) Another consequence of societal insignificance assigned to LAS is the high percentage of people (~55%) who sprain their ankle and do not seek treatment from a health care professional.(McKay, 2001) As a result, the true incidence of injury may be much greater than what has been previously reported.

Even more troubling is the fact that about 30% of those who suffer a first time LAS develop CAI; however this number has been reported as high as 75%.(Anandacoomarasamy & Barnsley, 2005; Peters, Trevino, & Renstrom, 1991; Smith & Reischl, 1986) This translates to at least 1 out of every 3 individuals who sprain their ankle will go on to suffer residual symptoms (i.e. CAI) indefinitely. Indeed, the residual symptoms that define CAI significantly alter an individual's health and function by causing them to become less active over their life span.(Verhagen et al., 1995) Further, a clear link has been established between CAI and post-traumatic ankle osteoarthritis (OA). Post-traumatic ankle OA is the most common cause, accounting for more than 70% of all ankle OA cases (Valderrabano, Hintermann, Horisberger, & Fung, 2006a) and both ankle joint fractures (Horisberger, Valderrabano, & Hintermann, 2009b) and ligament lesions associated with CAI (Hirose, Murakami, Minowa, Kura, & Yamashita, 2004; Valderrabano et al., 2006a) are a significant cause of post-traumatic ankle OA. Indeed, a high percentage (66-78%) of patients with CAI go on to develop post-traumatic ankle OA.(Hirose et al., 2004; Valderrabano et al., 2006a)

3. Pathophysiology: Perspectives of the patient, clinician, and laboratory scientist

3.1 Acute ankle sprains
3.1.1 Patient-oriented evidence
Anyone who has ever suffered a lateral ankle sprains knows that it is a painful and disabling injury. The published literature also supports this belief across a wide range of self-report questionnaires/scales.(de Vries, Kingma, Blakevoort, & van Dijk, 2010; Evans, Hertel, & Sebastianelli, 2004) For example, Brostrom (Brostrom, 1966) reported 20% of patients reported their ankle feeling unstable a year after an initial ankle sprain. Further, a prospective investigation performed by Evans et al.(Evans et al., 2004) indicated that self-assessed disability (as measured by two independent scales) did not return to baseline (i.e. pre-injury) levels until twenty-one days post injury.

3.1.2 Clinician-oriented evidence
The hypermobility associated with acute LAS can be assessed qualitatively and empirically using various clinical techniques such as manual stress tests, instrumented arthrometry and stress radiographs. Manual stress tests are one of the most common means to assess laxity

after an ankle sprain. To date, evidence indicates that 30% of patients have had a positive anterior drawer 2-weeks post injury and 11% had a positive anterior drawer 6-weeks post injury.(Avci et al., 1998) Additionally, 12% have been shown to have a positive anterior drawer at 8-weeks post injury. (Cetti et al., 1984) Similarly, significantly more anterior displacement and inversion rotation was shown via an ankle arhtrometer 8-weeks after an acute LAS.(Hubbard & Cordova, 2009a) Another study showed that 42% and 33% of subjects from separate treatment groups had an increased talar tilt compared to their uninvolved healthy ankle at 3-months post injury using stress radiography. (Freeman, 1965b) At 1-year post injury, ~30% of patients had a positive anterior drawer. (Brostrom, 1966) Using a more objective outcome, 5% of patients presented with pathologic stress radiography values 3-months post injury.(Konradsen et al., 1991) Further, over 50% of patients who sprained their ankle between 9-13 years prior, had mechanical laxity on stress radiographs.(Munk et al., 1995)

In addition to hypermobility, LAS can also cause hypomobility. Hubbard and Hertel (Hubbard & Hertel, 2008), using simple lateral radiographs of the ankle, found that the distal fibula has been pulled anteriorly, relative to the tibia, from a 'normal' position seen in healthy uninjured adults (i.e. a positional fault had occurred). Similarly, a decreased posterior talar glide (Denegar, Hertel, & Fonseca, 2002) has been observed in those with acute LAS suggesting that a talar positional fault may also be present. Since normal osteokinematic motion cannot occur without propoer arthrokinematics, these studies support the commonly observed limitations in ankle range of motion (ROM) following acute LAS.(Aiken, Pelland, Brison, Pickett, & Brouwer, 2008; Youdas, McLean, Krause, & Hollman, 2009) These studies have shown that: 1) active dorsiflexion ROM returns to 'normal' values between 4- and 6- weeks post injury (Youdas et al., 2009) and that clinical measures of ROM are not as sensitive as laboratory measures (e.g. isokinetic dynamometer).(Aiken et al., 2008)

3.1.3 Laboratory-oriented evidence

There have been numerous investigations that have quantified deficits in sensorimotor function in those with LAS using laboratory-oriented evidence. In short, grade II or III acute LAS have been reported to cause deficits in ankle inversion joint position sense for up to 12- weeks post injury when compared to the uninjured limb.(Konradsen, Olesen, & Hansen, 1998) In addition, isometric strength deficits have been reported, in multiple planes of motion, as long as 6-weeks post injury.(Holme et al., 1999; Koralewicz & Engh, 2000) The most commonly studied sensorimotor outcome is postural control. Recent systematic reviews demonstrated that postural control is impaired on the involved limb (McKeon & Hertel, 2008a; Wikstrom, Naik, Lodha, & Cauraugh, 2009) and uninvolved limb following acute LAS.(Wikstrom, Naik, Lodha, & Cauraugh, 2010c) These findings are supported by prospective data indicating that balance deficits on the uninjured limb resolve in about 7- days while balance deficits on the involved limb take about 21-28 days to fully resolve.(Evans et al., 2004) Given the above mentioned impairments, as well as the obvious pain and dysfunction associated with LAS, it is not surprising that both the temporal and spatial parameters of gait are also impaired.(Crosbie, Green, & Refshauge, 1999)

3.2 Chronic ankle instability

Based on the above presented information, it is clear that there a numerous consequences of acute LAS and that those consequences are multi-factorial in nature. While the exact physiological mechanism of CAI remains unknown, evidence suggests that it is multi-factorial in nature. Therefore, while ankle ligamentous damage is the most obvious result of a LAS, the laxity itself is not likely to be the sole cause of CAI. Rather, the true mechanism is most likely linked to a number of adaptations and impairments which cause a cascade of events that ultimately leads to CAI (Figure 1).(Hertel, 2008) One consequence that has been, for the most part, ignored is the loss of relevant sensory (i.e. afferent) information from those damaged ligaments, and surrounding tissue, that is associated with the continuum of disability.(McKeon, 2010; McKeon et al., 2010) As mentioned above, the deafferentation theory (Freeman, 1965a), has been refuted in the literature because of inconsistent support and because the link between local mechanical instability and global functional disability in those with CAI has not been clearly established. One factor that remains clear however, is that those with CAI have a decreased ability to cope with changes in task and environmental demands. This inability to effectively cope is thought to be most commonly manifested in episodes of giving way.

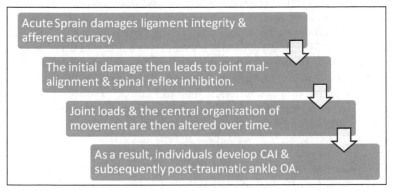

Fig. 1. Hypothetical cascade of events that causes the development of CAI and post-traumatic ankle OA based on the available evidence.

3.2.1 Patient-oriented evidence

The most commonly reported symptom across the continuum of disability associated with CAI is decreased functional performance due to repeated episodes of 'giving way'.(Hertel, 2002; 2008) It is crucially important to assess how impaired sensorimotor control due to CAI, often measured with laboratory-oriented outcomes, manifests into patient-reported activity limitations and participation restrictions. In other words, how does the instability a patient experiences at the ankle move from a local ankle instability to a global disability in function? Gaining the patient's perception of disability is very important in developing a thorough understanding of the impact of CAI on quality of life. These patient-oriented tools can be used to both assess the impact of CAI and the effects of rehabilitation strategies on function. Overall, patient-oriented measures of function provide the opportunity to gain insight into how the patient experiences disability due to ankle injuries.

Numerous scales/questionnaires have been developed in the sport injury literature to quantify the impact of CAI on patient-oriented function. Each scale assesses functional ability differently and has unique grading/weighting systems but all scales contain questions related to an individual's ability to complete both activities of daily living and sport. The Ankle Joint Functional Assessment Tool (AJFAT), Cumberland Ankle Instability Tool (CAIT), Foot and Ankle Outcome Score (FAOS), the Foot and Ankle Disability Instrument (FADI), and the Foot and Ankle Ability Measure (FAAM) are some of the more commonly reported scales in the literature. In 2007, Eechaute et al.(Eechaute, Vaes, Van Aerschot, Asman, & Duquet, 2007) performed a systematic review of the clinimetric qualities of these scales and found that the FADI and the FAAM are the most appropriate scales to use for the assessment of function in those with CAI. Further, a self-reported loss of at least 10% of function during activities of daily living and at least a 20% loss of function during sport-related activities are the current recommendations for classifying those with CAI when using the FADI and/or FAAM.(Hale & Hertel, 2005)

3.2.2 Clinician-oriented evidence
Capturing the deficits that patients report associated with CAI in measurable clinical tests is crucial for the development of objective outcomes for diagnosis, prognosis, and rehabilitation. Several clinical tests have been developed to assess the effects of CAI across a wide range of outcomes and some of the more commonly reported will be discussed below.
There have been numerous studies which have reported mechanical instability in those with CAI. Tropp et al.(Tropp, Odenrick, & Gillquist, 1985) reported 42% of subjects with CAI had a positive manual anterior drawer test. More recently, Hertel et al.(Hertel et al., 1999) illustrated ankles with CAI demonstrated significantly greater laxity during an anterior drawer test and greater talar tilt angles upon supination stress than did uninjured ankles. Significantly greater talar tilt values have also been shown in those with CAI compared with a healthy reference group.(Lentell et al., 1995; Louwerens, Ginai, Van Linge, & Snijders, 1995) Similar results have also been reported using an instrumented ankle arthrometer (i.e. more anterior translation and inversion stress in those with CAI relative to uninjured ankles).(Hubbard, Kramer, Denegar, & Hertel, 2007) Further, those with CAI, relative to uininjured controls, have been shown to have an anterior positional fault of the distal fibula (Hubbard, Hertel, & Sherbondy, 2006b) and talus.(Wikstrom & Hubbard, 2010b) These results using different techniques demonstrate that mechanical instability and structural adaptations are present in patients with CAI and similar to those reported following a LAS.
The weight-bearing lunge test (WBLT) is a clinical measure of the amount of dorsiflexion available in a weight-bearing environment.(Hoch & McKeon, 2011) It has been demonstrated that those with CAI have a dorsiflexion deficit on their affected limb during functional activities.(Drewes, McKeon, Kerrigan, & Hertel, 2009) The WBLT and the anterior reach of the Star Excursion Balance Test (SEBT) are highly correlated in healthy people, but not correlated as highly in those with CAI suggesting that those with CAI adopt a new movement strategy to complete the test. The SEBT has been the most extensively studied clinical measure of balance.(Gribble, Hertel, & Denegar, 2007; Hertel, 2008; Hertel, Braham, Hale, & Olmsted-Kramer, 2006; Olmsted, Olmsted, Carcia, Hertel, & Shultz, 2002) It has been consistently shown that those with CAI have a reduced ability to maintain balance on their injured leg and maximally reach with the opposite limb in different directions. Currently, it is recommended that the anterior, posteromedial, and posterolateral directions be used because each present a unique contribution to the assessment of dynamic postural control deficits and because these directions can elucidate postural control deficits associated with CAI.(Hertel, 2008; Hertel et al., 2006) Another test for the assessment of balance in those with CAI is the Balance Error Scoring System (BESS) (Docherty, McLeod, & Shultz, 2006). The premise of the

BESS is that individuals attempt to maintain balance under a series of postural challenges and the clinician counts the number of errors committed during the test. Further, the BESS provides a clinical assessment which utilizes the manipulation of different postural control tasks and environments to explore the sensorimotor system's ability to cope with changing demands. Out of the six conditions of the BESS, it has been found that the single limb stance on a firm surface and a foam surface provide the most relevant information associated with clinically relevant postural control deficits in those with CAI.(Docherty et al., 2006)

3.2.3 Laboratory-oriented evidence

Ankle instability has been shown to result in a host of functional impairments. These impairments have included local effects thought to be a direct consequence of the joint damage described above including deficits in ankle joint position sense and movement detection, evertor muscle strength, peroneal and soleus motor neuron pool excitability, and peroneal muscle reaction time in response to perturbation (see Hertel, 2008) for further review). In addition to local effects around the joint, CAI has also been associated with global deficits in sensorimotor function, specifically alterations in proximal muscle and joint control as well as alterations in stereotypical movement patterns. For example, those with CAI have decreased hip extension and abduction strength.(Hubbard et al., 2007) and have diminished levels of alpha motorneuron pool excitability at the knee.(Sedory, McVey, Cross, Ingersoll, & Hertel, 2007) The use of motion analysis systems has also identified an increased use of knee flexion ROM while landing from a jump (Caulfield & Garrett, 2002) and altered hip biomechanics during the SEBT in those with CAI.(Gribble, Hertel, & Denegar, 2007) Differences have also been seen in stereotypical movement patterns which are now believed to be the result of a constrained sensorimotor system. For example, those with CAI have altered movement patterns during the swing phase of walking gait (Delahunt, Monaghan, & Caulfield, 2006; Monaghan, Dean, & Caulfield, 2006) and throughout the entire running gait cycle.(Drewes et al., 2009) More recently neuromuscular and biomechanical control alterations have been seen during gait initiation (Hass, Bishop, Doidge, & Wikstrom, 2010) and gait termination.(Wikstrom, Bishop, Inamdar, & Hass, 2010a) These most recent investigations clearly demonstrate that the global deficits associated with CAI negatively affect the central nervous system as both gait initiation and termination are mediated via supraspinal motor control mechanisms.(Wang et al., 2009). Cumulatively, these deficits and/or alterations in proximal muscles and joint control as well as stereotypical movement patters indicate global deficits in sensorimotor function. However, the link between local and global impairments in sensorimotor control is poorly understood at this time and this link must be a focus of future investigations if more effective treatments are to be developed.

3.3 Post-traumatic ankle OA

Only recently has there been an impetus to investigate the impairments associated with post-traumatic ankle OA because the diagnosis of ankle OA is becoming more common (Saltzman et al., 2005) and because ankle replacement procedures are anticipated to increase at a rate of about 5% a year.(Jeng, 2006) However, there is a limited amount of information available regarding patient-, clinician-, and laboratory-oriented evidence for those with ankle OA at this time. The vast majority of post-traumatic ankle OA research has been focused on patient-oriented evidence and the results consistently show, regardless of the scale used, that those with post-traumatic ankle OA have greater levels of self-reported disability relative to age matched controls.(Horisberger, Hintermann, & Valderrabano, 2009a; Hubbard, Hicks-Little, & Cordova, 2009b; Khazzam, Long, Marks, & Harris, 2006; Messenger, Anderson, & Wikstrom, 2011; Valderrabano et al., 2007; Valderrabano et al., 2006b) Clinical-oriented evidence shows similar impairments as those associated with acute LAS and CAI. Specifically, decreases in ankle muscle strength and increased mechanical stiffness have been observed relative to age matched controls.(Hubbard et al., 2009b) Laboratory-oriented evidence is also similar to the impairments associated with acute LAS and CAI. For example, static postural control (i.e. plantar pressure distributions and COP displacements) have been reported to be altered and/or increased (Horisberger et al., 2009a; Hubbard et al., 2009b; Messenger et al., 2011) and walking gait velocity, cadence, and stride length are all reduced in those with ankle OA.(Khazzam et al., 2006; Valderrabano et al., 2007) Most recently, Messenger et al.(Messenger et al., 2011) illustrated that post-traumatic ankle OA alters gait initiation relative to uninjured age-matched controls. This evidence further illustrates that the long term sequela of LAS are global in nature and can negatively influence the central nervous system.

4. Finding context

Based on the information provided above from the PCL model, those with acute LAS, CAI, and post-traumatic ankle OA report significant and similar limitations in patient-, clinician-, and laboratory-oriented outcome measures. By examining all 3 sources of evidence, it is clear that an ankle sprain is more than just a peripheral musculoskeletal pathology with only local consequences. Further, examining the interaction of specific deficits on global function will help elucidate the cascade of events that leads to the development of CAI (Figure 1) and more importantly identify effective evidence-based treatment protocols that can address not only the isolated impairments but also the complex interactions among them. By developing context through the PCL model, a more thorough understanding of the consequences of injury and rehabilitation can be gained. What remains needed is a working theoretical construct to link these sources of evidence in a meaningful way. In the next section, we provide the theoretical construct that we believe will allow a more thorough understanding to be obtained.

5. Ankle instability and impaired sensorimotor control

The human body is a system composed of many interacting parts which can be organized in a variety of ways to accomplish movement goals.(Davids & Glazier, 2010) The hallmark of this system is its ability to adapt to changing demands both internally and externally. The sensorimotor control theory that captures the dynamic nature of this system is known as the dynamic systems theory of motor control.(Davids, Glazier, Araujo, & Bartlett, 2003) According to dynamic systems theory, the organization of the sensorimotor system is constrained, or shaped, by the interaction of 1) the health of the person (organismic constraint), 2) the task being performed (task constraint), and 3) the environment in which a movement goal is executed (environmental constraint) (Hoch & McKeon, 2010b; McKeon & Hertel, 2006) (Figure 2). Rather than having preprogrammed pathways to accomplish a movement goal, the dynamic systems theory states that the sensorimotor system is free to develop and change strategies based on its current state as it interacts with the environment.(Davids et al., 2010) For example, an individual will use different gait strategies when walking on a sidewalk compared to walking in soft sand on a beach because the individual is interacting with different environments. In this way, coordination within the sensorimotor system changes based on the constraints related to the movement goal. Because of this freedom of spontaneous (goal-oriented) self-organization, a healthy sensorimotor system can accomplish a movement goal in a variety of ways based on the interaction with the tasks performed and the environmental cues received.(Hoch et al., 2010b) If there are changes in the task or environment, the sensorimotor system can reorganize to adopt a new strategy to achieve the movement goal. More strategies translate to an enhanced ability to successfully accomplish the movement goal and cope with change. This has been referred to as invariant results through variant means, also known as functional variability.(Latash, Scholz, & Schoner, 2002)

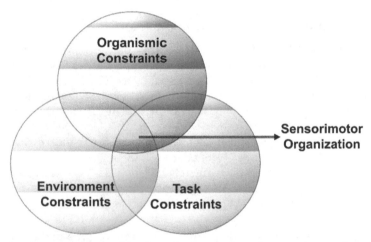

Fig. 2. Sensorimotor organization based on the interaction of constraints as described by the Dynamic Systems Theory

Ankle injury, which introduces organismic constraints, can significantly hinder the sensorimotor system in its ability to accomplish movement goals.(Hoch et al., 2010b) Ankle injuries result in mechanical and functional alterations within a component part of the sensorimotor system.(Hertel, 2002) Consequently, injured parts of the system cannot be used in movement solution development. This then reduces the functional variability of the sensorimotor system — in other words; it is constrained in its ability to cope with change. The result of this decrease in sensorimotor control is a reduction in functional performance. Ankle injury epidemiological evidence supports this framework in that the primary risk factor for an ankle sprain is a previous history of one. (Beynnon, Renstrom, Alosa, Baumhauer, & Vacek, 2001) Based on this information, it is apparent that there is the potential for a continuum of disability associated with CAI (McKeon, 2010) (Figure 3). Poor control may predispose a person to injury and injury significantly constrains sensorimotor control. To gain understanding into this continuum as it relates to CAI, we will discuss management strategies that address different points along the continuum and present recommendations to help improve treatment options that may attenuate the effects of organismic constraints on sensorimotor control.

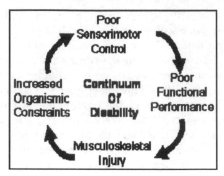

Fig. 3. Continuum of Disability

6. Management strategies through the continuum

Acute LAS management typically involves rest, ice, compression, elevation (RICE) and functional rehabilitation (i.e. early mobilization with support).(Mattacola & Dwyer, 2002) In more severe cases, LAS are treated with crutches and are typically immobilized for a short period of time.(Mattacola et al., 2002) To date, numerous investigations have assessed the efficacy of rehabilitation techniques on short-term patient-oriented outcomes including: pain, ROM, and return to work/activity. However, the high percentage of re-injury occurrence (up to 70%) and development of CAI (up to 75%) (Anandacoomarasamy et al., 2005; Peters et al., 1991; Smith et al., 1986) after an LAS, suggests that further research of both short and long-term outcomes following rehabilitation is needed to investigate not only specific mechanical and/or sensorimotor impairments but the interactions among them by examining patient-, clinician-, and laboratory-oriented evidence.

6.1 Acute care/immobilization – Overcoming the constraints of a damaged joint

Immediately after a LAS the primary goals are to manage pain, control inflammation and protect the joint. In the acute phase of healing, the most important structures to protect are the lateral ligaments of the ankle because the traumatic mechanism has caused increased laxity. In the past, the majority of the literature has focused on functional rehabilitation (i.e. early mobilization with support) but the high recurrence rates of LAS and development of CAI suggest that functional rehabilitation may not allow adequate time for the ligaments of the ankle to heal and stability to be restored. Indeed, increased laxity has been reported using both patient- (ankle giving way, or feelings of instability) and clinician-oriented (manual stress tests, radiographs) outcomes.(Hertel et al., 1999; Hubbard et al., 2007; Lentell et al., 1995; Louwerens et al., 1995)   Unfortunately, ankle laxity often persists despite treatment as positive anterior drawer tests were still present in 3%-31% of subjects 6-months after injury (Cetti et al., 1984; Konradsen et al., 1991) and feelings of instability were present in 7%-42% of subjects up to 1-year after injury.(Brostrom, 1966; Munk et al., 1995) Cumulatively, these studies provide strong evidence that better and longer protection of the ankle joint after an acute LAS is needed to help restore mechanical stability. If mechanical stability is not restored, increased laxity could lead to further mechanical adaptations, deficits in sensorimotor control, recurrent injury and decreases in global function as a maladaptive compensation of the changes in joint laxity and/or sensorimotor control.

To help examine the effects of immobilization, a multi-center prospective randomized control trial was conducted examining three different mechanical supports (Aircast brace, Bledsoe boot, and 10-day below the knee cast) compared with that of a double-layer tubular compression bandage (current standard of care) in promoting recovery after severe LAS.(Lamb, Marsh, Nakash, & Cooke, 2009) A total of 584 patients with LAS were followed over nine months with the primary outcome being the quality of ankle function measured using the Foot and Ankle Score (i.e. a patient-oriented outcome). The below-knee cast caused a more rapid recovery than the tubular compression bandage with clinically important benefits in quality of ankle function at 3-months post injury.(Lamb et al., 2009) Based on the data, a short period of immobilization in a below-knee cast or Aircast ankle brace (2nd best results) may result in faster recovery than the current standard of care. Additionally, the authors recommended the below-knee cast because it showed the widest range of benefit. However, future research is needed to determine if similar benefits will be found in clinical and laboratory measures such as ligament laxity and postural control.

An earlier study (Beynnon, Renstrom, Haugh, Uh, & Barker, 2006) also examined the type of immobilization that had the best outcomes. The authors stratified acute LAS based on the grade (I, II, or III) and randomized patients to undergo functional treatment with different types of ankle immobilization. They compared an elastic wrap (current standard of care), Air-Stirrup ankle brace, Air-Stirrup ankle brace with an elastic wrap and fiberglass walking cast. They reported treatment of grade I and II ankle sprains with Air-Stirrup brace combined with elastic wrap allowed patients return to pre-injury function, as measured by both patient- and clinical-oriented evidence, quicker than the other immobilizers.(Beynnon et al., 2006) For grade III sprains, there were no differences between the Air-Stirrup brace and the fiberglass walking cast. The subjects in the Lamb et al.(Lamb et al., 2009) study were considered to have severe ankle sprains, which may be why the below-knee cast was more favorable.

Based on the research available to best treat acute LAS, some form of immobilization needs to be used to help protect the joint and allow ligament healing to occur. Thus, elastic or tubular wraps are not recommended because research suggests that they do not provide adequate protection to allow restoration of function. An Air-Stirrup brace with elastic wraps for grade I and grade II, and below-knee casts for grade III appear to be the best treatment strategy based on the current literature. After a period of controlled immobilization functional exercises are necessary to rehabilitate the joint and two of the more commonly used adjunctive therapies are discussed below.

6.2 Joint mobilizations

To date manipulative therapy techniques; including Maitland's mobilizations,(Maitland, 1985) Mulligan's mobilizations with movement,(Mulligan, 2004) and High-Velocity Low-Amplitude (HVLA) thrusts,(Bleakley, McDonough, & MacAuley, 2008; van der Wees et al., 2006) have all been postulated to be effective treatments for acute LAS. Indeed, manipulative therapy techniques are theorized to reduce pain (patient-oriented), improve function and increase ROM via the restoration of arthrokinematic motions (i.e. roll, glide, spin) (clinician-oriented),(Maitland, 1985) and improve spatiotemporal postural control in single limb stance (laboratory-oriented); thus recommendations to use these techniques make intuitive sense.

Patient-oriented outcome measures have improved following manipulative therapy. For example, multiple manipulative therapy treatment sessions result in improvements in self-report levels of pain and function.(Coetzer, Brantingham, & Nook, 2001; Green, Refshauge,

Crosbie, & Adams, 2001; Pellow & Brantingham, 2001; Whitman et al., 2009) Further, a single treatment session, involving multiple osteopathic and manipulative techniques, immediately reduced self-reported pain in patients with acute LAS.(Eisenhart, Gaeta, & Yens, 2003) Based on this evidence, it appears that multiple treatment sessions are needed to consistently see improvements in a variety of patient-oriented outcomes, regardless of the specific manipulative therapy technique used, in patients with acute LAS. However, the exact number of treatments and dosage within each treatment session remains unknown.

The available literature also indicates that both active and passive ROM (clinician-oriented evidence) are improved following the delivery of multiple treatment sessions.(Green et al., 2001; Pellow et al., 2001) Additionally, significant improvement in non-weight bearing range of motion (ROM) was reported after the delivery of a variety of manipulative therapy techniques over a 2-week intervention.(Coetzer et al., 2001) Thus, the cumulative data suggest that multiple treatment sessions are needed to see ROM improvements in patients with acute LAS. However, significant improvements in dorsiflexion ROM have been reported after just a single treatment session of Maitland's (AP talocrural) mobilizations in patients who underwent a prolonged period of ankle immobilization for a variety of pathological conditions.(Landrum, Kellen, Parente, Ingersoll, & Hertel, 2009) Thus, it appears that even if acute LAS patients are immobilized (i.e. casted) following injury, ankle joint mobilizations could be used to help restore ROM.

Similarly, a single treatment session consisting of two manipulative therapy techniques lead to an immediate redistribution of foot loading patterns (laboratory-evidence) during static stance relative to a placebo laying of hands procedure in patients with acute grade II LAS.(Lopez-Rodriguez, Fernandez de-las-Penas, Alburquerque-Sendin, Rodriguez-Blanco, & Palomeque-del-Cerro, 2007) There is also evidence to suggest that a single bout of anterior-to-posterior talocrural joint mobilizations (Maitland Grade 3 oscillations) improves ROM measured by the WBLT (clinician-oriented evidence) and spatiotemporal measures of postural control (laboratory-oriented evidence) in those with CAI.(Hoch & McKeon, 2010a; c) By combining these results with the patient-oriented evidence above, there appears to be strong indications that joint mobilization has the potential to be an excellent rehabilitation intervention for those with acute LAS and CAI. However, no investigation has directly compared the effectiveness of different manipulative therapy techniques on any outcome measures in patients with acute LAS or those with CAI. Thus direct comparisons of manipulative therapy techniques should be the focus of future research endeavors.

6.3 Balance exercises

One of the most commonly examined sensorimotor outcome measures following a LAS is single leg postural control and recent systematic reviews have demonstrated that postural control is impaired on both the involved limb (Arnold, De La Motte, Linens, & Ross, 2009; McKeon et al., 2008a; Wikstrom et al., 2010c) and the uninvolved limb (Wikstrom et al., 2010c) relative to an uninjured control group within six weeks of a LAS. The presence of bilateral balance impairments (Wikstrom et al., 2010c) suggest that global impairments as a result of a peripheral injury have occurred. Further, impaired postural control is associated with an increased risk of ankle injury (McGuine, Greene, Best, & Leverson, 2000; McKeon et al., 2008a) and because of this strong association, balance training is a common component of therapeutic intervention programs used by allied health care practitioners to treat acute LAS. Fortunately, balance training is effective at improving postural control scores in subjects with acute LAS (McKeon & Hertel, 2008b; Wikstrom et al., 2009) and at reducing the risk of recurrent LAS.(McKeon et al., 2008b; McKeon & Mattacola, 2008d) The effectiveness of balance training is hypothesized to be due to the modality's ability to restore and/or correct feed-forward and feedback neuromuscular control alterations that have occurred as a result of a LAS. Indeed, neural adaptations occur at multiple sites within the central nervous system as a result of balance training intervention programs.(Beck et al., 2007; Taube et al., 2007) In other words, balance training capitalizes on the incredible plasticity of the central nervous system and enhances a patient's ability to react to both internal and external perturbations.

Balance training programs have been shown to improve self-reported function (patient-oriented), enhance the performance on the SEBT (clinician-oriented), and improve center of pressure and spatiotemporal measures of postural control (laboratory-oriented).(Hale, Hertel, & Olmsted-Kramer, 2007; McKeon et al., 2008c) While balance training improves postural control, the exact treatment dosage needed to cause balance improvements and reduce the risk of recurrent injury remains unknown. However, the generally accepted timeframe for improvements to be observed is 4-6 weeks of balance training.(McKeon et al., 2008b; McKeon et al., 2008d). Bahr et al. (Bahr, Lian, & Bahr, 1997) reported that the longer a balance training program is implemented the greater preventative effects accrue from the program. To date, published balance training investigations primarily use prospective cohort designs where the baseline measures represent postural control prior to the intervention but not pre-injury postural control values. So while the literature indicates that balance training improves postural control, it is not clear if balance training restores postural control to pre-injury balance values.

When designing a balance training program, it is important to consider the dynamic systems theory of motor control (Figure 2). Specifically, this chapter has focused on the organismic constraints as defined by both mechanical adaptations and sensorimotor dysfunction associated with LAS, CAI, and post-traumatic ankle OA. In order to overcome the effects of these constraints on the sensorimotor system, a systematic process of purposefully manipulating task and environmental constraints must be employed.

6.3.1 Cultivating functional variability

In rehabilitation, it becomes imperative that the clinician is very specific when identifying the desired movement goal for the patient.(McKeon, 2009) Rather than focusing on the task to be performed (task-oriented rehabilitation), the functional activities should be associated with the quality of the movement goal execution (goal-oriented rehabilitation). The most important elements for the development of functional variability are to incorporate: 1) a systematic progression through the exercises, 2) a logical manipulation of task and environmental constraints at each level of the progression, 3) specific outcomes that capture improvements and help the clinician determine when patient progression is appropriate, 4) an ability to reduce the outcomes into a decision as to whether the patient has overcome the continuum of disability, and 5) ensure that the process is replicable by documenting the systematic, logical, empirical, and reductive elements.

In order to present the systematic and logical process of program development, we have included examples of a published balance training protocol used for patients with CAI.(McKeon et al., 2008c) Further information associated with this program, including the full description of activities, progressions, outcomes used, and results can be found in the published manuscript.

6.3.2 Task constraints in balance training

Changing the demands of the balance training task results in changes within the component parts of the sensorimotor system to accomplish the movement goal.(McKeon, 2009) The complexity of the task will govern the variability of movement solutions the sensorimotor system can use. An example of this is balancing in single limb stance. In order to accomplish this movement goal (i.e. maintain single limb stance), the sensorimotor system can develop several movement solutions from its many component parts (e.g. ankle muscles, knee muscles, hip muscles, etc.) and is readily afforded the freedom to correct for any errors introduced in executing the movement goal. However, when a person lands from a jump on one leg and attempts to regain balance there are fewer solutions available to accomplish the movement goal, because of the increased task demands (e.g. increased 3-dimensional forces, momentum acting on the body, etc.). As a result, there is an increased likelihood of errors being committed. If an error in postural control is introduced during physical activity and/or athletic event, it can potentially have severe consequences, such as an ankle injury. As stated above, an ankle injury would result in increased organismic constraints and subsequently increase the likelihood of errors in the future, starting a vicious cycle. However, the introduction of errors in a controlled training environment gives the sensorimotor system time to develop either 1) more/new movement solutions or 2) enhance the efficacy of existing movement solutions so that the likelihood of committing errors and the consequences of those errors can be diminished over time.

6.3.3 Purposeful manipulation of task constraints

When progressing an individual through a balance training program, it becomes essential for the movement goals to be meaningful to the individual.(McKeon, 2009) Balance training has been shown to be beneficial at improving functional outcomes associated with CAI.(Holmes & Delahunt, 2009; McKeon et al., 2008b; McKeon et al., 2008d) From the dynamic systems perspective, the most important consideration in functional rehabilitation program development is the clarity of the movement goal.(McKeon, 2009) The task constraints then can be structured to challenge the sensorimotor system as it spontaneously organizes (i.e. develops new solutions) to accomplish the movement goal.

An example of the strategic manipulation of task constraints in the referenced balance training program is the "Hop to Stabilization" activity compared to the "Hop to Stabilization and Reach" activity (McKeon et al., 2008c). For both activities, the movement goal was to regain single limb stance as fast and effectively as possible after landing from a hop. In the first activity, subjects performed single limb hops to a target, stabilized single limb stance, and then hopped back to their starting position. In the "Hop to Stabilization and Reach" activity, subjects hopped to the target, stabilized, and reached back to the starting position with their opposite leg. Although the movement goal was the same, the tasks resulted in the development of different solutions for goal achievement. In order to keep patients on the cusp of failure (i.e. continuously challenge the sensorimotor system), the task constraints were increased when each patient could perform 10 error-free repetitions in the current task constraints. An important note is that each patient in the program progressed to higher levels based on their ability to execute the movement goals. This was done by increasing the distance of the hop target. To add additional task constraints for each activity, the patients hopped in eight different directions. Each direction presented unique task constraints that challenged the sensorimotor system to develop movement solutions to accomplish the movement goal and ultimately make the patient more adaptable to unexpected perturbations (e.g. a mid-air collision with another player) that occur during athletic events.

6.3.4 Environmental constraints in rehabilitation

Environmental constraints (or cues) are essential components for the organization of the sensorimotor system.(McKeon, 2009) Rather than viewing the environment as such things as grass versus sidewalk, the cues from the environment should be considered for the predictability they offer to the sensorimotor system.(McKeon, 2009) More predictable environmental cues allow for greater freedom for the development of strategies to accomplish movement goals. Less predictable environment cues constrain the sensorimotor system's ability to develop movement goal strategies. An example of this is performing sport-specific activities in a rehabilitation environment compared to sport-specific activities during actual participation in athletic events. In the rehabilitation environment, environmental cues are based on the room, the performance of the activities, and the interaction with the therapist, and are much more predictable compared to real life performance. Once the patient returns to participation in athletics, the interaction with the playing surface, teammates, and opponents provide significantly more unpredictable environmental cues. This is one of the reasons that an athlete might pass a functional screen performed by a health care provider, but still struggle upon their return to actual competition.

With increased exposure to task and environmental constraints, the sensorimotor system can develop new strategies to accomplish movement goals and cope with change over time. Therefore, to maximize the efficacy of the sensorimotor system in those with ankle inversion trauma, it is essential to adjust the environmental and task constraints to keep the patient on the cusp of failure (i.e. continually manipulate the constraints so that patients have to provide near maximum physical and psychological effort to complete the assigned activities) throughout the rehabilitation program. When challenged in this way, the sensorimotor system develops greater flexibility in achieving its motor goals, and this translates into better outcomes of the movement goal and potentially a decreased risk of injury.(McKeon, 2009; McKeon et al., 2008c)

6.3.5 Purposeful manipulation of environmental constraints

The environmental constraints used in balance training should also be associated with specific movement goals.(McKeon, 2009) Initially, a predictable environment allows the sensorimotor system the freedom to explore a variety of strategies to accomplish a specified movement goal. The more unpredictable the environment becomes, the less free the sensorimotor system becomes to explore strategies. Consequently, a valuable balance training activity has a systematic progression from hopping to a predictable target, as described above, to an unpredictable one. In the example above of the hopping activities, patients started by hopping to a predictable target. The environmental constraints were then manipulated by having the subjects perform the same types of hops in an unpredictable environment in the "Unanticipated Hop to Stabilization" activity. In the Unanticipated Hop to Stabilization, patients were presented with a random sequence of numbers on a grid set up like a large phone pad that represented the order of targets to which they would hop and stabilize in single limb stance. For each number sequence, the subjects had a specified amount of time to get the next target before the next number in the sequence was shown to them and the sequence changed each time they performed this activity. As performance improved and subjects began to make their target times, the environmental constraints were increased by decreasing the amount of time allotted to complete the task. From the dynamic systems perspective, this change in the number sequence is a form of environmental constraint. The cues subjects received from the environment (the number in the hopping sequence) shaped the strategies that the sensorimotor system needed to use to accomplish the movement goal. The reduction in time challenged the sensorimotor system to adapt to the unpredictable environment in which the movement goal was being executed.

It is important to note that with the systematic and logical progression, each patient progresses through the balance training program at their own rate based on their individual ability to accomplish the movement goal in each activity. Upon completion of the program, patients reported significant improvements in their ability to engage other task and environmental constraints in activities such as running, cutting, and participating in their desired activities.(McKeon et al., 2008c) The goal of balance training and functional rehabilitation from the dynamic systems perspective is to restore the sensorimotor system's ability to cope with change during the execution of movement goals, thus improving sensorimotor control and functional performance. Once a movement/rehabilitation goal can be accomplished without error, the constraints can again be systematically increased. Purposeful and logical manipulation of task and environmental constraints include the logical progression from single limb balance activities to more functional activities such as hopping, landing, rapidly changing direction, etc. In order to accomplish more advanced movement goals effectively, more degrees of freedom (i.e. using more joints, muscles, etc.) are necessary to correct for errors introduced during goal execution. By freeing more degrees of freedom to correct errors, the Continuum of Disability (Figure 3) can be broken. The clinician can utilize the principles of the purposeful manipulation of task and environmental constraints to guide the progression of rehabilitation. By doing so, it is possible to tailor a program to a patient's ability to achieve movement goals and restore sensorimotor system freedom.

Lastly, it is imperative to utilize outcome tools that have been shown to capture patient-oriented, clinician-oriented, and laboratory-oriented aspects of changes within the sensorimotor system. In the study referenced in this section, (McKeon et al., 2008c) those in the balance training group experienced significant improvements in self-reported function (patient-oriented evidence), dynamic postural control as assessed through the SEBT (clinician-oriented evidence), and spatiotemporal postural control (laboratory-oriented evidence). By assessing self-reported function through the FADI or FAAM, dynamic balance through the BESS or SEBT, and potentially instrumented measures of postural control and/or gait when available, it is possible to determine if a rehabilitation program has an impact on taking a patient out of the Continuum of Disability.

7. Summary

When evaluating patients with ankle inversion trauma and/or instability, clinicians should consider the Continuum of Disability rather than simply local instability. Buchanan et al.

(Buchanan, Docherty, & Schrader, 2008) has provided the best example of why the PCL model is more appropriate than the examination of deficits in isolation to date. The authors had individuals with CAI and healthy controls complete clinical measures of functional performance (i.e. hop tasks) and asked the subjects if their ankle "felt" unstable during the tasks. The initial results indicated no group differences in performance but a secondary analysis compared those with CAI that "felt" unstable to those with CAI that "felt" stable and healthy controls. This secondary analysis, that combined patient- and clinical-oriented outcomes, revealed that the CAI subjects who "felt" unstable during the tasks had performance deficits relative to the other groups. This investigation demonstrates how the combination of a patient- and clinician-oriented outcomes are more revealing than either outcome in isolation. We recommend using the constraints-led approach to guide decisions about comprehensive sensorimotor system evaluation, the development of rehabilitation progressions, and safe return to participation. Most importantly, as presented throughout this chapter, an ankle sprain is not simply a local joint injury; it results in a constrained sensorimotor system that leads to a continuum of disability and life-long consequences such as high injury recurrence and decreased quality of life.

8. References

Admirall, WM, van Valkengoed, IG, L de Munter, JS, Stronks, K, Hoekstra, JB, Holleman, F. The association of physical inactivity with type_2 diabetes among different ethnic groups. Diabet Med 2011; 28(6): 668-672.

Aiken, AB, Pelland, L, Brison, R, Pickett, W, Brouwer, B. Short-term natural recovery of ankle sprains following discharge from emergency departments. J Orthop Sports Phys Ther 2008; 38(9): 566-571.

Anandacoomarasamy, A, Barnsley, L. Long term outcomes of inversion ankle injuries. Br J Sports Med 2005; 39(3): 1-4.

Arnold, BL, De La Motte, S, Linens, S, Ross, SE. Ankle instability is associated with balance impairments: a meta-analysis. Med Sci Sports Exerc 2009; 41(5): 1048-62.

Avci, S, Sayh, U. Comparison of the results of short-term rigid and semi-rigid cast immobilization for the treatment of grade 3 inversion injuries of the ankle. Injury 1998; 29: 581-584.

Bahr, R, Lian, O, Bahr, IA. A twofold reduction in the incidence of acute ankle sprains in volleyball after the introduction of an injury prevention program: a prospective cohort study. Scand J Med Sci Sports 1997; 7(3): 172-7.

Baumhauer, J, Alosa, D, Renstrom, A, Trevino, S, Beynnon, B. A prospective study of ankle injury risk factors. Am J Sports Med 1995; 23(5): 564-570.

Beck, S, Taube, W, Gruber, M, Amtage, F, Gollhofer, A, Schubert, M. Task-specific changes in motor evoked potentials of lower limb muscles after different training interventions. Brain Res 2007; 1179: 51-60.

Beckman, SM, Buchanan, TS. Ankle inversion injury and hypermobility: effect on hip and ankle muscle electromyography onset latency. Arch Phys Med Rehabil 1995; 76(12): 1138-1143.

Beynnon, BD, Renstrom, PA, Alosa, DM, Baumhauer, JF, Vacek, PM. Ankle ligament injury risk factors: a prospective study of college athletes. J Orthop Res 2001; 19(2): 213-20.

Beynnon, BD, Renstrom, PA, Haugh, L, Uh, BS, Barker, H. A prospective, randomized clinical investigation of the treatment of first-time ankle sprains. Am J Sports Med 2006; 34(9): 1401-1412.

Bleakley, CM, McDonough, M, MacAuley, DC. Some conservative strategies are effective when added to controlled mobilization with external support after acute ankle sprain: a systematic review. Aust J Physiother 2008; 54: 7-20.

Brostrom, L. Sprained ankles: I, anatomic lesions on recent sprains. Acta Chir Scand 1964; 128: 483-495.

Brostrom, L. Spraiuned ankles V: Treatment and prognosis in recent ligament ruptures. Acta Chir Scand 1966; 132: 537-550.

Buchanan, AS, Docherty, CL, Schrader, J. Functional performance testing in participants with functional ankle instability and in a healthy control group. J Athl Train 2008; 43(4): 342-346.

Bullock-Saxton, JE, janda, V, Bullock, MI. The influence of ankle sprain injury on muscle activation during hip extension. Int J Sports Med 1994; 15: 330-334.

Caulfield, BM, Garrett, M. Functional instability of the ankle: differences in patterns of ankle and knee movement prior to and post landing in a single leg jump. Int J Sports Med 2002; 23(1): 64-8.

CDC. National Center for Injury Prevention and Control. CDC Injury Research Agenda, 2009-2018., Atlanta, GA: US Department of Health and Human Services, Centers for Disease Control and Prevention, 2009.

Cetti, R, Christensen, SE, Corfitzen, MT. Ruptured fibular ankle ligmanet plaster or pliton brace? Br J Sport Med 1984; 18: 104-109.

Coetzer, D, Brantingham, JW, Nook, B. The relative effectiveness of piroxicam compared to manipulation in the treatment of acute grades 1 and 2 inversion ankle sprains. J Neruomusculoskelet Syst 2001; 9: 1-12.

Crosbie, J, Green, T, Refshauge, K. Effects of reduced ankle dorsiflexion following lateral ligament sprain on temporal and spatial gait parameters. Gait Posture 1999; 9: 167-172.

Davids, K, Glazier, P. Deconstructing neurobiological coordination: the role of the biomechanics-motor control nexus. Exerc Sport Sci Rev 2010; 38(2): 86-90.

Davids, K, Glazier, P, Araujo, D, Bartlett, R. Movement systems as dynamical systems: the functional role of variability and its implications for sports medicine. Sports Med 2003; 33(4): 245-60.

de Vries, JS, Kingma, I, Blakevoort, L, van Dijk, CN. Difference in balance measures between patients with chronic ankle instability and patients after an acute ankle inversion trauma. Knee Surg Sports Traumatol Arthrosc 2010; 18(5): 601-606.

Delahunt, E, Monaghan, K, Caulfield, B. Altered neuromuscular control and ankle joint kinematics during walking in subjects with functional ankle instability of the ankle joint. Am J Sports Med 2006; 34(12): 1070-1976.

Denegar, CR, Hertel, J, Fonseca, J. The effect of lateral ankle sprain on dorsiflexion range of motion, posterior talar glide, and joint laxity. J Orthop Sports Phys Ther 2002; 32(4): 166-173.

Docherty, CL, McLeod, TCV, Shultz, SJ. Postural Control Deficits in Participants with Functional Ankle Instability as Measured by the Balance Error Scoring System. Clinical Journal of Sports Medicine 2006; 16: 203-208.

Drewes, LK, McKeon, PO, Kerrigan, DC, Hertel, J. Dorsiflexion deficit during jogging whith chronic ankle instability. J Sci Med Sport 2009; 12(6): 685-687.

Eechaute, C, Vaes, P, Van Aerschot, L, Asman, S, Duquet, W. The clinimetric qualities of patient-assessed instruments for measuring chronic ankle instability: a systematic review. BMC Musculoskelet Disord 2007; 8: 6.

Eisenhart, AW, Gaeta, TJ, Yens, DP. Osteopathic manipulative treatment in the emergency department for patients with acute ankle injuries. Journal of the American Osteopathic Association 2003; 103(9): 417-421.

Evans, T, Hertel, J, Sebastianelli, W. Bilateral deficits in postural control following lateral ankle sprain. Foot Ankle Int 2004; 25(11): 833-839.

Fernandez, WG, Yard, EE, Comstock, RD. Epidemiology of lower extremity injuries among U.S. high school athletes. Acad Emerg Med 2007; 14(7): 641-5.

Freeman, MA. Instability of the foot after injuries to the lateral ligament of the ankle. J Bone Joint Surg Br 1965a; 47(4): 669-677.

Freeman, MA. Treatment of ruptures of the lateral ligament of the ankle. J Bone Joint Surg 1965b; 47B: 661-668.

Green, T, Refshauge, K, Crosbie, J, Adams, R. A randomized controlled trial of a passive accessory joint mobilization on acute ankle inversion sprains. Phys Ther 2001; 81: 984-994.

Gribble, PA, Hertel, J, Denegar, CR. Chronic ankle instability and fatigue create proximal joint alterations during performance of the star excursion balance test. Int J Sports Med 2007; 28(3): 236-242.

Hale, SA, Hertel, J. Reliability and Sensitivity of the Foot and Ankle Disability Index in Subjects With Chronic Ankle Instability. J Athl Train 2005; 40(1): 35-40.

Hale, SA, Hertel, J, Olmsted-Kramer, LC. The effect of a 4-week comprehensive rehabilitation program on postural control and lower extremity function in individuals with chronic ankle instability. J Orthop Sports Phys Ther 2007; 37(6): 303-11.

Hass, CJ, Bishop, M, Doidge, D, Wikstrom, EA. Chronic ankle instability alters central organization of movement. Am J Sports Med 2010; 38(4): 829-834.

Hertel, J. Functional anatomy, pathomechanics, and pathophysiology of lateral ankle instability. J Athl Train 2002; 37(4): 364-375.

Hertel, J. Sensorimotor deficits with ankle sprains and chronic ankle instability. Clin Sports Med 2008; 27(3): 353-70, vii.

Hertel, J, Braham, RA, Hale, SA, Olmsted-Kramer, LC. Simplifying the star excursion balance test: analyses of subjects with and without chronic ankle instability. J Orthop Sports Phys Ther 2006; 36(3): 131-7.

Hertel, J, Denegar, CR, Monroe, MM, Stokes, WL. Talocural and subtalar joint instability after lateral ankle sprain. Med Sci Sports Exer 1999; 31(11): 1501-1508.

Hirose, K, Murakami, G, Minowa, T, Kura, H, Yamashita, T. Lateral ligament injury of the ankle and associated articular cartilage degeneration in the talocrural joint: anatomic study using elderly cadavers. J Orthop Sci 2004; 9(1): 37-43.

Hoch, MC, McKeon, PO. The effectiveness of mobilization with movement at improving dorsiflexion after ankle sprain. J Sport Rehabil 2010a; 19(2): 226-32.

Hoch, MC, McKeon, PO. Integrating contemporary models of motor control and health in chronic ankle instability. Athletic Training and Sports Health Care 2010b; 2(2): 82-88.

Hoch, MC, McKeon, PO. Joint mobilization improves spatiotemporal postural control and range of motion in those with chronic ankle instability. J Orthop Res 2010c; 29(3): 326-32.

Hoch, MC, McKeon, PO. Normative range of weight-bearing lunge test performance asymmetry in healthy adults. Man Ther 2011; 1-4,doi:10.1016/j.math.2011.02.012

Holme, E, Magnusson, SP, Becher, K, Bieler, T, Aargaar, P, Kjar, M. The effect of supervised rehabilitation on strength, postural sway, position sense and reinjury risk after acute ankle ligament sprain. Scand J Med Sci Sports 1999; 9(2): 104-109.

Holmes, A, Delahunt, E. Treatment of common deficits associated with chronic ankle instability. Sports Med 2009; 39(3): 207-24.

Hootman, JM, Dick, R, Agel, J. Epidemiology of collegiate injuries for 15 sports: summary and recommendations for injury prevention initiatives. J Athl Train 2007; 42(2): 311-9.

Horisberger, M, Hintermann, B, Valderrabano, V. Alterations of plantar pressure distribution in posttraumatic end-stage ankle osteoarthritis. Clin Biomech 2009a; 24(3): 303-307.

Horisberger, M, Valderrabano, V, Hintermann, B. Posttraumatic ankle osteoarthritis after ankle-related fractures. J Orthop Trauma 2009b; 23(1): 60-67.

Hubbard, TJ, Cordova, ML. Mechanical instability after an acute lateral ankle sprain. Arch Phys Med Rehabil 2009a; 90(7): 1142-1146.

Hubbard, TJ, Hertel, J. Mechanical contributions to chronic lateral ankle instability. Sports Med 2006a; 36(3): 263-277.

Hubbard, TJ, Hertel, J. Anterior positional fault of the fibula after sub-acute lateral ankle sprains. Man Ther 2008; 13(1): 63-67.

Hubbard, TJ, Hertel, J, Sherbondy, P. Fibular position in those with self-reported chronic ankle instability. J Orthop Sports Phys Ther 2006b; 36(1): 3-9.

Hubbard, TJ, Hicks-Little, CA, Cordova, ML. Mechanical and sensorimotor implications with ankle osteoarthritis. Arch Phys Med Rehabil 2009b; 90: 1136-1141.

Hubbard, TJ, Kramer, LC, Denegar, CR, Hertel, J. Contributing factors to chronic ankle instability. Foot Ankle Int 2007; 28(3): 343-354.

Jeng, C. One step ahead. Advance for Directors in Rehabilitation 2006; 15: 49-52.

Kannus, P, Renstrom, PA. Treatment for acute tears of the lateral ligaments of the ankle. J Bone Joint Surg Am 1991; 73: 305-312.

Khazzam, M, Long, JT, Marks, RM, Harris, GF. Preoperative gait characterization of patients with ankle arthrosis. Gait Posture 2006; 24: 85-93.

Konradsen, L, Holmer, P, Sondergaard, L. Early mobilizing treatment for grade III ankle ligmanet injuries. Foot Ankle 1991; 12: 660-668.

Konradsen, L, Magnusson, P. Increased inversion angle replication error in functional ankle instability. Knee Surg Sports Traumatol Arthrosc 2000; 8: 246-251.

Konradsen, L, Olesen, S, Hansen, H. Ankle sensorimotor control and eversion strength after acute ankle inversion injuries. Am J Sports Med 1998; 26: 72-77.

Koplan, JP, Powell, KE, Sikes, RK, Campbell, CC. An epidemiologic study of the benefits and risks of running. JAMA 1982; 248: 3118-31212.

Koralewicz, LM, Engh, GA. Comparison of proprioception in arthritic and age-matched normal knees. J Bone Joint Surg Am 2000; 82-A(11): 1582-8.

Lamb, SE, Marsh, JL, Nakash, R, Cooke, MW. Mechanical supports for acute, severe ankle sprain: a pragmatic, multicentre, randomised controlled trial. Lancet 2009; 373: 575-581.

Landrum, EL, Kellen, BM, Parente, WR, Ingersoll, CD, Hertel, J. Immediate effects of anterio-to-posterior talocrural joint mobilization after prolonged ankle immobilization. J Man Manip Ther 2009; 16(2): 100-105.

Latash, ML, Scholz, JP, Schoner, G. Motor Control Strategies Revealed in the Structure of Motor Variability. Exercise & Sport Sciences Reviews 2002; 30: 26-31.

Lentell, G, Baas, B, Lopez, D, McGuire, L, Sarrels, M, Snyder, P. The contributions of proprioceptive deficits, muscle function, and anatomic laxity to functional instability of the ankle. J Orthop Sports Phys Ther 1995; 21(4): 206-15.

Liu, H, Paige, NM, Goldzweig, CL, Wong, E, Zhou, A, Suttorp, MJ, Munjas, B, Orwoll, W, Shekelle, PG. Screening for osteoporosis in men: a systematic review for an American College of Physicians guideline. Ann Intern Med 2008; 148(9): 685-701.

Lopez-Rodriguez, S, Fernandez de-las-Penas, C, Alburquerque-Sendin, F, Rodriguez-Blanco, C, Palomeque-del-Cerro, L. Immediate effects of manipulation of the talocrural joint on stabilometry and baropodometry in patients with ankle sprain. J Manipulative Physiol Ther 2007; 30: 186-192.

Louwerens, JWK, Ginai, AZ, Van Linge, B, Snijders, CJ. Stress radiography of the talocrural and subtalar joints. Foot Ankle 1995; 16: 148-155.

Maitland, GD. Passive movement techniques of intra-articular and periarticular disorders. Aust J Physiother 1985; 31(1): 3-8.

Mattacola, CG, Dwyer, MK. Rehabilitation of the ankle afteracute sprain or chronic instability. J Athl Train 2002; 37(4): 413-429.

McGuine, TA, Greene, JJ, Best, T, Leverson, G. Balance as a predictor of ankle injuries in high school basketball players. Clin J Sport Med 2000; 10(4): 239-44.

McKay, GD. Ankle injuries in basketball: injury rate and risk factors. Br J Sports Med 2001; 35: 103-108.

McKeon, PO. First Words: Cultivating Functional Variability: The Dynamical Systems Approach to Rehabilitation. Athletic Therapy Today 2009; 14(4): 1-3.

McKeon PO, Medina McKeon JM, Mattacola CG, Lattermann C. Finding Context: A New Model for Interpreting Clinical Evidence. International Journal of Athletic Therapy and Training. 2011;16(5):10-13.

McKeon, PO. A new twist on ankle sprains: Sensorimotor rehab keeps a local injury from developing into a cascade of disability. Advance for Physical Therapy and Rehabilitation 2010; 21(13): 29-32.

McKeon, PO, Booi, MJ, Branam, B, Johnson, DL, Mattacola, CG. Lateral ankle ligament anesthesia significantly alters single limb postural control. Gait Posture 2010; 32(3): 374-7.

McKeon, PO, Hertel, J. The dynamical-systems approach to studying athletic injury. Athletic Therapy Today 2006; 11(1): 31-33.

McKeon, PO, Hertel, J. Systematic Review of postural control and lateral ankle instability, Part 1: can deficits be detected with instrumented testing? J Athl Train 2008a; 43(3): 293-304.

McKeon, PO, Hertel, J. Systematic review of postural control and lateral ankle instability, part II: is balance training clinically effective? J Athl Train 2008b; 43(3): 305-15.

McKeon, PO, Ingersoll, CD, Kerrigan, DC, Saliba, E, Bennett, BC, Hertel, J. Balance training improves function and postural control in those with chronic ankle instability. Med Sci Sports Exerc 2008c; 40(10): 1810-9.

McKeon, PO, Mattacola, CG. Interventions for the prevention of first time and recurrent ankle sprains. Clin Sports Med 2008d; 27(3): 371-82, viii.

Messenger, RD, Anderson, RB, Wikstrom, EA. Post-traumatic ankle osteoarthritis alters the central organization of movement. Med Sci Sports Exer 2011; 43(5): S-641.

Meyer, JM, Garcia, J, Hoffmeyer, P, Fritschy, D. The subtalar sprain: a roentgenographic study. Clin Orthop 1986; 226: 169-173.

Mokdad, AH, Marks, JS, Stroup, DF, Gerberding, JL. Actual causes of death in the United States. JAMA 2004; 291: 1238-1245.

Monaghan, K, Dean, E, Caulfield, B. Altered neuromuscular control and ankle joint kinematics during walking in subjects with functional ankle instability of the ankle joint. Clin Biomech 2006; 21: 168-174.

Mulligan, BR. Manual Therapy: "Nags", "Snags", "MWMS" etc, 5th ed. Wellington, NZ: APN Print Limited, 2004; 87-116

Munk, B, Holm-Christensen, K, Lind, T. Long-term outcome after ruptured lateral ankle ligaments. Acta Orthop Scand 1995; 66: 452-454.

Myers, JB, Riemann, BL, Hwang, JH, Fu, FH, Lephart, SM. Effect of peripheral afferent alteration of the lateral ankle ligaments on dynamic stability. Am J Sports Med 2003; 31(4): 498-506.

Olmsted, LC, Carcia, CR, Hertel, J, Shultz, SJ. Efficacy of the star excursion in balance tests in detecting reach deficits in subjects with chronic ankle instability. Journal of Athletic Training 2002: 37(4): 501-506.

Pate, RR, Pratt, M, Blair, SN, al., e. Physical activity and public health: a recommendation from the Centers for Disease Control and Prevention and the American College of Sports Medicine. JAMA 1995; 273: 402-407.

Pellow, JE, Brantingham, JW. The efficacy of adjusting the ankle in the treatment of subacute and chronic grade I and grade II ankle inversion sprains. J Manipulative Physiol Ther 2001; 24(1): 17-24.

Peters, JW, Trevino, SG, Renstrom, PA. Chronic lateral ankle instability. Foot Ankle 1991; 12(3): 182-91.

Saltzman, CL, Salamon, ML, Blanchard, GM, Huff, T, Hayes, A, Buckwalter, JA, Amendola, A. Epidemiology of ankle arthritis: report of a consecutive series of 639 patients from a tertiary orthopaedic center. Iowa Orthop J 2005; 25: 44-46.

Sedory, EJ, McVey, ED, Cross, KM, Ingersoll, CD, Hertel, J. Arthrogenic muscle response of the quadriceps and hamstrings with chronic ankle instability. J Athl Train 2007; 42(3): 355-360.

Sesso, HD, Paffenbarger, RS, Lee, IM. Physical activity and coronary heart disease in men - the harvard alumni health study. Circulation 2000; 102: 975-980.

Smith, RW, Reischl, SF. Treatment of ankle sprains in young athletes. Am J Sports Med 1986; 14(6): 465-71.

Soboroff, SH, Pappius, EM, Komaroff, AL. Benefits, risks, and costs of alternative approaches to the evaluation and treatment of severe ankle sprain. Clin Orthop Relat Res 1984; (183): 160-8.

Steanovv, TS, Vekova, AM, Kurktschiev, DP, Temelkova-Kurktschiev, TS. Relationship of physical activity and eating behaviour with obesity and type 2 diabetes mellitus: sofia lifestyle (SLS) study. Foloa Med (Plovidiv) 2011; 53(1): 11-18.

Taube, W, Gruber, M, Beck, S, Faist, M, Gollhofer, A, Schubert, M. Cortical and spinal adaptations induced by balance training: correlation between stance stability and corticospinal activation. Acta Physiol (Oxf) 2007; 189(347-358).

Troiano, RP, Berrigan, D, Dodd, KW, Masse, LC, Tilert, T, McDowell, M. Physical activity in the United States measured by accelerometer. Med Sci Sports Exer 2008; 40: 181-188.

Tropp, H, Odenrick, P, Gillquist, J. Stabilometry recordings in functional and mechanical instability of the ankle joint. Int J Sports Med 1985; 6(3): 180-182.

Valderrabano, V, Hintermann, B, Horisberger, M, Fung, TS. Ligamentous posttraumatic ankle osteoarthritis. Am J Sports Med 2006a; 34(4): 612-620.

Valderrabano, V, Nigg, BM, von Tscharner, V, Stefanyshyn, DJ, Goepfert, B, Hintermann, B. Gait analysis in ankle osteoarthritis and total ankle replacement. Clin Biomech 2007; 22: 894-904.

Valderrabano, V, von Tscharner, V, Nigg, BM, Hintermann, B, Goepfert, B, Fung, TS, Frank, CB, Herzog, W. Lower leg muscle atrophy in ankle osteoarthritis. J Orthop Res 2006b; 24: 2159-2169.

van der Wees, PJ, Lenssen , AF, Hendriks, EJM, Stomp, DJ, Dekker, J, de bie, RA. Effectiveness of exercise therapy and manual mobilization in acute ankle sprain and functional instability: a systematic review. Aust J Physiother 2006; 52: 27-37.

Verhagen, RA, de Keizer, G, Van Dijk, CN. Long-term follow-up of inversion trauma of the ankle. Arch Orthop Trauma Surg 1995; 114: 92-96.

Wang, J, Wai, Y, Weng, Y, Ng, K, Huang, YZ, Liu, H, Wang, C. Functional MRI in the assessment of cortical activation during gait-related imaginary tasks. J Neural ransm 2009; 116(9): 1087-92.

Weiderpass, E. Lifestyle and cancer risk. J Prev Med Public Health 2010; 43(6): 459-471.

Whitman, JM, Cleland, JA, Mintken, P, Keirns, M, Bienek, ML, Albin, SR, Magel, J, McPoil, TG. Predicting short-term response to thrust and nonthrust manipulation and exercise in patients post inversion ankle sprain. J Orthop Sports Phys Ther 2009; 39(3): 188-200.

Wikstrom, EA, Bishop, M, Inamdar, AD, Hass, CJ. Gait termination control strategies are altered in chronic ankle instability subjects. Med Sci Sports Exer 2010a; 42(1): 197-205.

Wikstrom, EA, Hubbard, TJ. Talar positional fault in person with chronic ankle instability. Arch Phys Med Rehabil 2010b; 91(8): 1267-1271.

Wikstrom, EA, Naik, S, Lodha, N, Cauraugh, JH. Balance capabilities after lateral ankle trauma and intervention: a meta-analysis. Med Sci Sports Exerc 2009; 39(6): 1287-1295.

Wikstrom, EA, Naik, S, Lodha, N, Cauraugh, JH. Bilateral balance impairments after lateral ankle trauma: a systematic review and meta-analysis. Gait Posture 2010c; 32(2): 82-86.

Wilkerson, GB, Nitz, AJ. Dynamic ankle stability: mechanical and neuromuscular interrelationships. J Sport Rehab 1994; 3: 43-57.

Youdas, JW, McLean, TJ, Krause, DA, Hollman, JH. Changes in active ankle dorsiflexion range of motion after acute inversion ankle sprain. J Sport Rehab 2009; 18: 358-374.

10

Proprioception and the Rugby Shoulder

Ian Horsley

Regional Lead Physiotherapist, English Institute of Sport
Manchester
UK

1. Introduction

Rugby union is an international sport played by two teams of 15 players (8 forwards and 7 backs) over two 40 minute halves. It is ranked internationally, as a football code, second to soccer, and is the most popular world wide team contact sport involving collision (IRB, 2004). Professional rugby league is a contact sport involving two teams of 13 players (6 forwards and 7 backs), also played over two 40 minute halves. Each tem has a set of six tackles to advance the ball downfield (Gissane *et al.*, 2003).

Little is known about the level and pattern of injuries occurring since rugby union became a professional sport, and the number of prospective studies among elite players is small (Brooks, *et al.*, 2005). Prior to Brooks et al., (2005), there have been several prospective cohort epidemiological studies of injuries sustained in professional Rugby Union (Bathgate, *et al.*, 2002; Garraway, *et al.*, 2000. Targett, 1998).

The mean incidence of injuries recorded from three studies within professional rugby union is 86.4 injuries per 1000 player hours (Holtzhausen, 2001). Pooled data analysis of injury incidence in rugby league, found an overall injury rate of 40.3 injuries per 1000 player hours (Gissane *et al.*, 2002).

Brooks et al., (2005) conducted the England Rugby Injury and Training Audit, which included all 12 Premiership rugby union teams, and England, England 'A', Under 21 and England 7's teams, during the 2002-2003 and 2003-2004 seasons. They used the operation definition which had been used previously by one of the authors in research into injuries in professional football; "any injury which prevented a player from taking a full part in all training activities typically planned for that day and match play for a period equal to or greater than 24 hours, from midnight of the day the injury was sustained" (Hawkins, and Fuller, 1999).

Detailed analysis of this audit, with respect to shoulder injuries, reports that the average number of tackles carried out during a Premiership match is 250, and that 65% of all shoulder injuries occurring during a match are to the shoulder. During the 2005-2006 season the number of days lost to training or playing due to reported shoulder dislocation or instability was 176 days per 1000 hours play (Heady et al., unpublished). Thus the tackle appears to be the phase of play associated with the greatest risk of injury overall. (Brooks et al., 2005; Bird et al.,1998; Garraway and Macleod ,1995; yet there appears to be scant published research regarding the affect on shoulder joint position sense within rugby players, in general, and the effect that tackling has on it.

Stability within the glenohumeral joint is maintained via anatomical factors such as the degree of bony congruity, integrity of the capsuloligamentous structures and neuromuscular feedback loops involving the joint and musculotendinous mechanoreceptors that are integrated within the central nervous system (Suprak, Osternig, van-Donkelaar, & Karduna, 2006).

Despite this highly integrated passive and active control system the glenohumeral joint is regarded as one of the least stable joints within the body.

The passive ligamentous and capsular structures are often exposed to deleterious loads due to the failure of the active muscular control systems of the glenohumeral joint. This failure of active muscular control system reported in the literature has in part at least been blamed on a failure of proprioception (Janwantanakul, Magarey, Jones, & Danise, 2001).

The term "proprioception" was introduced by Sherrington in 1906 who described it as a type of feedback loop from the limbs to the central nervous system; afferent information arising from peripheral areas of the body contribute to joint stability, postural control and motor recruitment patterns. It has more recently been described as a combination of joint position sense (JPS, the ability of a person to identify the position of a limb in space) and kinaesthesia (the perception of active and passive motion) (Aydin, Yildiz, & Yanmis, 2001).

The awareness of the position of the joint (JPS) is obviously an important aspect of proprioception. An intact JPS has been shown to be necessary for normal muscle coordination and timing, and this has been shown to be especially evident where active muscle forces play a significant role, as in glenohumeral joint stability Blasier, Carpenter, & Huston, 1994; Cain, Mutschler, Fu, & Lee, 1987). JPS contributes to the maintenance of muscle stiffness and coordination about t a joint to produce smooth limb movements, and has been found to be affected by ligamentous trauma, surgical intervention, and rehabilitation programmes (Lephart, Warner, Borsa, & Fu, 1994) Muscle fatigue, trauma and hyper laxity can be responsible for damage to the mechanoreceptors (deafferentation), which can reduce the afferent supply so that the central nervous system receives inaccurate information, and hence, responds with inaccurate output responses.

In the current literature it is generally agreed that tension in muscles, capsuloligamentous structures, and skin at a joint varies at the different points in the joint's range of movement (Allegrucci, Whitney, Lephart, & Fu, 1995; Dover, Kaminski, Maister, Powers, & Horodyski, 2003) Janwantanakul et al., 2001; Sullivan, Hoffman, & Harter, 2008). Because mechanoreceptors in tissues are activated by tension exerted on them, their activation would be expected to vary at different points in range as the tension in tissues around the joint varied. Consequently, position sense acuity may alter from one joint position to another. The accuracy of joint position reproduction at different criterion angles during JPS testing has been found to vary in studies involving the shoulder (Janwantanakul et al., 2001). In addition, Allegrucci et al. (1995) and Blasier et al. (1994) noted greater movement sense acuity at the shoulder complex, measured by the threshold for detection of movement test, at the end of range than in the mid joint range.

Joint position sense has been demonstrated to differ between participants in different sports and non-sporting individuals. Dover et al. (2003) showed baseball pitchers to have significantly decreased JPS at the extreme of external shoulder rotation than controls. This lack of awareness of joint position could potentially expose the glenohumeral joint to deleterious loading and result in injury.

Several factors have been reported to influence JPS including training, joint range, and fatigue (Myers & Lephart, 2000). Herrington, Horsley and Rolf (2007) and others (e.g.,

Dover, Kaminski, Meister, Powers, & Horodyski, 2003) have shown the level of training or nature of sports performance has a significant effect on JPS, with for instance, rugby players showing superior shoulder JPS to matched controls (Herrington et al., 2007). Janwantanakul et al. (2001) found that the joint angle set as the criterion angle to be matched had a Significant effect on JPS, with JPS improving towards the end of the range position as the capsular structures became taut. Several authors (Carpenter, Blasier, & Pellizzon, 1996; Tripp, Boswell, Gansneder, & Schultz, 2004: Voight, Hardin, Blackburn, Tippett, & Canner, 1996) found fatiguing activities to have a significant effect on shoulder JPS, causing a decrease following fatiguing activity. The consensus from these papers was that muscle fatigue somehow decreases the sensitivity of the capsular receptors and thus decreases proprioception indirectly. Fatigue, as in the decreased ability to generate the required force, leads to a production of substances, such as lactic acid and bradykinins, which exhibit affects via the nervous system which lengthen the muscle spindles. Hence, when the stretch stimulus arrives, the muscle spindle is not at the expected length, and affects the spindle output. If this situation is repeated, then the resulting sub-optimal motor response may be responsible for anatomical injury. This injury may itself contribute to deafferentation in a cyclic response (Voight, Hardin, Blackburn, Tippett, Canner, 1996). It has yet to be investigated if fatiguing tasks influence the angle-specific effect outlined above. It could be hypothesised from the above studies that end of range JPS could be preferentially decreased following a fatiguing task. This would then potentially expose the passive structures of the shoulder to increased loading and injury. Herrington, Horsley and Rolf (2007) assessed the effect of a simulated tackling task on shoulder joint position sense in rugby players, and also attempted to assess if differences in JPS occurring between mid range and end of range JPS, and if the tackling task had angle-specific effects on these values, utilizing a repeated measures design with 22 asymptomatic professional rugby players. JPS was assessed using two criterion angles in the 90degrees shoulder abduction position (45degrees and 80 degrees external rotation) prior to and following a simulated tackling task against a tackle bag.

They concluded that JPS was significantly reduced following a fatiguing task. But this change was only true for the end of range position, with JPS in the mid range not changing. If the mechanoreceptors are unable to accurately report shoulder position in the outer range (stretch) position due to repetitive tackling, then there is a potential for the anterior structures to become stressed before any compensatory muscle contraction can take place. These results highlight the presence of sensorimotor system deficits following repeated tackling. These deficits were proposed to contribute to overuse injuries and micro-instability of the glenohumeral joint which may be related to the increasing rate of shoulder injuries in rugby.

Following this, the same authors repeated a similar study using 15 asymptomatic professional rugby union players, 15 previously injured professional rugby union players, 15 asymptomatic matched non-rugby playing controls and assessed their joint position sense, with the aim of identifying whether joint position sense (JPS) in the shoulder differed between un-injured rugby players, matched control subjects and previously injured rehabilitated rugby players. The study found a significant difference between groups in error score (p = 0.02). The testing angle also had a significant effect on error score (p = 0.002), with greater error scores occurring in the mid range position. They concluded that rugby players have better JPS than controls, indicating JPS might not be related to injury risk. Poor JPS appears to be related to injury, players having sustained an injury have decreased JPS despite surgery and/or rehabilitation and returning to sport without incident.

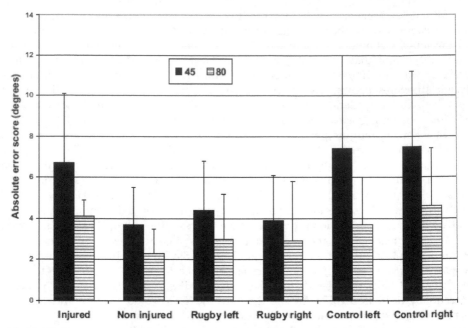

Fig. 1. Absolute error scores for the three groups.

Joint position sense can be defined as the ability to appreciate and recognise where a joint or a limb is in space (Ellenbecker, 2004). It has been reported in literature that joint position sense has great importance in avoiding non-physiological joint movements, such as extremes of movement – thus providing injury prevention and co-ordinates complex movement patterns (Jerosch and Prymka, 1996).

The mechanoreceptors found with in the capsule of the glenohumeral joint aid in providing afferent proprioceptive input via both slowly and rapidly adapting receptors (Vangsness et al. (1995). The rapidly adapting receptors respond to sudden changes in tension within the passive joint structures, although decrease their input into the central nervous system if the tension remains the same, in order to process acceleration and deceleration within the glenohumeral joint.

Proprioceptive feedback in not only produced from the passive restraints of the shoulder but from contractile structures too (Myers and Lephart, 2000; Nyland et al., 1998). The muscles which span the joint have three methods of assisting with joint stability by activation of various muscular contraction reflexes (Jerosch et al., 1997) (Jerosch et al., 1993), regulation of muscular contraction (Speer and Garrett 1993). The feedback is via the muscle spindles and golgi tendon organs. The muscle spindles provide feedback to enable effective motion execution via the monitoring of muscle length and joint position, and the sensitivity of the muscle receptors can be altered via efferent input from higher brain centres (Nyland, et al., 1998). The feedback from the golgi tendon organs registers changes in muscle tension and joint position, which induces agonist relaxation and contemporary increased activity within the antagonist, as a method of protection.

Processing of this information is carried out within the central nervous system at spinal level, brain stem, cerebellum, or cerebral cortex (Lephart and Henry 1996) and affects the function of the dynamic restraints surrounding the glenohumeral joint. This is via feed forward (anticipatory) and feed back (reactive) loops (Ghez, 1991). These two loops work in harmony, within the healthy shoulder, to indicate the actions of the dynamic restraints, which themselves are responsible for maintaining appropriate force couples across the joint, reflex action and regulating muscle stiffness (Myers and Lephart, 2000).

During the rugby tackle high trauma, or repeated minor trauma, could compromise the stability of the shoulder joint via increased joint laxity has decreased proprioceptive acuity compared to subjects with less joint laxity (Blaiser et al 1994). This laxity could bring about a cycle of events; described by Lephart and Henry (1996) as shoulder functional joint stability paradigm. Figure 2

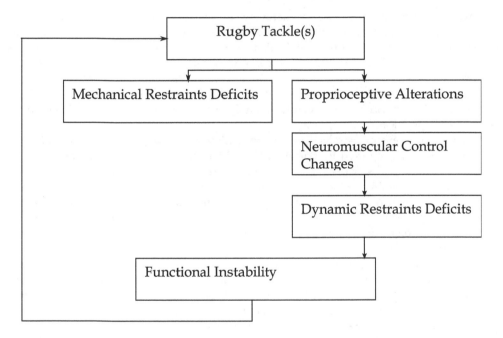

Adapted from Lephart and Henry (1996)

Fig. 2. Functional joint instability due to a Rugby Tackle.

Patients lacking proprioception have demonstrated an inability to perform multi-joint movements, suggesting that deficits in joint position sense detrimentally affects the co-ordinated movements at other joints along the kinetic chain (Riemann and Lephart, 2002) Following trauma to the shoulder joint through a heavy tackle of repeated contacts to the shoulder, proprioceptive input appears to be disrupted – which in turn affects neuromuscular co-activation deficits (Myers and Lephart, 1994).

Rehabilitation following injury to the glenohumeral joint should take into consideration not only pain relief, reduction of inflammation and restoration of optimal muscle strength and joint range of motion, but should include functional movements which replicate the demands of the sport in order to increase proprioceptive awareness, dynamic stabilization, feed forward mechanism (through anticipatory muscle responses), and sound reactive muscle function to athletic demands (Lephart and Henry, 1995). Proprioceptive training has been suggested as re-connecting the afferent pathways from the joint to the central nervous system with the production of complimentary afferent responses as a compensation for the joint position deficits produced by fatigue and/or injury (Myers and Lephart, 2000).

With shoulder joint injury there is much more than the soft tissues which are damaged; the sensorimotor system which is responsible for motor control and proprioception, and as has been demonstrated following shoulder injuries in rugby (Herrington, Horsley, Rolf, 2007).

2. Restoration of the sensorimotor system

Following disruption of the sensorimotor system it is imperative that restoration of functional joint stability is carried out as quickly as possible, in order to minimise the deleterious consequences. This rehabilitation needs to be able to replicate the demands placed on the joint, under controlled conditions but identifying deficits within the sensorimotor system in a clinical setting is not easy. Within scientific literature many sophisticated devices such as isokinetic dynamometers and motion analysis have been utilised. But these devices are not readily available in a clinical setting and thus render these techniques impractical.

The assessment of proprioception using "reproduction of passive positioning" is a valid and established method reported by Barrett (1991) Clinically joint angular replication tests – whereby the shoulder is placed in a position and the patient holds it in that position and consciously registers this position, then the arm is returned to a resting position. The subject is then asked to return the arm to the test position. This test has been described by Davies and Hoffmann (1993) and assesses both the static and dynamic shoulder joint stabilisers providing a thorough afferent pathway assessment (Lephart & Fu, 2000). Other examples of open kinetic chain exercises are;

Joint angle repositioning, whereby the shoulder joint is taken to a specific position in space (generally a combination of abduction and external rotation) by the examiner. The subject (who has their eyes closed in order to negate visual cues) is asked to hold this position for 5 seconds, then the limb is moved to the starting position, and the subject is asked to move to the test position. The degree of error from the stated position is recorded.

Contra lateral limb mirroring; the subject's uninvolved shoulder is placed in a position in space (whilst they have their eyes closed) and the subject is asked to mirror that position with the "involved" limb. Once again the degree of error between the two sides is noted.

Rehabilitation:

The goals of neuromuscular rehabilitation according to Borsa et al., (1994) are:

- To improve cognitive appreciation of the shoulder relative to position and motion.
- To enhance muscular stabilisation of the joint in the absence of passive restraints.
- Restore synergistic muscular firing and coordinated movement patterns.

The progression of the rehabilitation programme should progress along continuum (table 1) of difficulty with respect to the sport or desired activity (Guido and Stemm, 2007) and evolve from bilateral to unilateral, supported to unsupported (Kennedy et al., 1982), utilising active and passive movement, with and without load. The act of gripping has been shown to activate reflex contraction of the rotator cuff muscles which will stimulate glenohumeral mechanoreceptors. (Shumway-Cook and Woollacott, 2001).

	Early Stress	End Stage
Support	Supported Bilateral	Unsupported Unilateral
Surface Stress	Stable Minimal Capsular Stress Mid Range	Unstable Maximal Capsular Stress Outer Range
Speed	Slow	Fast
Stress Application	Predetermined Stress	Random/ Sudden Stress
Movement Pattern	Simple Co-ordination	Complex Co-ordination

Table 1. Rehabilitation Continuum

Weight bearing exercises through the limb (closed kinetic chain exercises) facilitates the activity of the rotator cuff muscles, and can be utilised in positions of forward lean standing or in four point kneeling from a four point kneeling position joint position reproduction can be utilised (figure 3). These can be progressed to a three point position (by extending the other arm or either leg) and further progressed to two point weight bearing which will facilitate the posterior chain to aid with scapular stabilisation.

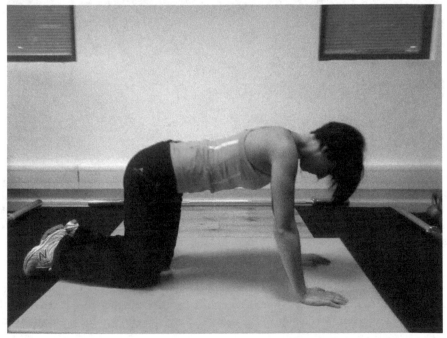

Fig. 3.

Further progression would be to change the surface from solid surface, to a wobble board or Swiss ball. The quality of the movement and exact local joint control needs to be monitored, as it is important to remember that arm movement, reflex stabilisation, postural control, and somatosensory perception are not separate events but rather different parts of an integrated action. (Guido and Stemm, 2007). Only the number of repetitions that the patient can carry out correctly with consistency should be carried out, rather that dictating a pre-determined number of repetitions and sets. Thus each exercise repetition is bespoke for that patient to avoid fatigue – as motor control decreases rapidly with fatigue, as does joint position awareness.

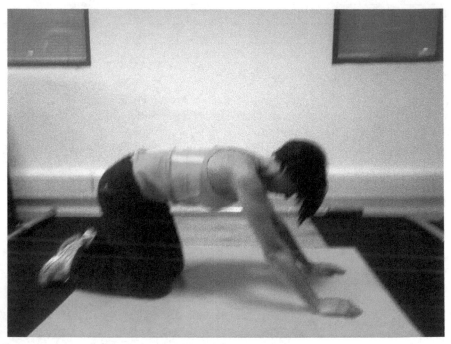

Fig. 4.

Another possibility of improving the cognitive awareness of shoulder JPS, is to challenge the patient to find the balance point (figure5) whereby in side lying, they are challenged to place their arm directly perpendicular to the glenoid and, initially, maintain this position against gravity. Dynamic balance can be further enhanced by asking the patient to maintain this position with a Swiss ball balanced on their hand (figure 6). To progress this exercise the patient is asked to stand from this position maintaining balance of the Swiss ball overhead.

The addition of externally applied forces (perturbations) will promote glenohumeral joint co-contraction, and rhythmic stabilisation (where by the patient's shoulder joint is place in position and isometrically resists externally applied focus of the therapist , take advantage of the stretch reflex creating a change in the desired muscle length producing local muscular splinting.

As soon as it is applicable the exercises need to be carried out in more functional positions such as sitting and standing (rather than the early stage of lying positions), as body position has a significant influence on a patient's ability to replicate a target position and to be aware of upper limb movement (Janwantanakul et al., 2003).

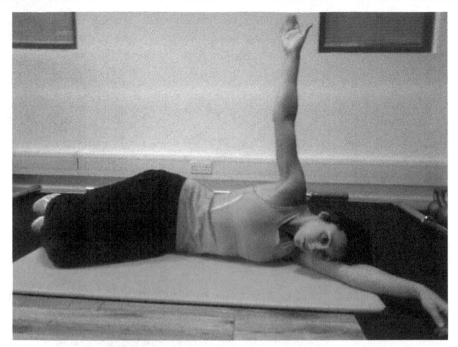

Fig. 5.

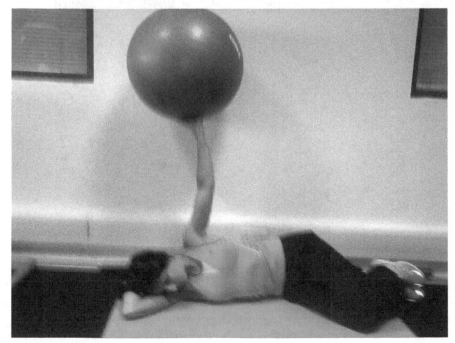

Fig. 6.

Another alternative to assess and rehabilitate proprioceptive acuity is to utilise a laser pointer. Targets can be placed on a wall, and a laser pointer attached to the arm that is being rehabilitated (fig 7). The patient is instructed to either follow a set path (such as a line) or land the pointer on a predefined mark.

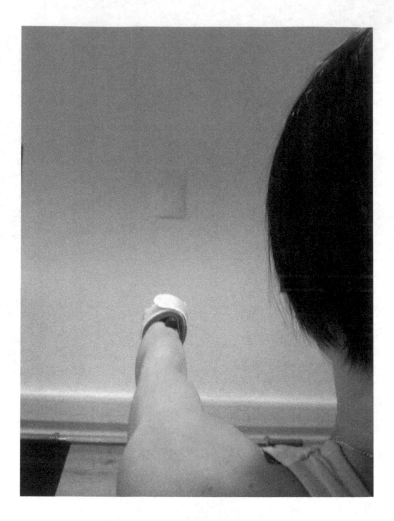

Fig. 7.

3. Proprioceptive neuromuscular facilitation (PNF)

Improvements in the neuromuscular response can be improved by utilising PNF exercises to stimulate the muscle spindles and golgi tendon organs. (Borsa et al., 1994). These movements occur in diagonal plans, against some form of external resistance, and require movement at the glenohumeral joint at all three planes (Voss and Ionta, 1985) and are designed to stimulate normal physiological movement.

Shoulder	Flexion External Rotation Adduction
Forearm	Supination
Wrist	Radial Deviation
Fingers	Flexion

Table 2. D1 flexion Joint Specific Movements

Shoulder	Extension Internal Rotation Abduction
Forearm	Pronation
Wrist	Ulnar Deviation
Fingers	Extension

Table 3. D1 Extension Upper Extremity Joint Specific Movements

Shoulder	Flexion External Rotation Abduction
Forearm	Supination
Wrist	Radial Deviation
Fingers	Extension

Table 4. D2 Flexion Upper Extremity Joint Specific Movements

Shoulder	Extension Internal Rotation Adduction
Forearm	Pronation
Wrist	Ulnar Deviation
Fingers	Flexion

Table 5. D2 Extension Upper Extremity Joint Specific Movements

The basic principles of PNF include utilisation of manual resistance (which varies throughout the range in response to the muscle strength), verbal cues, visual stimulus, and proprioceptive input via specific hand placement on the skin, stretch and timing order.

4. Plyometric exercises

Polymeric exercises involve an eccentric load or pre- stretch followed by a concentric contraction, (Borsa et al., 1994) which is induced via the myotactic reflex. This, then, facilitates reflex joint stabilisation. It has been proposed that movement towards the end of the shoulder range stimulates joint mechanoreceptors, as well as facilitating muscle spindle activity and decreasing GTO activity from the length – tension changes occurring at the musculotendinous structures (Swanik et al., 2002)

Common plyometric exercises include throwing motions trunk motions, resistive band exercises ball/ wall drills and plyometric push ups (Borsa et al., 1994).

A plyometric push up involves starting from the lower position of the press up, with the chest neat the floor, and rapidly extending the elbows with force, so that both hands leave the floor, then controlling the movement back to the start position eccentrically.

It is essential to demonstrate excellent dynamic control around the shoulder, through full range, with good proprioceptive acuity before progressing to these demanding exercises. (Gibson, 2004).

5. Compression

It has been reported that tactile sensations (along with vestibular and visual) aid with joint repositioning (Allegruci et al., 1995). Compression garments are believed to enhance sensory and proprioceptive awareness leading to an increase in proximal stability (Gracies et al., 1997) and stimulate mechanoreceptors to enhance joint positioning sense and body awareness (Hylton and Allen, 1997) (Ulkar et al., 2004). There is a reduced contribution of cutaneous proprioceptive information in proximal areas such as the glenohumeral joint (Grigg 1994) and the provision of compressive force stimulates mechanoreceptors within the skin to provide joint position sense to the central nervous system (Barrack et al., 1983) and has been reported to promote the cognitive feeling of joint stability (Jerosch and Prymka, 1996; Barrack 1983).

Functional stability of the shoulder is dependent on co activation of the musculature as well as reactive neuromuscular characteristics. Injury to any of the soft tissue structures has been postulated as a cause of disruption of this neuromuscular mechanism. Treatment of such a dysfunction needs to consider proprioceptive training and rehabilitation, since the function of the shoulder joint is optimal when proprioception is normalized.

6. Summary

Injuries to the shoulder are becoming increasingly more frequent in professional rugby. It has been cited that this is due to the increased intensity and frequency of the contact/tackle phase (Brookes et al., 2005). Recent studies have provided at least a partial explanation of why this is occurring. professional rugby players to have superior JPS than controls, indicating JPS might not be related to injury risk, when assessed in a rested state Following a tackling task JPS was significantly decreased in the outer range position potential exposing to the anterior structures of the shoulder to increased loading. JPS would appear to be significantly affected by injury, players who have sustained an injury having inferior JPS, compared to their peers These results highlight the presence of sensorimotor system deficits following repeated tackling. These deficits are proposed to contribute to overuse injuries and micro-instability of the glenohumeral joint (Lephart & Henry, 1996). Thus, it would appear advisable, when appropriate, to restrict shoulder joint activity following repeated tackling. One way of achieving this would be to place tackling drills at the end of the training sessions and not to match tackling with heavy upper body weight training sessions.

7. References

Gissane C, Jennings D, Kerr K, White J. (2003) Injury rates in rugby league football: impact of change in playing season. Am J Sports Med. Nov-Dec; 31(6):954-8.]

Brooks J, Fuller C, Kemp S, Reddin D. Epidemiology of injuries in English Professional Rugby Union: Part I match injuries. British Journal of Sports Medicine. 2005; 39:757-766]

Bathgate A, Best JP, Craig Jamieson M. A Prospective Study of Injuries to the Elite Australian Rugby Union Players. British Journal of Sports Medicine. 2002; 36:265-269]

Garraway WM, Lee AJ, Hutton SJ, Russell EBAW, Macleod DAD. Impact of professionalism on injuries in rugby union. Br J Sports Med 2000; 34: 348-351]

Holtzhausen L J (2001). The epidemiology of injuries in professional rugby union. Int SportMed J, 2(2): 1-13]

Targett SG. Injuries in professional Rugby Union. Clin J Sport Med. 1998; 8(4):280-5.]

Gissane C, Jennings D, Kerr K, White J. (2003) Injury rates in rugby league football: impact of change in playing season. Am J Sports Med. Nov-Dec; 31(6):954-8.]

Hawkins, R.D. and Fuller C.W. (1999) A prospective epidemiological study of injuries in four English professional football clubs. British Journal of Sports Medicine Volume 33, page 196 – 203]

Bird YN, Waller AE, Marshall SW, et al. The New Zealand rugby injury and performance project. V. Epidemiology of a season of rugby injury. Br J Sports Med 1998; 32:319-25

Garraway M, Macleod D. Epidemiology of rugby football injuries. Lancet 1995; 345:1485-7.]

Hughes DC, Fricker PA. A prospective survey of injuries to first-grade rugby union players. Clin J Sports Med 1994; 4:249–56]

Suprak, D., Osternig, L., van-Donkelaar, P., & Karduna, A. (2006). Shoulder joint position sense improves with elevation angle in a novel, unconstrained task. Journal of Orthopaedic Research, 24, 559–568.

Janwantanakul, P., Magarey, M., Jones, M., & Danise, B. (2001). Variation in shoulder position sense at mid and extreme range of motion. Archives of Physical Medicine and Rehabilitation, 82, 840–844.

Aydin, T., Yildiz, Y., Yanmis, I., Yildiz, C., & Kalyon, T. (2001). Shoulder proprioception: a comparison between the shoulder joint in healthy and surgically repaired shoulders. Archives of Orthopaedic and Trauma Surgery, 7, 422–425.

Blasier, R., Carpenter, J., & Huston, L. (1994). Shoulder proprioception: effect of joint laxity, joint position and direction of motion. Orthopaedic Reviews, 23, 45–50.

Cain, P., Mutschler, T., Fu, F., & Lee, S. (1987). Anterior instability of the glenohumeral joint: A dynamic model. American Journal of Sports Medicine, 15, 144–148.

Lephart, S., & Henry, T. (1996). The physiological basis for open and closed kinematic chain rehabilitation for the upper extremity. Journal of Sports Rehabilitation, 5, 71–87.

Allegrucci, M., Whitney, S., Lephart, S., & Fu, F. (1995). Shoulder kinaesthesia in healthy unilateral athletes participating in upper extremity sports. Journal of Orthopaedic and Sports Physical Therapy, 21, 220–226.

Dover, G., Kaminski, T., Maister, K., Powers, M., & Horodyski, M. (2003). Assessment of shoulder proprioception in the female softball athlete. American Journal of Sports Medicine, 31, 431–437.

Sullivan, J., Hoffman, M., & Harter, R. (2008). Shoulder joint position sense after thermal, open and arthroscopic capsulorrhaphy for recurrent anterior instability. Journal of Elbow and Shoulder Surgery, 17, 389–394.

Myers, J., & Lephart, S. (2000). The role of the sensorimotor system in the athletic shoulder. Journal of Athletic Training, 35, 351–363.

Herrington, L., Horsley, I., & Rolf, C. (2007) Evaluation of joint position sense in professional rugby players. Journal of Sports Science and Medicine, under review.

Carpenter, J., Blasier, R., & Pellizzon, G. (1996). The effects of muscle fatigue on shoulder joint position sense. American Journal of Sports Medicine, 26, 262–265.

Ellenbecker, T.S., In Clinical Examination of the Shoulder – Elsevier Saunders, St Louis, Missouri 2004.

Jerosch, J., Prymka, M., (1996) Proprioception and joint stability. Knee Surgery. Sports Traumatol. Arthroscopy: 4; 171-9.

Vangsness, C.T., Ennis, M., Taylor, J.G., et al (1995) Neural anatomy of the glenohumeral ligaments, labrum and subacromial bursa. Arthroscopy 11(2): 180-184.

Myers, J.B., Lephart, S.M. (2000) The role of the sensorimotor system in the athletic shoulder. J. Athletic Training; 35 (3):351-362.)

Nyland, J.A., Caborn, D.N.M., Johnson, D.L., (1998) The glenohumeral joint; a proprioceptive and stability alliance; Knee Surgery Sports Traumatology Arthroscopy 6:50-61.

Jerosch, J., Steinbeck, J., Schroder, M., Westhues, M., Peer, R. (1997). Intra-operative EMG response of the musculature after stimulation of the glenohumeral joint capsule. Acta Orthop. Belg; 63: 8-13.

Jerosch, J., Castro, W.H.M., Holm, H., Drescher, H., (1993). Does the glenohumeral joint capsule have proprioceptive capability? Knee Surgery sports Traumatol. Arthroscopy; 1: 80-4.

Speer, K.P., Garrett, W.E., (1993). Muscular control of motion and stability about the pectoral girdle in (Matsen. F.A., Fu, F.H., Hawkins, R.J., editors. The Shoulder a balance of mobility and stability. Rosemont (IL) American Academy of Orthopaedic Surgeons: P159-72) coordination (Speer and Garrett, 1993.

Lephart, S.M., Henry, T.J. (1996): The physiological basis for open and closed kinetic chain rehabilitation for the upper extremity. J. Sports Rehabil; S: 71-87.

Ghez, C, (1991); The control of movement in Kendel, E., Schwartz, J., Schwartz, J., Jessell, T. (eds): Principles of neural Science, 3rd ed. New York, Elsevier Science

Blaiser, R.B., Carpenter, J.E., Huston, L.J. (1994). Shoulder proprioception effect of joint laxity, joint position, and direction of motion. Orthop Rev; 23: 45-50).

Riemann, B.L., Lephart, S.M., (2002). The sensorimotor system, part II: The role of proprioception in motor control and functional joint stability J. Athl Training; 37 (1): 71-9

Barrett, D.S. (1991) Proprioception and function after anterior cruciate reconstruction. J. Bone Joint Surgery (Br); 73; 833-7.

Davies, G.J., Hoffman, S.D. (1993): Neuromuscular testing and rehabilitation of the shoulder Complex, J. Orthop Sports Phys Ther 18: 449-458

Lephart, S.M., Fu. F.H., (2000): Proprioception and neuromuscular control in joint stability, Champaign, IL. Human Kinetics Publishers.

Borsa, P.A., Lephart, S.M., Kocker, M.S., Lephart, S.P. (1994): functional assessment and rehabilitation of shoulder proprioception for glenohumeral instability. Journal of Sports Rehabilitation; 3: 84-104

Guido, J.A., Stemm, J. (2007) Reactive neuromuscular training: a multi-level approach to rehabilitation of the unstable shoulder. North American Journal of Sports Physical Therapy; 2 (2): 97-103.

Kennedy J.C. Alexander, I.J., Hayes, K.C. (1982). Nerve supply to the human knee and its functional importance. Am J. Sports Med; 10: 329-335.

Shumway-Cook, A., Woollacott, M.H. (2001) Motor Control: Theory and practical applications 2nd edition. Lippincott; Philadelphia, P.A; Baltimore, M.D.

Janwantanakul, P. (2003). The effect of body orientation on shoulder proprioception. Phys. Ther. Sport; 4: 67-73.

Tripp, B., Boswell, L., Gansneder, B., & Shultz, S. (2004). Functional fatigue decreases 3-dimensional multijoint position reproduction acuity in the overhead throwing athlete. Journal of Athletic Training, 39, 316–320.

Voight, M., Hardin, J., Blackburn, T., Tippett, S., & Canner, G. (1996). The effect of muscle fatigue on and the relationship of arm dominance to shoulder proprioception. Journal of Orthopaedic and Sports Physical Therapy, 23, 348–352.

Lephart, S.M., Henry, T.J., (1995). Functional rehabilitation of the upper and lower extremity. Ortho Clin N Am; 26(3):579-92

Myers, J.B., Lephart, S.M., (2000). The role of the sensorimotor system in the athletic shoulder. Journal of Athletic training; 35(3):351-63

Swanik, K.A., Lephart, S.M., Swanik, C.B., Lephart, S.P., Stone, D.A., Fu, F.H., (2002). The effects of shoulder Plyometric training on proprioception and selected muscle performance characteristics. Journal of shoulder and Elbow Surgery: 11 (6):579-86]

Stone, J.A., Partin, N.B., Leuken, J.S., Timm, K.E., Ryan, E.J., (1994).Upper extremity proprioceptive training. Journal of Athletic Training; 29 (1):15-18].

Voss DE, Ionta MK, Myers BJ. Proprioceptive Neuromuscular Facilitation: Patterns and Techniques. Philadelphia: Harper & Row, Publishers; 1985; 302-303.].

Gibson, J.C. (2004), Mini symposium: Shoulder Instability (III) Rehabilitation after shoulder instability surgery. Current Orthopaedics; 18: 197-209.

Allegruci, M., Whitney, S.L., Lephart, S.M., et al (1995) Shoulder kinaesthesia in healthy unilateral athletes participating in upper extremity sports. J. Orthop Sports Phys Ther; 69: 220-6.

Gracies, J., Fitzpatrick, R., Wilson, L., Burke, D., Gandevia, S.C., 1997). Lycra garments designed for patients with upper limb spasticity: Mechanical effects in normal subjects. Archives of Physical Medicine and Rehabilitation; 78: 1066-1071.

Hylton, N., Allen, C., (1997) The development and use of SP10 Lycra compression bracing in children with neuromotor deficits. Paediatric Rehabilitation; 1 (2): 109-116.

Ulkar, B., Kunduracioglen, B., Cetin, C., Guner, R.S. (2004) Effect of positioning and bracing on passive position sense of the shoulder joint. British Journal of Sports Medicine; 38: 549-552.

Grigg, P. (1994) Peripheral neural mechanisms in proprioception. Journal of Sports Rehabilitation: 3: 2-17.

Barrack, R.L., Skinner, H.B., Brunel, M.E. (1983). Joint laxity and proprioception in the knee. Phys Sports Med; 11: 130-5.

11

Treatment of Talar Osteochondral Lesions Using Local Osteochondral Talar Autograft – Long Term Results

Thanos Badekas, Evangelos Evangelou and Maria Takvorian
Department of Foot and Ankle Surgery, Metropolitan Hospital, Athens, Greece

1. Introduction

Osteochondral lesion of the talus (OLT) is a broad term used to describe an injury or abnormality of the talar articular cartilage and adjacent bone. A variety of terms have been used to refer to this clinical entity including osteochondritis dissecans, osteochondral fracture, and osteochondral defect. Whether OLT of the talus is a precursor to more generalized arthrosis of the ankle remain unclear, but the condition is often symptomatic enough to warrant treatment. Above one third of cases conservative treatment is not successful and a surgery is indicated. Several surgical options have been described including: debridement, isolated or combined with drilling, excision and curettage, abrasion arthroplasty, microfracture technique arthroscopically or not, internal fixation with screws, autologous chondrocyte implantation and implantation of osteochondral autograft using single or multiple cylinders of articular cartilage and subchondral bone. The optimal solution remains uncertain. Furthermore smaller lesions are symptomatic and untreated OCDs can progress, current treatment strategies have not solved the problem

The goal of this study was to retrospectively evaluate the long-term results of 23 patients who underwent local osteochondral talar autograft for the treatment of OLT.

2. Materials and methods

From March 2005 to December 2008 a series of 58 patients were retrospectively evaluated. Thirty seven male and twenty one female with age ranged from 19 to 53 (mean 38) years. Sports related injury concerned 37 patients and the duration of symptoms was mean 65 months (range 6 to 98). Mean follow-up was 22,1 months (range 14 to 32). Preoperative evaluations included a clinical history, physical examination of the foot and recording of American Orthopaedic Foot and Ankle Society (AOFAS) Ankle- Hindfoot score. Special radiological studies performed preoperative, MRI (58 patients), CAT (58 patients), Bone Scan 3 patients (ordered by other doctors, because we don't need it for detection OLT) and weight-bearing radiographs to all of them to evaluate the injury. The majority of lesions n=41 were on the medial aspect of talus, 17 on the lateral talar dome and 4 medial and lateral lesions. The graft was harvested from the medial or lateral talar articular facet on the same side of the lesion depended by the geometry of the lesion. Graft sizes ranged from four to eight millimeters in diameter. More specific 4 mm 6, 6mm 28, 8mm 24. So, this operation is used for stages 3 and 4 lesions according to Berndt and Hardy classification and for stages 1 and 2 in symptomatic patients that failed previous surgical treatment. (table 1).

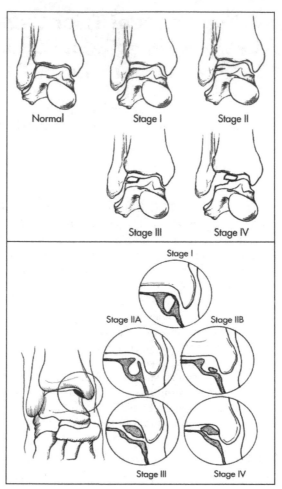

Table 1. Berndt and Hardy classification

Associated findings after the preoperative control (table2) was 17patients with Pes Planus, 11 patients with arthritis, 8 patients with Achilles tendinopathy, 3 with Tibialis Posterior Dysfunction, 3 with Hallux Rigidus, 13 with lateral ankle instability and 2 patient with previous pinning controlateral ankle. Additional procedures were an FHL tenosynovectomy and repair, excision of a lipoma, lateral ligaments reconstruction (Brostrom modification), TAL lengthening, synovectomy and AAI removal. Preoperative and postoperative results evaluated used the AOFAS hindfoot score. The result of the score was classified in excellent, good, fair and poor and additionally patients have been asked about their satisfaction following the procedure. Statistical analyses were performed using SPSS software.

Pes planus	17
Arthritis	11
Achilles tend	8
Tib.Post Dysf.	3
Hallux Rigidus	3
Lateral Ankle Instability	13
Previous pinning contr	2

Table 2. Associated Findings & History

3. Surgical technique

All procedures were performed with the patient in the supine position under tourniquet control. An arthrotomy was performed through a 7cm antero-medial or antero-lateral incision as required. The lesion is approached by removing a bone block from the tibia including the articular surface. To accomplish with this a wedge shaped bone block, 10mm wide, 20mm deep and 30mm in height is made at the distal anterior tibia articular surface on the side of the osteochondral lesion. Vertical parallel saw cuts are made with a high-speed micro oscillating saw. Care is taken to avoid injuring the uninvolved talar articular surface. The saw was then used to connect the two vertical parallel cuts proximally in the metaphysis. A 10mm wide thin osteotome is then driven from the superior portion of the transverse saw cut inferiorly to the articular surface of the tibial plafond 10 to 20mm deep depending on the location of the lesion on the talar dome. The tibial fragment is removed and set aside to be replaced later (figure 1). The defect created in the tibia following removal of the bone fragment permits direct access to the lesion from above. The lesion is delivered into the field by plantar-flexing the ankle. It is prepared by first debriding the loosened cartilage fragments. The lesion is then drilled using the appropriate size drill. Care is taken to ensure that the drill is perpendicular to the articular surface of the talus directly over the lesion. Drill sizes are matched to the diameter of the defect 4, 6 or 8mm to the size of the defect determined from the MRI. The osteochondral graft is harvested from the anterior aspect of the ipsilateral talar articular facet. A total of 15 grafts were harvested: two 4mm, six 6mm and seven 8mm (figure 2). This is performed through the same incision as the tibial osteotomy. The graft is harvested using the core-harvesting device (figure 3). The cutter was positioned over the talar facet near the anterior border ensuring that it was perpendicular to the articular surface. The inferior border of the talar facet flares outward slightly and the harvesting tube is oriented so that the flared margin can be identified and oriented toward the medial or lateral talar dome respectively. This ensures that the graft shape will approximate the saddle shape of the talar dome more closely. It is then tapped with a mallet until the cutter reaches the desired depth. The harvester is then rotated and removed with graft held in the harvester tube. The outer cutter is removed leaving the graft plug inside the harvester tube and a delivery guide is screwed onto the harvester tube. A plunger is inserted into the proximal end of the tube. The assembled harvester tube, guide and plunger are positioned perpendicular to the talar done over the prepared site in the talus orienting the outer flair of the graft toward the outer edge of the dome. The plunger is tapped gently pressing the osteochondral graft plug into the hole (Figure 4). The graft is inserted until it is flush slightly proud to the surrounding cartilage overhanging. For the true medial lesions a Chevron-type medial malleolar osteotomy was performed at the end the osteotomy fixed with 2 screws. The approach to lateral lesions performed with anterolateral incision by taking down the ATFL and CFL. At the end a modified Brostrom performed. The postoperative treatment was immobilization for 4 weeks, walker boot for next 4 weeks and weight bearing at six weeks. Range of motion exercises was allowed once the surgical incision healed.

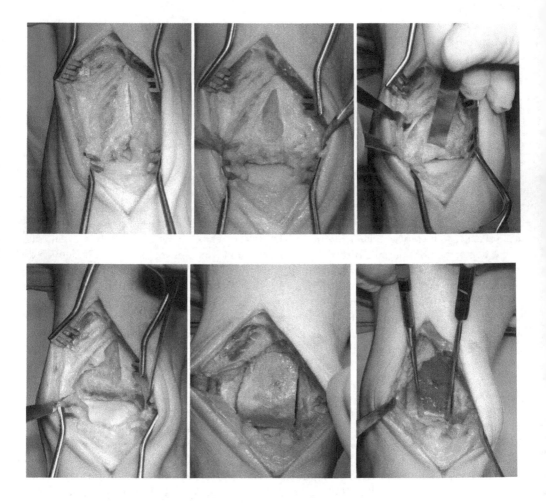

Fig. 1. Tibial osteotomy trapezoid wedge shape for perpedicular access to the recipient sit

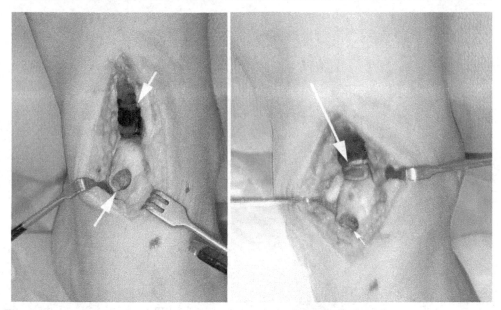

Fig. 2. Donor medial talar facet-recipient site with the local garft altready inserted

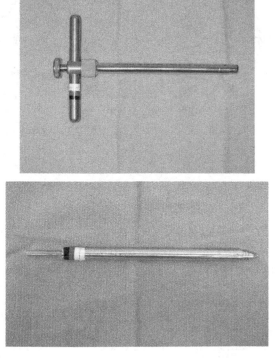

Fig. 3. Instrumention

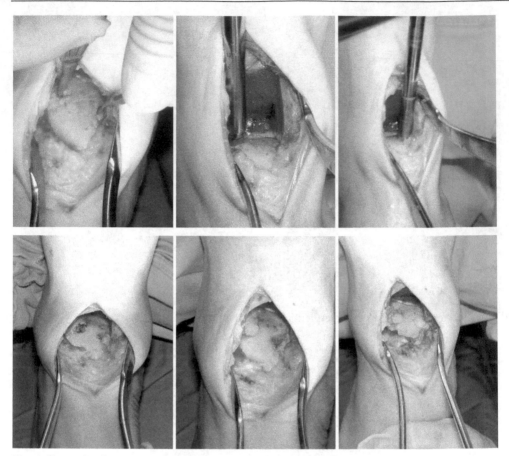

Fig. 4. Perpedicular access to the recipient site a case with 2 lesions

4. Results

Patients were evaluated both intraoperatively and postoperatively. Operative findings included: degenerative joint disease in six cases, lipoma in two cases and lateral ankle ligament instability in two cases.

Preoperative AOFAS scoring using the ankle and hindfoot score was 65 average. At follow up, 41 months (average). Postoperative was 89 average. The patients under the age of 40 had higher average AOFAS scores postoperatively, compared to the patients over the age of 40. (table 3) The presence of degenerative arthritis yielded a lower AOFAS score in. However, the difference between these small subgroups was not significant. No reciprocal "kissing lesions" were encountered on the tibial articular surface opposite the osteochondral lesion. There was no deterioration in the overall functional improvement in patients underwent additional procedures. There were no perioperative complications. Long term, the most common complaint in patients over time was mild aching over the anterior aspect of the ankle, although this did not decrease activities of daily living or sports. All patients stated they would undergo the procedure again.

	Pre-operative	Post-operative
AOFAS	65	89
Under 40 years	69	92
No Arthritis	68	91
Arthritis	63	86

Table 3.

Evaluation of postoperative x-rays revealed no evidence of decreased joint space in the ankle. X-ray findings also revealed that the cyst visible preoperatively was no longer visible at the last follow up visit. No increase in arthritis was noted. Clinical examination postoperatively revealed improved range of motion, muscle strength, gait pattern and endurance. Patients returned to their work 8 months following surgery, without restrictions. Two patients underwent surgery subsequent to the index procedure, one had arthroscopy and removal of impinging osteophytes from the lateral malleolus six months following surgery and one had arthroscopy with debridement of the anterior tibial margin at the site where the tibial bone block had been removed twelve months following surgery (Figure 5). In both cases the cartilage of the graft appeared to have grown into the surrounding cartilage of the talar dome. The tibial articular cartilage on the tibial plafond had also healed without articular surface defects. It appeared that the use of talar osteochondral graft does not adversely affect the joint surface and easily incorporates into the surrounding surface cartilage.

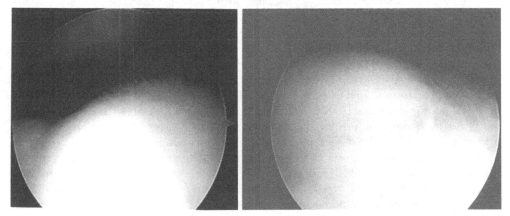

Fig. 5. Second look arthroscopy with a good incorporation of the local graft same quality and thickness cartilage

5. Discussion

The result of non-operative treatment of stage III and IV osteochondral lesions of the talus have been poor[1, 3]. Berndt and Harty reviewing 200 cases from the literature and adding 24 of their own found 73.9% poor results with non-surgical treatment. Of the fifty-six treated surgically 78.6% had good results[3]. O`Farrell and Costello (1982)[9] reported on 24 patients treated surgically and found the results were better with early diagnosis and treatment. This report was further substantiated by Pettine and Morrey (1987)[10] who retrospectively reviewed 68 patients at average follow-up of 7.5 years and concluded that a delay in diagnosis and surgery resulted in a poor outcome. Whilst a high percentage of satisfactory results can be obtained with non-surgical treatment for Stage I and II lesions most stage III and IV lesions require surgery. Canale and Belding (1980)[4] recommended stage IV and III lateral lesions be treated surgically but that III medial lesions be treated non-surgically initially. All lesions in our study were stage III or IV and two/thirds were related to sports injuries. The surgical treatment for osteochondral lesions of the talus includes excision, excision and curettage with or without drilling, microfracture, cancellous bone grafting, internal fixation and osteochondral grafting. Review of the literature suggests a higher percentage of good and excellent results with excision and curettage with or without drilling the base of the lesion[14]. Mosaicplasty autogenous osteochondral grafting has been recently introduced and has evolved from treatment of osteochondral lesions of the knee. Hangody et al (1997)[7] reported their results in 11 patients treated with mosaicplasty autogenous osteochondral grafting for talar dome lesions using the knee as a donor site with a high success rate. However donor site morbidity can occur in up to 15% -16% of cases in an asymptomatic joint[8]. We feel this increased morbidity can be avoided. By harvesting the graft from a location on the talar dome, which carries minimal loads, the risks of the procedure are reduced. The graft is taken from the anterior part of the medial or lateral talar facet. Since the graft size is relatively small the integrity anterior dome is maintained. There was no incidence of collapse of the talus either at the donor site or at the site of the lesion. The two patients on whom arthroscopy was performed revealed the graft well incorporated on the surface of the joint. The chondral border of the graft revealed no line of degeneration or necrosis. Also, there was no additional change noted on the medial or lateral facet either at the site of the lesion or at the donor site.

The removal of a portion of the anterior tibial plafond to access this lesion has been previously described[6]. However, osteochondritic lesions are often large and located farther back in the talar dome so that they are inaccessible unless a large portion of tibia is removed. This makes the method described by Flick and Gould[6] impractical since the amount of bone needed to be removed is significant, ten mm. and will decrease the tibial load bearing capacity of tibial plafond if it not replaced. Moreover the location of such lesions is often so far posterior that removal without replacing tibial bone to access the lesion would significantly weaken the tibial plafond and medial malleolus. In addition, this method cannot be used laterally unless the lesion is located anteriorly. The use of a medial malleolar osteotomy carries the risk of nonunion and malunion and the results may deteriorate with time[2]. The securing of the malleolus with screws leaves the heads of the screws at the tip of the malleolus and these may require removal later. Our method allows access to either side of the ankle directly even if the lesion is located toward the posterior third of the dome. The defect is visualized from above after the bone block has been removed. The bone block is then replaced and secured with an absorbable pin. There is no risk of malunion since the block is replaced in the same position from which it was removed. No fractures occurred in the tibia. The tibial graft held in place without any fixation only by gentle tapping, since it holds the bone block in place but not carry any loads.

Moreover we use same quality osteochondral graft, the cartilage of the knee is thicker than the talus cartilage hence cannot incorporate precisely like the talus cartilage.

There are some lesions that are difficult to access even with this method. These are located in the posterior 20 to 30% of the talar dome, particularly in the lateral posterior region of the talus. For these less common lesions, not included in this report, we expose the talus through a posterolateral incision and performed the grafting using a second anterior incision to harvest the graft.

Additionally for the true medial lesions we still perform an osteotomy of the medial malleolus(figure 6) because it is difficult to have perpedicular access to the recipient site through the wedge shaped bone block, at the distal anterior tibia articular surface on the side of the osteochondral lesion.

For the true lateral lesions sometimes is needed to approach the lesion through an anterolateral incision we have to take down the anterior tibiofibular ligament (ATFL) and the calcaneofibular ligament (CFL) in order to have perpendicular access again to the recipient site (figure7), then we have to reconstruct the ligament with a standard modified Brostrom technique.

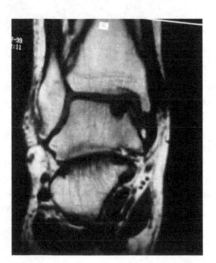
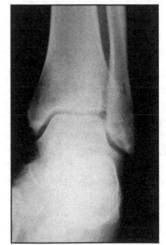

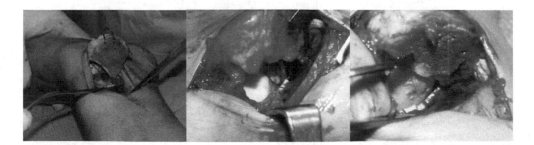

Fig. 6. Medial malleolus osteotomy for true medial site lesions

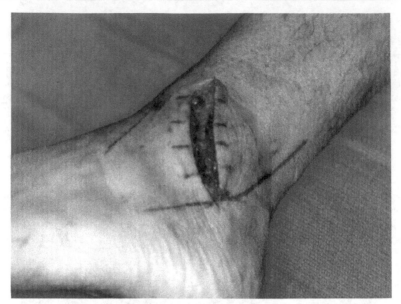

Fig. 7. Lateral OLT Approached through an anterolateral incision, with takedown of ATFL and CFL. Reconstruction with modified Brostrom

The overall improvement in the AOFAS score in our study was 24 points at an average follow up of 41 months. Improvement can be expected for as long as eighteen months postoperatively[12]. Canale and Belding (1980)[4] found 15 out of 31 cases (50%) developed degenerative joint changes at an average 11.2 years. The long-term success of preventing late joint degenerative changes has yet to be determined using our technique.

In this study our mid term results suggest that stage III and IV talar dome lesions can be treated successfully using local autogenous osteochondral grafts from the medial or lateral talar articular facet This procedure is combined with removal of a tibial bone block and its subsequent replacement and does not yield complications experienced with other procedures.

6. References

[1] Al Shaikh, RA; Chou, LB; Mann, JA; Dreeben, SM; Prieskorn D: Autologous osteochondral grafting for talar cartilage defects. Foot Ankle Int. 23(5): 381 – 389, 2002.

[2] Baker, CL; Andrews, JR; Ryan JB: Arthroscopic treatment of transchondral talar dome fractures. Arthroscopy. 2(2): 82 – 87, 1986. http://dx.doi.org/10.1016/S0749-8063(86)80017-2.

[3] Barnes, CJ; Ferkel RD: Arthroscopic debridement and drilling of osteochondral lesions of the talus. Foot Ankle Clin. 8(2): 243 – 257, 2003. http://dx.doi.org/10.1016/S1083-7515(03)00016-0.

[4] Bartlett, W; Skinner, JA; Gooding, CR; et al.:Autologous chon-drocyte implantation versus matrix – induced autologous chondrocyte implantation for osteochondral

defects of the knee: a prospective, randomised study.J Bone Joint Surg Br. 87(5):640 – 645, 2005. http://dx.doi.org/10.1302/0301-620X.87B5.15905.

[5] Bauer, M; Jonsson, K; Lind´ en, B: Osteochondrosis dissecans of the ankle: A 20-year followup study. J Bone Joint Surg Br. 69(1): 93 – 96, 1987.

[6] Brittberg, M; Sj¨ ogren-Jansson, E; Lindahl, A; Peterson, L:Influence of fibrin sealant (Tisseel) on osteochondral defect repair in the rabbit knee. Biomaterials.18(3): 235 – 242, 1997. http://dx.doi.org/10.1016/S0142-9612(96)00117-2.

[7] Browne, JE; Branch, TP: Surgical alternatives for treatment of articular cartilage lesions. J Am Acad Orthop Surg. 8(3): 180 – 189, 2000.

[8] Campbell, CJ; Ranawat, CS: Osteochondritis dissecans: the question of etiology. J Trauma. 6(2): 201 – 221, 1966. http://dx.doi.org/10.1097/00005373-196606020-00007.

[9] Cherubino, P; Grassi, FA; Bulgheroni, P; Ronga, M: Autologous chondrocyte implantation using a bilayer collagen membrane: a preliminary report. J Orthop Surg (Hong Kong). 11(1): 10 – 15, 2003.

[10] Chiroff, RT; Cooke, CP 3rd: Osteochondritis dissecans: a histologic and microradiographic analysis of surgically excised lesions. J Trauma. 15(8): 689 – 696, 1975.

[11] Ewing, JW: Arthroscopic management of transchondral talar-dome fractures (osteochondritis dissecans) and anterior impingement lesions of the ankle joint. Clin Sports Med. 10(3): 677 – 687, 1991.

[12] Finsen, V; Saetermo, R; Kibsgaard, L; et al.: Early postoperative weight-bearing and muscle activity in patients who have a fracture of the ankle. J Bone Joint Surg Am. 71(1): 23 – 27, 1989.

[13] Hangody, L; Kish, G; Krp´ati, Z; Szerb, I; Eberhardt, R: Treatment of osteochondritis disseuse of the mosaicplasty technique — Acans of the Ttalus: Uàa Int.18(10): 628 – 634, 1997. preliminary report. Foot Ankle

[14] Hangody, L; Kish, G; M´odis, L; et al.: Mosaicplasty for the treatment of osteochondritis dissecans of the talus. : two to seven year results in 36 patients. Foot Ankle Int. 22(7): 552 – 558, 2001.

[15] Kitaoka, HB; Alexander, IJ; Adelaar, RS; et al.: Clinical rating systems for the ankle-hindfoot, midfoot, hallux, and lesser toes. Foot Ankle Int. 15(7): 349 – 353,1994.

[16] Koulalis, D; Schultz, W; Heyden M: Autologous chondrocyte transplantation for osteochondritis dissecans of the talus. Clin Orthop Relat Res.395:186 – 192, 2002. http://dx.doi.org/10.1097/00003086-200202000-00021.

[17] Kumai, T; Takakura, Y; Higashiyama, I; Tamai, S: Arthroscopic drilling for the treatment of osteochondral lesions of the talus. J Bone Joint Surg Am. 81(9): 1229 – 1235, 1999.

[18] Lee, CH; Chao, KH; Huang, GS; Wu, SS: Osteochondral autografts for osteochondritis dissecans of the talus. Foot Ankle Int. 24(11): 815 – 822, 2003.

[19] Myles, P; Gin, T: Statistical Methods for Anaesthesia and Intensive Care. First Edition, Butterworth Heinemann Oxford, 2000.

[20] Robinson, DE; Winson, IG; Harries, WJ; Kelly, AJ: Arthroscopic treatment of osteochondral lesions of the talus. J Bone Joint Surg Br. 85(7): 989 – 993, 2003.http://dx.doi.org/10.1302/0301-620X.85B7.13959.

[21] Schenk, RC; Goodknight, JM: Current concepts review: Osteochon-dritis dessicans. J Bone Joint Surg. 78A: 439 – 456, 1996.

[22] Taranow, WS; Bisignani, GA; Towers, JD; Conti, SF: Retrograde drilling of osteochondral lesions of the medial talar dome. Foot Ankle Int. 20(8): 474 – 480, 1999.

[23] Thompson, JP; Loomer, RL: Osteochondral lesions of the talus in a sports medicine clinic. A new radiographic technique and surgical approach. Am J Sports Med.12(6): 460 – 463,1984. http://dx.doi.org/10.1177/036354658401200611

[24] Tol, JL; Struijs, PA; Bossuyt, PM; Verhagen, RA; van Dijk, CN: Treatment strategies in osteochondral defects of the talar dome: a systematic review: Foot Ankle Int. 21(2): 119 – 126, 2000.

[25] Whittaker, JP; Smith, G; Makwana, N; et al.: Early results of autologous chondrocyte implantation in the talus. J Bone Joint Surg Br. 87(2): 179 – 183, 2005. http://dx.doi.org/10.1302/0301-620X.87B2.15376.

[26] Willers, C; Wood, DJ; Zheng, MH: A current review of the biology and treatment of articular cartilage defects (part I &part III). J Musculoskeletal Res. 7:157 – 181, 2003. http://dx.doi.org/10.1142/S0218957703001125

[27] Zheng, MH; King, E; Kirilak, Y; et al.: Molecular characterisation of chondrocytes in autologous chondrocyte implantation. Int J Mol Med. 13(5):623 – 628, 2004.

12

Tibial Stress Injuries: Aetiology, Classification, Biomechanics and the Failure of Bone

M. Franklyn[1] and B. Oakes[2]

[1]*Department of Mechanical Engineering, The University of Melbourne, Melbourne,*
[2]*Cheltenham Sports Medicine Clinic, Cheltenham, Melbourne*
Australia

1. Introduction

Stress fractures (SFs) were originally recognised in 1855 by Breithaupt, a Prussian military surgeon, who noticed that young military recruits suffered painful swelling of the forefoot after long marches (Carlson and Wertz, 1943). Initially called March Fractures, he believed the condition to be inflammatory, but in 1897 the bony nature of the affliction was identified when Stechow performed Roentgen studies on the metatarsals (Carlson and Wertz, 1943).

During World War II, the incidence of March fractures was prominent in new military recruits who were unaccustomed to long route marches with heavy packs (Carlson and Wertz, 1943; Bernstein and Stone, 1944). When the training programme became more intense, it was noticed that the frequency of the injury increased (Bernstein and Stone, 1944; Bernstein et al., 1946). By this time, 'March' fractures were also known as insufficiency, exhaustion, fatigue and creeping fractures (Hullinger, 1944). Although diagnosed in bones other than the metatarsals, they were still called March fractures (Carlson and Wertz, 1943; Hullinger, 1944; Bertram, 1944). The classic military type March fractures, however, are found in the neck and the mid-shaft of the second metatarsal.

Medial Tibial Stress Syndrome (MTSS) was probably first identified in 1913 when Hutchins discovered what he called 'spike soreness' in runners (as they were wearing running spikes). He described it as an area of tenderness in the posteromedial distal tibial region sustained in new athletes learning running techniques, or athletes altering their training regimens. Although there was no name for the injury at the time, Hutchins noticed the involvement of the periosteum and attributed the cause of pain to the flexor digitorum longus (FDL) tibial origin (Hutchins, 1913).

MTSS was not originally recognised as a separate entity to an overt stress fracture (SF) of the tibia, which is not surprising as at the time, patient examination and radiographs were the only clinical tools available for the diagnosis of these injuries. Usually MTSS patients demonstrated no abnormal signs on plane X-rays, but this common observation was due to lack of refinement of the imaging technology available at the time.

Devas (1958) was one of the first clinicians to extensively study tibial SFs and 'shin soreness' in athletes by using clinical observations in conjunction with plane radiographic interpretations. Assuming only one type of injury under study, Devas (1958) described a 'shin soreness type of SF involving a disruption of the periosteum over a varying distance' and described other symptoms i.e. tibial tenderness with soft tissue 'thickening' of the subcutaneous surface of the tibia and periosteal oedema. He also noted that plane radiological changes in this type of so-called SF were either of late onset, or not seen at all.

The term *shin splints* was originally used as a non-specific clinical term to describe distal tibial pain caused by repeated impact in the absence of any other injuries to the region. However, an improved understanding of the aetiology in conjunction with advances in nuclear medicine diagnostic techniques led researchers and clinicians to realise that shin splints, later defined more specifically as MTSS, was a separate condition which could be differentiated from other forms of distal leg pain such as SFs or compartment syndrome.

The distinction between tibial SFs and MTSS was becoming clearer and in 1966, the American Medical Association (AMA) defined the shin splint syndrome as "pain and discomfort in leg from repetitive running on hard surface or forcible excessive use of foot flexors; diagnosis should be limited to musculotendinous inflammations, excluding fatigue fracture or ischemic disorder" (AMA, 1966). It was not until the late 1960s and in the 1970s that a large range of Technitium-99 labelled radiopharmaceuticals were developed (Seibert, 1995), making Triple Phase Bone Scintigraphy (TPBS) available as a diagnostic tool. TPBS was initially believed by some clinicians to be of no advantage in the diagnosis of MTSS as it was claimed that the uptake of radionuclide was related to increased activity of the patient rather than being specific to a particular pathology (Rorabeck et al., 1983; Wallensten, 1983; Allen, 1996). However, abnormal scintigraph findings in patients with clinical signs of MTSS who did not subsequently develop a SF lead to the scintigraph definition of MTSS (Holder and Michael, 1984).

About this time, probably the first comprehensive and now classic clinical study of SFs was published (Matheson et al., 1987). Using plane film radiography coupled with nuclear medicine imaging, the pattern of SFs in athletes was found to differ from military recruits, with the most common SF type in athletes being the tibia (49.9%). This was followed by the tarsus (25.3%), metatarsus (8.8%), femur (7.2%), fibula (6.6%), pelvis (1.6%), sesamoids (0.9%) and lastly, the spine (0.6%). Bilateral stress fractures were observed in 16.6% of the cases. The femoral and tarsal SFs were more frequent in older athletes, whilst the fibula and tibial stress fractures were more common in the younger athletes. Matheson et al. (1987) radiographed 43.3% of these cases at presentation, and only 9.8% were abnormal. They recognised tibial periostitis ('tibial stress syndrome') as a separate entity to a tibial SF. This supported earlier studies such as Mubarak et al. (1982), who found that MTSS was due to periostitis rather than elevated compartment pressure or an overt tibial SF.

In the 1980's, a series of nuclear medicine studies on MTSS was published, leading to more specific diagnostic criteria for the injury. These criteria included recognising that MTSS had a characteristic scintigraphic appearance comprising of an elongated linear deposition of medium intensity radionucleotide along the posterior medial cortex of the tibia (Deutsch et al., 1997; Holder and Michael 1984; Matin, 1988). This differed from the more intense localised fusiform pattern typical of a SF (Matin, 1988), and highlighted that MTSS was a specific injury rather than just a precursor to a SF (Macleod, 1999). Despite these advances in nuclear medicine, MTSS is still used as a generic term for distal tibial pain. However, this perception is changing as more studies are published on the nature of this injury.

2. Diagnosis and classification

2.1 Definitions

From an aetiologic perspective, stress fractures can be divided into two types: insufficiency/pathological fractures and fatigue fractures. An insufficiency fracture occurs when normal loads are applied to bone which has mineral or elastic resistance deficiencies, such as in the case of osteoporosis, where there is a loss of normal bone per unit volume of bone tissue. On the other hand, fatigue fractures develop in normal bone which is exposed to atypical and/or more frequent loading. It is believed that this load alteration causes muscular fatigue, which then results in an altered stress state in the bone, initiating a microfracture. The muscular fatigue assumption is supported by the fact that non-weight bearing bones such as the ribs, humerus, radius and ulna, e.g. in tennis players, can sustain SFs (Devas, 1975; Bruckner, 1998).

Less is known about the aetiology of MTSS. Initially believed to be only tibial periostitis, current evidence indicates it is, at least in many cases, also a bone injury (Johnell et al., 1982; Magnusson et al., 2001; Magnusson et al., 2003, Franklyn et al., 2008). Additionally, clinical data indicates that there is more than one type of MTSS, with specific aetiology and injury mechanisms for each type. This is discussed further later.

2.2 Diagnosis and classification of tibial SFs

All tibial SFs fall into several different categories depending on location and fracture type/injury mechanism (Table 1). This was first recognised by Devas (1975), who initially categorised tibial SFs into two different types, compression and distraction (i.e. tensile) SFs, based on X-ray findings and clinical studies. Tensile tibial SFs were then further subdivided into transverse, oblique and longitudinal fractures.

Tibial SF type	Incidence	Most common age	Most common location
Compression	50%	Children or elderly	Upper third in children or lower third in elderly
Transverse	2.5%	Young adults, particularly physically active ones	Shaft
Oblique	42.5%	Young adults, particularly athletes and military recruits	Lower third
Longitudinal	5%	Mature adults	Shaft

Table 1. Various classifications of tibial stress fractures as defined by their characteristics, incidence and location (reproduced from material contained in Devas, 1975).

Devas found that young active individuals are likely to sustain either transverse or oblique tibial SFs. The transverse SFs, which he observed in the tibial shaft, were prevalent in athletes who performed plyometric activities, e.g. ballet or jumping sports, where powerful plantar-flexion of the foot occurs. He attributed these SFs to the dynamic pull of the calf muscles (Soleus and Gastrocnemius) loading the tibia, causing the tibia to bend and become more convex anteriorly; subsequently producing high tensile stresses on the anterior tibial mid-shaft. On the other hand, Devas (1975) believed oblique SFs of the distal third of the tibia, found in athletes and military recruits, to be the result of bending forces which subject the injury site to excessive tension. He found that the propagation of the oblique crack generally begins at the posteromedial border of the tibia and occurs in conjunction with mild inflammation around the bone and a small swelling on the medial tibia. He also noted that thickening of the cortex may occur around the SF site due to an associated attempted healing periostitis.

Much of Devas's original observations form the basis for the current knowledge regarding SFs. In the current clinical setting, focal tenderness (due to periosteal swelling and probable attempted bone repair with cortical thickening) is the key for diagnosis of a SF. In the tibia, the whole anteromedial surface of the bone is subcutaneous; hence, there may be overt anteromedial subcutaneous pitting oedema on firm digital palpation reflecting the underlying response of the periosteum to micro-fracture formation (Johnell et al., 1982; Matin, 1988). Additionally, there is sometimes linear tenderness along the whole anterior margin of the tibia to which the deep fascia of the leg has a strong attachment for the anterior compartment. The tenderness sometimes also extends to the posteromedial longitudinal tibial margin or border, where the deep fascia also attaches in addition to the origin of the FDL. Medial tenderness may also arise from the medial belly of the Soleus, which is attached to the proximal medial tibial and the deep fascia. Intense localised posteromedial margin tenderness in addition to significant oedema and early callus formation may be palpable in athletes who have a delayed presentation of several weeks.

In addition to the above observations, the clinical exam of a potential tibial SF patient should also include an examination of lower limb alignment and foot types. The presence of foot pronation, and in particular, weak inverter muscles (Hinterman et al., 1998; Oakes, 1993), has been shown to predispose the running athlete's tibia to excessive medial torque during weight bearing, thus potentially altering the stress distribution in the tibia (Figure 1).

2.3 Diagnosis and classification of MTSS

MTSS has been defined as a condition resulting in intermittent pain in the lower extremities, in particular, tibial periostitis associated with a specific scintigraphic appearance (Macleod, 1999; Macleod et al., 1999). Probably the most widely accepted definition of MTSS is a condition comprising of tibial anteromedial surface subcutaneous periostitis in the vicinity of the junction of the middle and distal thirds on the medial border (Holder and Michael, 1984; Macleod, 1999) due to an osteoblastic irritation and stimulation of the periosteum (Deutsch et al., 1997). Oakes proposed that this was also potentially associated with outer cortical bone microfractures (Oakes, 1988).

The research of Holder and Michael (1984), which was later verified by other studies (e.g. Matin, 1988) is used by most medical imaging specialists as the standard reference for the correct definition and diagnosis of MTSS, and was supported by the British Medical Journal (Macleod, 1999). Holder and Michael (1984) described shin splints to be exercise-induced pain and tenderness to palpation along the posterior medial border of the tibia. In a study of 10 patients (5 males and 5 females), they described the injury as:

1. Exercise-induced pain initially relieved by rest and exacerbated by exercise;
2. Usually subacute onset of pain, initially dull and aching;
3. Pain and palpable tenderness along the posterior medial border of the tibia in the distal region of the middle third; diffuse and less focal than with an acute SF;
4. Hindfoot abnormality with heel valgus and excess pronation of the forefoot.

Foot pronation has been consistently identified as a significant risk factor for MTSS (Matheson et al., 1987; Moen et al., 2009), although not in all affected patients. As discussed by Hinterman et al., (1998), individuals with overuse lower limb injuries typically have a 2-4 degrees greater pronation than those with no injuries, although 40-50% of runners with excessive pronation have no overuse injuries.

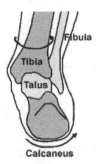

Fig. 1. Posterior view of the right foot. Notice the calcaneal eversion, which is associated with forefoot pronation and principally occurs at the subbtalar and midtarsal joints. This movement of the forefoot is associated with medial tibial rotation.

Using Cybex isometric leg muscle testing, Oakes demonstrated that MTSS patients had weaker inverter muscles than uninjured control subjects. He hypothesised that the weak inverters lead to excessive foot pronation due to eversion of the foot at the subtalar joint and subsequent medial rotation of the tibia (Oakes, 1993). Other authors have supported this injury mechanism (e.g. Hinterman et al., 1998), stating that the tibial rotation leads to injuries on the medial aspect of the tibia. This rotation would result in altered stress distribution in the bone, potentially increasing the tension on the medial border.

In-shoe orthotics can be beneficial for MTSS patients as they attempt to statically raise the medial arch of the foot, thereby preventing excess medial tibial torque or rotation by attempting to minimise forefoot pronation. However, orthotics have not consistently shown to be effective (Craig, 2008), which is not surprising, as not all MTSS patients show excessive pronation. This highlights the importance for the treating physician to identify the type of MTSS and therefore ensure correct management. It also emphasises that medial arch maintenance is mainly under the dynamic muscle control of the tibialis posterior and cannot be corrected optimally in the athlete by the use of simple static medial arch orthotics.

2.4 Nuclear medicine and imaging tibial SFs and MTSS

SFs and MTSS have been classified by both nuclear medicine and by clinical findings. Matin (1988) used a five-stage classification, where the initial two stages are defined as MTSS and the final three stages are a SF (Table 2). It is important to note that although there is bone involvement in Stages I and II, MTSS is not considered to be a precursor to a tibial SF in this system. Accuracies of 75% or greater have been found for scintigraphy (Lieberman and Hemingway, 1980; Allen, 1996; Gaeta et al., 2005), although false positives do occur, thus highlighting the need for a clinical diagnosis in conjunction with nuclear imaging.

Stage of injury	Percentage of bone cross-section involved	Description
I	0-20%	Minimal periosteal reaction
II	20-40%	Moderate periosteal reaction
III	40-60%	Early stress fracture
IV	60-80%	True stress fracture
V	80-100%	Full thickness stress fracture

Table 2. Classification of a stress fracture and MTSS using nuclear medicine techniques (Matin, 1988).

Figure 2 demonstrates a TPBS image from a patient showing three features of interest: a SF of the fourth metatarsal, MTSS, and bone bruising (i.e. increased bone oedema due to greater water content as a result of bone micro-damage or micro-fracture) of the calcaneus, where the patient had pronounced clinical symptoms of the SF and MTSS. The focal uptake at the location of the SF and the diffuse uptake at the MTSS site are readily apparent. Although the uptake at the calcaneus is considerable, the patient only experienced periodic mild tenderness at this site.

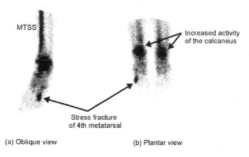

Fig. 2. Patient scintigraph illustrating three conditions (1) MTSS, (2) stress fracture of the fourth metatarsal and (3) mildly symptomatic bone bruising of the calcaneus.

Based on extensive clinical observations, Oakes (1988) proposed there were two distinct types of MTSS, where they can occur in isolation, or in conjunction to form a third type:
1. Tenderness on the distal tibia which when overt, can result in subcutaneous oedema or periostitis on the anteromedial surface of the distal third of the tibia. He proposed this was a result of tibial flexion from contraction of the two heads of the Gastrocnemius and the Soleus muscle causing tibial bending moments during the push-off stage of running. This type of MTSS subsequently results in microtrauma (microcracks between Haversian systems or osteons) to the underlying cortical superficial cortical bone and potentially a tibial SF at the thinnest tibial profile (i.e. the lowest tibial total cortical cross-sectional area).
2. Posteromedial linear pain and tenderness, predominantly due to the strong deep fascia of the posterior calf muscle compartment attaching to the linear posteromedial border of the tibia, but also from the tibial origin of the FDL. The cause of this longitudinal pain is tension in the tibial attachment of the deep fascia in conjunction with the origins of the powerful action of the Gastrocnemius and Soleus muscles proximally.
3. A combination of the above seen in serious long and middle distance runners.
As discussed further later, the authors have observed that some cases of MTSS may lead to a tibial SF, while most cases will not.

In two complementary studies, the first involving ten athletic patients diagnosed with MTSS by a TPBS and the second where anatomical dissection was performed on the lower limb of fourteen cadavers; Holder and Michael (Holder and Michael, 1984; Michael and Holder, 1985) found both pain and abnormal tracer accumulation were present at the origin of the Soleus. This study supports the Soleus involvement in MTSS, although Holder and Michael believed this to be the only cause of the injury. They further postulated the periosteal irritation stimulated afferent pain nerve fibres and activated an osteoblastic response. This can be observed clinically from distal tibial tenderness, and possibly oedema, over the subcutaneous surface of the tibia.

Matin (1988) attributed the bony changes in MTSS to the insertion of Sharpey's fibres. He suggested that abnormal stress on the Sharpey's fibres not only led to the periosteal reaction with an elongated radionucleotide pattern, but also resulted in increased bone remodelling. He further postulated that Sharpey's fibres, which originate from muscles and other fasciae, increase stress on the superficial region of the tibial cortex as the fibres extend through the periosteum into the mineralised bone matrix of the outer circumferential cortical lamellae.

Radiographic findings are likely to be absent in the case of MTSS (Matin, 1988; Deutsch et al., 1997) with some clinicians stating they will always be radiographically occult (Matin, 1988). As opposed to a TPBS where bone turnover/remodelling is positively imaged due to increased bone vascularity, radiography relies on bone density changes for visualisation of pathology. Therefore, a tibial SF will be several millimetres in length and thus provides sufficient density contrast for radiographic visualisation, but only with optimal imaging conditions required for 'early' SF identification. On the other hand, even when MTSS is associated with microfractures, it is likely that they will never be large enough to be visible on plane radiography.

More recently, CT and MRI have been used to classify both SFs (Bergman and Fredericson, 1999; Deutsch et al., 1997; Feydy et al., 1998; Matin, 1988; Reeder et. al., 1996) and MTSS (Matin, 1988; Deutsch et al., 1997; Beck, 1998; Bergman and Fredericson, 1999). The main advantage of CT is that it provides a good delineation of fine bone detail (Feydy et al., 1998) so both SFs and partial SFs can be more easily observed. Unlike X-ray scans, cross-sectional images are possible using CT as this imaging modality uses a large number of X-ray beams to reconstruct a slice of bone. However, like radiography, the fracture line cannot always be observed readily as visualisation of the fracture line depends critically on the views imaged.

Fredericson et al. (1995) first reported MRI to be significantly better than other techniques for the early diagnosis of tibial and other SFs. They performed a study on 14 runners with 18 symptomatic legs within 10 days of referral for radiology. A TPBS and an MRI exam were also performed and the three imaging modes were compared. From this small number of patients, they concluded that MRI was more sensitive and more accurate in its correlation with the clinical symptoms and signs than a TPBS.

The main limitation with MRI is the lack of sensitivity in the assessment of cortical bone. Although Fredericson et al. (1995) found MRI to be superior to other imaging techniques in their 1995 study, SFs are often present without the fissure being observable, and the absence of a fracture line is considered a negative diagnosis (Bergman and Fredericson, 1999). The main advantages with MRI are that the patient is not subjected to ionising radiation and soft tissue changes can be easily depicted (Deutsch et al., 1997) as well as 'bone-bruising'. However, like TPBS, positive MRI images are possible in the absence of clinical symptoms (Kiuru et al., 2005). Additionally, oedema visible on MRI can be due to other conditions e.g. osteomyelitis.

In the original MRI study by Fredericson et al. (1995), the images were graded into four groups (Table 3). This was further modified by Pomeranz (2011) by dividing Group 4 into two separate categories: Group 4a (partial cortical fracture) and Group 4b (complete cortical fracture.

Grade	Clinical Exam	MRI
1	Periosteal tenderness at the distal 1/3-1/2 of the anteromedial tibial surface. Requires **firm** palpation with thumb.	Periosteal oedema: mild to moderate on T2 weighted images. Marrow normal on T1 and T2-weighted images.
2	Tenderness as above. Requires **less firm** palpation with thumb & may have linear tenderness along the posteromedial tibial border.	Periosteal oedema: moderate to severe on T2 weighted images. Marrow oedema on STIR or T2-weighted images. T1 normal.
3	Tenderness as above. Requires **less firm** palpation and may have linear tenderness as above. May have subcutaneous anteromedial tibial oedema.	Periosteal oedema: moderate to severe on T2 weighted images. Marrow oedema on T1 & STIR-T2-weighted images.
4	Tenderness as above. Requires **less firm** palpation and may have linear tenderness as above. A discrete region of maximal tenderness/thickening (early callus formation) over the fracture site will be palpable. Obvious tibial subcutaneous oedema is usually present.	Periosteal oedema: moderate to severe on T2 weighted images. Marrow oedema on T1-STIR or T2-weighted FS images. Fracture line clearly visible as low fuzzy incomplete (4a) or complete (4b) line. May see oedema in proximal tibial origins of Tibialis Posterior, FDL and Soleus.

Table 3. Modified by Oakes from Fredericson et al. (1995) and Pomeranz (2011).

As shown by the categories in Table 3, MRI can be used for the early detection of periosteal oedema, which is a reflection of microcracks between and through the Haversian systems in cortical bone in the region subjected to excessive repetitive loading. Fredericson et al. (1995) noted that the average marrow oedema extended over 5.2 cm and penetrated the outer one third of the marrow diameter. This indicated endosteal oedema as well as periosteal oedema.

For the managing physician, MRI can also be used to determine rehabilitation protocols and return to activity time without fear of reoccurance of a further episode of disabling bone pain due to inappropriate premature activity by often over-enthusiastic athletes, especially high-earning athletes. The soft-tissue sensitivity in detecting oedema due to microfractures can be used to determine the level of injury, as the extent of the bone oedema is a direct reflection of the strain damage to the tibial cortical bone. As a guide, Grade 1 injuries may be able to return to activity within 4-6 weeks if the aetiology of their stress reaction or SF is rectified. The most severe injuries, Grade 4a and 4b, can take as long or even longer to heal than the more conventional tibial fractures depending on the cause. For example, if the patient has poor biomechanical lower limb alignment coupled with excessive pronation due to unilateral weak inverter muscle groups (i.e. Tibialis Anterior and Posterior), 12 weeks or more might be needed for full recovery as the muscles will need strengthening prior to full safe return to activity or competition. Shoe orthotics can be beneficial in partial prevention of excess forefoot pronation and therefore excess medial tibial torque or rotation; however, the weak inverter musculature must also be addressed as outlined above.

2.5 Differential diagnosis

As a positive scintigraph is a non-specific finding (i.e. fracture lines cannot be observed) and MRI has a number of limitations, a differential diagnosis should be considered:

1. Insufficiency fracture: described earlier, in this case the bone has normal loading or low-level repetitive loading but is weak due to loss of bone mass, mineral or elastic resistance. The prime aetiological cause is osteoporosis (i.e. a loss of normal bone volume), and it should be considered as a potential diagnosis, particularly in older female patients.

2. Anterior tibial compartment syndrome: this condition is not common; however, it should be suspected when the pain is localised to the proximal anterior muscle compartment following intense exercise. This injury is aggravated by impact exercise and relieved when the exercise ceases. A measurement of compartment pressure during leg exercise can be used to confirm this diagnosis.

3. Popliteal artery entrapment syndrome (rare): muscle ischaemia from stenosis of the popliteal artery, which may pass through the medial head of Gastrocnemius. As with anterior tibial compartment syndrome, this condition also worsens during exercise. Dopler flow studies of the popliteal artery may help confirm the diagnosis prior to the use of femoral artery angiography.

4. Tibial tumours: Both benign and malignant tumours are possible. These tumours can usually be identified by X-ray; therefore, in order to exclude bone tumour, X-ray should be performed prior to scintigraphy.

5. Bone infection/osteomyelitis: This should be suspected in young athletes, especially if it involves the proximal tibial epiphysis. MRI can be used to establish the diagnosis and its exact location and extent.

Clinical symptoms and patient history should be used in conjunction with medical imaging for correct diagnosis of these injuries.

3. Mechanics of the tibia and bone failure

Numerous risk factors have been associated with tibial SFs (e.g. Burr, 1997; Bennell et al., 1999; Brukner et al., 2000), and to a lesser extent, MTSS (e.g. Moen et al., 2009). As these have been extensively published in the literature, they are not discussed here. The following sections focus on the biomechanical cortical bone parameters relating to tibial stress injuries, bone failure under various loading conditions, and *in-vivo* tests on humans and animals.

3.1 Tibial cortical bone parameters

The preponderance of the literature on cortical bone parameters originates from research on Israeli and US military recruits, with some studies having been performed on athletes. Most of this work has focused on male rather than female populations; hence the significant bone geometry related factors in females are less well understood. In male military cohorts, parameters which have been associated with tibial SFs include a narrow mediolateral (ML) width at the narrowest tibial cross-section (Giladi et al., 1991; Giladi et al., 1987) and small diaphyseal dimensions relative to body weight (Beck et al., 1996). In both male military cohorts and male athletes, a low cortical bone cross-sectional area (Beck et al., 1996; Crossley et al., 1999; Franklyn et al., 2008), small second moments of area (Milgrom et al., 1989;

Franklyn et al., 2008) and a small section modulus (Beck et al., 1996; Franklyn et al., 2008) have been associated with increased tibial SF risk.

A major limitation with many of these studies is that only basic cross-sectional dimensions have been measured from the images, and when they are then used to calculate parameters such as the cross-sectional area, introduce significant error for an irregularly shaped object such as a tibial section. Additionally, in some instances, the correct mechanical parameter has not been measured. This is most obvious in the case of the section modulus, which is often described as the cross-sectional area divided by the half-width of the cross-section. Lastly, using a formula to approximate tibial cross-sections to a shape such as en ellipse introduces a similar error; this error is compounded by the fact that tibial cross-sections can differ considerably from subject to subject (Figure 3).

Using a sample of 130 tibial CT cross-sections derived from a population of athletic and sedentary subjects, both male and female, Franklyn (2004) demonstrated that for irregularly-shaped sections such as tibial cross-sections, use of a formula involves a highly statistically significant degree of error. In this study, a series of cross-sectional parameters were calculated using various formulae from the literature and compared to the values of the parameter computed numerically by a validated code. For example, Milgrom et al. (1989) used a formula to calculate second moments of area about two planes; these moments are cross-sectional properties related to bending strength. Franklyn (2004) found that the formula for the second moment of area about the ML axis resulted in an overestimation by 1.09 (p = 3.15E-19), while the formula for the second moment of area about the anteroposterior (AP) axis resulted in an underestimation of 1.23 (p = 9.87E-32) when compared to the values of parameters computed numerically, with the error being larger for bigger sections. Other formulae in the literature tested resulted in similar levels of error. As these errors depend on both the parameter and the formula used, there was no one mathematical transformation which could be used to correct these values for all cross-sectional parameters.

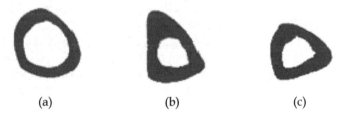

(a)   (b)   (c)

Fig. 3. Normal variation observed in cross-sections of the human tibia at the same cross-sectional level (a) elliptical, (b) triangular and (c) a hybrid of both shapes.

If basic methods are used to calculate tibial parameters, the error introduced is generally not a problem if, for example, cross-sectional areas are compared between groups of subjects within a specific study. However, problems arise when specific values need to be compared (i.e. values compared between two different studies) or the magnitude of the parameter is needed to better understand the injury mechanisms. It introduces doubt as to whether, for instance, an accurate cross-sectional area or section modulus is actually being calculated. Conclusions drawn from a particular study should be considered in light of the error implicit in the method used.

A further concern is the type of imaging modality used to scan the bone. Some imaging types, e.g. DEXA (Dual Energy X-ray Absorptiometry), have poor cortical bone resolution, but the technique has previously been used in a number of military or marine studies to calculate bone dimensions (e.g. Beck et al., 1996). DEXA was designed for bone mineral density (BMD) computation; hence dimensions measured from these images are likely to involve considerable error. DEXA can be used to directly compute geometric properties, but this technique also has error: a series of scan lines is performed through the bone at a specific cross-section, producing a profile of bone content in that section. For each line, the bone content is summed over the region; hence the distribution of bone cannot be determined (see Figure 4).

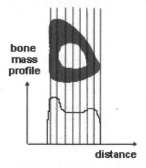

Fig. 4. DEXA uses a series of scan lines to produce a profile of bone content.

In order to overcome some of the abovementioned limitations, the current authors examined tibial geometry in athletes using CT imaging in conjunction with numerical methods to compute the true mechanical parameters (Franklyn et al., 2008). Bone geometry of MTSS patients was also analysed in order to make comparisons with the tibial SF patients. These results are discussed in detail later.

4. Bone alterations due to injury

It is now evident that MTSS involves alterations to at least the cortical bone of the tibia (Johnell et al., 1982; Magnusson et al., 2001; Magnusson et al., 2003; Franklyn et al., 2008; Murrihy, 2009), although whether the trabecular bone is also involved is unknown. This was first evident in the study by Johnell et al. (1982), where cortical bone and soft tissue biopsies were obtained from control (non-injured) patients and patients with chronic MTSS. The MTSS patients, who had one month's rest prior to the biopsies, were diagnosed by patient history and clinical examination in conjunction with radiography to exclude those with a stress fracture (scintigraphy was not widely available at the time).

Johnell et al. (1982) found there were no bone or inflammatory changes in any of the control subjects, while patients with MTSS had alterations such as increased osteoblastic activity at the medial surface of the tibia (where the biopsies were performed) and vascular ingrowth in conjunction with the soft tissue inflammatory changes. These findings were consistent with nuclear medicine studies at the time which demonstrated that MTSS patients had positive scintigraphy, indicating changes in bone metabolism (Matin, 1988). However, not all bone biopsies demonstrated changes: from a total of 35 cortical bone biopsies, 22 specimens had at least one sign of bony changes, but 13 did not. Consequently, they concluded that microfractures were a cause of MTSS, but not necessarily in all cases.

In other research performed since this time, BMD and cortical bone geometry in MTSS and tibial SF patients have been examined. These studies provide corroboration that MTSS involves alterations to the cortical bone, at least in many cases of MTSS, but not necessarily identical changes to those seen in tibial SF patients.

4.1 Bone mineral density in tibial SF and MTSS patients

In previous studies, BMD has been found to not differ between tibial SF patients and exercising controls subjects in most cases. This has been shown in male military recruits (Giladi et al., 1991; Milgrom et al., 1989), male marine recruits (Beck et al., 2000), male athletes (Crossley et al., 1999) and female athletes (Bennell et al, 1999). However, BMD differences have been found between female marine recruits with and without a tibial SF, (Beck et al., 2000). Nevertheless there is strong evidence to suggest the differences found in female subjects are due to hormonal effects such as menstrual irregularities or use of oral contraceptives (Myburg et al., 1990).

There are only a few studies where BMD has been analysed in MTSS patients. Magnusson et al. (2001) measured BMD in 18 male athletes sustaining clinically and scintigraphy-diagnosed MTSS, 18 competitive athletic controls (exercising 3-15 hours/week) and 16 control subjects who exercised at the non-professional level (0 to 5 hours per week). The authors demonstrated that at the injury site, male athletes with chronic MTSS had localised decreased BMD, and this reduction was bilateral even when the injury was unilateral. Additionally, they found that BMD normalises after recovery from the injury (Magnusson et al., 2003). At other sites of the tibia, the MTSS patients had higher BMD than the control group but lower BMD than the athletic control group.

The Magnusson study was limited by several factors. Firstly, subjects in the control group performed some exercise and were comprised of both manual and non-manual workers; hence they were not a true sedentary control group. A second limitation was the large range in number of hours of exercise per week, and both control groups contained a combination of subjects with manual and sedentary occupations; hence the groups were not uniform with regards to exposure. It is known that BMD increases due to impact exercise (e.g. Etherington et al., 1996), but these results show that BMD is reduced at the injury site in MTSS patients. It is likely that the reduced BMD is not inherent but develops in conjunction with the symptoms.

Differences in BMD at the injury site have not only been found between (male) MTSS and non-injured control subjects, but also between (female) MTSS and SF patients at the injury site. The authors of this chapter measured BMD from DEXA scans on 5 SF patients ($n = 10$ scans) and 10 MTSS patients ($n = 20$ scans), all of whom performed impact exercise a minimum of 3 to 4 times per week and had a minimum training history of 2 years (study criteria was described in Franklyn et al., 2008). All scans were performed at the same medical clinic with a Norland XR-36 scanner (Norland Medical Systems Inc.), and each subject was scanned in three regions 2.1 cm in length. Although only a small number of subjects, it was found that MTSS patients had significantly lower localised BMD (1.46 g/cm^2) than tibial SF patients (1.63 g/cm^2) at the injury site, but not at sites in the proximal and distal tibia (Table 4 and Figure 5).

Hence, from these studies, it can be concluded that male MTSS patients have localised low BMD at the injury site compared to non-injured exercising controls, and the BMD returns to normal after the symptoms have resolved. Also, at the injury site, female MTSS patients have lower BMD than female tibial SF patients. As subjects with a tibial SF have been shown to have normal BMD, MTSS patients clearly have reduced BMD at the injury site.

BMD (g/cm²)	SF (n = 10)	MTSS (n = 20)	Significance
Proximal	1.2757	1.2139	0.136
33% level (injury site)	1.6354	1.4598	0.013[a]
Distal	0.9439	0.9023	0.403

[a] Statistically significant p < 0.05

Table 4. Statistical analysis of BMD in female tibial SF and MTSS patients (Oakes and Franklyn, 1998).

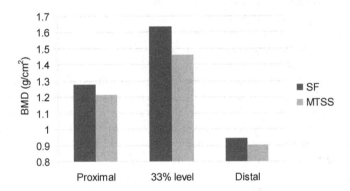

Fig. 5. BMD in female tibial SF and MTSS patients at three tibial sites (Murrihy, 2009).

4.2 Bone geometry in tibial SFs and MTSS patients

It has been shown that tibial SF and MTSS athletes have lower values of some cortical bone geometrical properties when compared to uninjured aerobic control subjects (Franklyn et al., 2008). These findings may imply that MTSS and tibial SFs are a continuum of injury, with MTSS being the precursory state of a tibial SF, and some researchers and clinicians believe this is the case. However, it is the belief of the authors that tibial SFs and MTSS are two separate injuries with some common aetiology and mechanisms. This is probably most strongly evidenced by the fact that not all cases of MTSS lead to a tibial SF. If they were one injury on a continuum, all MTSS patients would eventually sustain a tibial SF with continued exposure to the same impact forces, yet this does not occur. Additionally, tibial SFs are a localised injury whereas MTSS is diffuse. Lastly, it has never been demonstrated that MTSS and tibial SFs fall on a continuum of injury.

The results of the study by Franklyn et al. (2008) showed that the tibiae of male athletes with a tibial SF or MTSS have less cortical bone cross-sectional area (A) than uninjured athletes, resulting in lower values of some other mechanical parameters such as the polar moment of area (J), the maximum and minimum second moments of area (I_{max} and I_{min} respectively) and the section modulus (Z). These mechanical parameters determine the strength of a beam, such as bone, under different types of loading (see Table 5).

Parameter	Symbol	Type of loading it represents
Cross-sectional area	A	Axial loading
Polar moment of area	J	Torsion
Maximum second moment of area	I_{max}	Maximum bending rigidity
Minimum second moment of area	I_{min}	Minimum bending rigidity
Section modulus	Z	Pure bending

Table 5. Geometric parameters with engineering denotations and meanings.

Thus, injured males are less adapted to axial loading, torsion, maximum and minimum bending rigidity and pure bending (a state where there are no axial, shear or torsional forces). The lower values of these parameters in the injured males were due to less cortical bone in the medullary region (primarily in the AP medullary region) rather than from differences in external tibial widths. These results suggest that in males, cortical bone loss occurs from the medullary region prior to, or as a result of, these injuries.

In this study discussed above (Franklyn et al., 2008), it was found that females with a tibial SF or MTSS had smaller section moduli than uninjured females, but as other cross-sectional parameters did not differ, it was not due to less cortical bone area. Instead, injured females are less adapted to pure bending, but the results show that this occurs by a redistribution of the cortical bone about the centroid (centre of mass) so that bending forces are less tolerated by the tibia. Figure 6 shows typical tibial cross-sections from injured male and female subjects compared to uninjured control subjects.

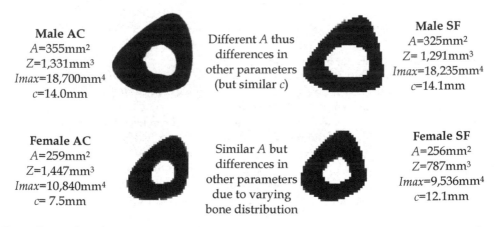

Male AC
A=355mm²
Z=1,331mm³
$Imax$=18,700mm⁴
c=14.0mm

Different A thus differences in other parameters (but similar c)

Male SF
A=325mm²
Z= 1,291mm³
$Imax$=18,235mm⁴
c=14.1mm

Female AC
A=259mm²
Z=1,447mm³
$Imax$=10,840mm⁴
c= 7.5mm

Similar A but differences in other parameters due to varying bone distribution

Female SF
A=256mm²
Z=787mm³
$Imax$=9,536mm⁴
c=12.1mm

Fig. 6. Examples of typical male and female cross-sections from the mid-distal junction of the tibia showing the characteristic differences in geometry AC = aerobic control.

In mechanics, Z is a measure of a specific type of bending (pure bending). It depends on both the amount of material (cortical bone area) as well as its distribution, and is defined as:

$$Z = I_{max} / c$$

where c is the distance from the centre of mass to the outmost fibre of the cross-section (on the anterior border or tensile side). This outermost point is important as it is where the stress is highest under bending and therefore where failure is predicted to occur. If Z is larger, the structure can support a greater load under bending. This can occur due to a higher value of I_{max} (due to more bone) or lower value of c (the bone is closer to the centre of mass). In the study by Franklyn et al. (2008), the lower values of Z in the injured males were predominately due to lower values of I_{max}, whereas in the females, it was from higher values of c, consistent with the fact that injured males had less cortical bone area, but injured females had a different bone distribution less favourable for bending forces.

Alterations in bone shape can occur as osteoblasts in the periosteum create compact bone around the external bone surface while osteoclasts in the endosteum remove bone on the internal medullary cavity. Two mechanisms in which bone can adapt to mechanical loading have been proposed in the literature: (1) periosteal expansion (reshaping) and (2) redistribution of bone mineral from trabecular to cortical components (Adami et al., 1999), although the validity of the former has been disputed (Jarvinen et al., 1999). Although not a longitudinal study, the results from Franklyn et al. (2008) suggest in injured males, cortical bone could be lost to trabecular bone either before or during the injury, whereas in females, cortical reshaping may occur in conjunction with the injury. It is difficult to hypothesise further on these mechanisms; however, it is apparent that longitudinal studies examining cortical bone alterations prior to and during injury progression are needed.

4.3 Conclusions on bone characteristics and tibial stress injuries

These more recent studies on cortical bone and tibial stress injuries clearly demonstrate MTSS is, in many cases, an injury involving microfractures in the cortical bone in addition to low BMD, and cortical bone geometry which is less adapted to some mechanical modes of failure such as bending. Matin (1988) suggested that in MTSS patients, the deposition of radionuclide around the injured region was due to the response of the periostium to the developing abnormality in the cortical bone. However, he also proposed that abnormal stress on the Sharpey's fibres from the tissues increases stress on the outer circumferential lamellae of cortical bone, implying the tissue response may occur first. It seems unclear as to whether the cortical bone alterations occur before the inflammatory response of the tissue. In cases of MTSS which do not involve microfractures (Oakes Type II), the periosteal response would have to be due to, or a result of, a factor other than bone microfractures.

Most previous studies have shown BMD does not differ between uninjured control subjects and tibial SF patients. However, patients sustaining MTSS have reduced BMD at the site of the injury, and lower BMD than tibial SF patients at the injury site (consistent with tibial SF patients having normal BMD). This provides further evidence that MTSS and tibial SFs are two distinct injuries. Both MTSS and tibial SF patients have cortical bone geometry which is less adapted to dynamic mechanical loads imparted by the musculature. In males, there is less cortical bone area, which results in a decreased ability to tolerate different loading conditions such as axial load, torsion and various bending loads. In injured females, cortical bone area is not affected but there is decreased ability to tolerate pure bending. More work is needed in this area as there is a lack of longitudinal studies to provide more information on cortical bone changes and development of both MTSS and tibial SFs.

5. Cortical bone failure and fatigue

5.1 Bone as an engineering material

Bone is composed of two types of osseous tissue: cortical bone and trabecular bone, where the main distinction between the two is the density and the degree of porosity (Carter and Hayes, 1977). Compared to trabecular bone, cortical bone is quite stiff. Hence it is able to endure greater stress (force per unit area) but less strain (deformation) before failure. On the other hand, trabecular bone can withstand greater deformation before failure, and as a result, has a large capacity for energy storage (Keaveny and Hayes, 1993). In a long bone, a SF occurs in cortical bone as this tissue type is subjected to higher stresses, particularly around the external or superficial surface. Under the right conditions, this eventually leads to cracks (failure).

In engineering, materials can be classified as ductile i.e. have the ability to deform, such as in a soft metal, or brittle i.e. breaks with little deformation, for example, glass. As shown in Figure 7, each type of material has a typical fracture type: a ductile material has a characteristic 'cup and cone' fracture shape, while a brittle material has little yield and then fractures at an oblique angle.

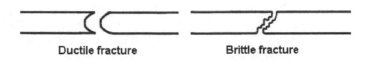

Ductile fracture   **Brittle fracture**

Fig. 7. Typical fractures of a ductile material and a brittle material.

Cortical bone does not act like a typical engineering material; it fractures in an oblique plane like a brittle material, but it also displays ductile behaviour. In addition, cortical bone demonstrates anisotropic properties i.e. the properties vary in different directions. For example, when subjected to tension transversely, cortical bone displays brittle behaviour, while if it is subjected to tension longitudinally, it appears to be ductile. Therefore, the type of behaviour depends on the loading conditions and the bone microstructure.

Although mechanical failure theories can be used to understand bone behaviour, like most biological materials, cortical bone exhibits unique characteristics that are different to standard engineering materials, and as such there are no mechanical theories of failure. Additionally, as the skeleton is subjected to complex loading conditions, it can be difficult to predict when and where failure will occur.

5.2 The biological basis for bone failure

According to the clinical evidence presented by Burr (1997), the most likely biological explanation for the initiation and/or propagation of a stress fracture is adaptive bone remodelling. This strain-mediated process is outlined below:

1. The stress is applied to the bone;
2. Osteoclastic resorption, which occurs as a part of the normal bone remodelling process, creates a reabsorption space that increases the bone porosity, reduces bone mass and exponentially decreases bone strength and stiffness. Osteoclasts reabsorb areas of bone, thereby forming hollow channels;
3. There is less bone, hence the strains on remaining bone increase;
4. The increased stress on the bone causes a new remodelling cycle to commence.

At Stage IV, there are two possibilities (Matin, 1988). First, the bone is allowed to rest so that osteoblastic bone regeneration can occur, with more dense bone replacing the lost bone so that the stress site is strengthened. Alternatively, at Stage IV, if there is no rest, the bone becomes weaker after the period of strain and resorption. This leads to the individual bone trabeculae eventually collapsing, subsequently causing microfractures in the bone which then may eventually lead to an overt SF.

In the initial osteoblastic stage, immature bone is laid down and eventually matures over time. Johnson (1963) found that it takes 90 days to fill a reabsorption space with mature bone. According to Reeder et al. (1996), the cross-sectional area decreases during this time period, which consequently subjects the bone to a potentially higher local stress. As a result, it is probable that the weakened state of the bone during the 90-day reparative period is when the bone is most susceptible to an injury such as a SF. Robling et al. (2001) demonstrated the importance of recovery time in restoring mechanosensitivity (i.e. the capability of sensing and responding to mechanical forces) to bone cells. Loading rat bones *in situ* using a four-point bending apparatus, tissue histology was examined when the rats were killed at various days after the loading commenced. They found that approximately 8 hours of recovery was required in the rat tibia to restore full mechanosensitivity to the cells after the cells had been desensitised from the application of repetitive mechanical loads for an extended period.

The theory outlined above is supported by other research. For example, Li et al. (1985) conducted an experiment where 20 rabbits were induced to run and jump by subjecting them to an electrical impulse at various intervals for a period of 60 days. Using radiographic and histological analyses on this group and a control (non-exercising) group, the authors found that osteoclastic reabsorption occurred before the presence of any cracks in the cortical bone. Furthermore, only some rabbits developed cracks in the bone after the period of exercise, suggesting that in the majority of cases, the rabbit tibiae adapted to changes in the applied stress.

Martin et al. (1997) performed a study *ex vivo* on deceased racehorses using the common SF site of the third metacarpal. Using the contralateral bone as a control, they found that if three-point cyclic bending loads were applied to the right bone for as many cycles as a racehorse would experience during its training and racing lifetime, then the elastic modulus and yield strength were not affected. This suggested that equine bone was not weakened by this loading *ex vivo*, and that SFs are not simply fatigue failure, but a result of the inability of the repair mechanism (remodelling) to sustain a level of equilibrium with the damage produced by fatigue. This implies that another mechanism, such as adaptive bone remodelling, is involved in SF development *in vivo*.

5.3 Fatigue failure in cortical bone specimens

In mechanics, ductile materials generally fail from a tensile load rather than a compressive load. Similarly, bone can withstand greater loads under compression than under tension; therefore, bone generally fails due to tensile stress. Hence, under *static* bending of a symmetrical specimen, bone will yield from tensile stresses rather than compressive stresses as bone is weaker in tension (Evans, 1957).

Currey and Brear (1974) tested cortical bone specimens under (non-fatigue) loading at different strain rates; some of the samples were subjected to compressive loads, while others were subjected to different types of bending loads. They demonstrated that cortical bone can fail under both tension and compression, but the modes of failure differed. When cortical bone is compressed longitudinally, shear lines develop at an angle of approximately 30 degrees with respect to the load line (rather than 45 degrees, as in a normal isotropic material) due to the anisotropy of bone). These shear lines are believed to be due to buckling of the bone lamellae. However, cortical bone under tensile stress does not develop shear lines (Currey and Brear, 1974), but instead tensile lines that show yield (Caler and Carter, 1989).

In mechanics, failure of a structure is often from a time-varying load rather than from a constant load; this type of failure is known as *fatigue failure*. In this case, failure of the structure will occur at a *lower* stress level than would otherwise be the case for a standard static load. Most materials under cyclic loading fail as a result of a crack which develops from *tensile* stress. This crack then leads to stress concentrations, which subsequently initiate unstable crack propagation in the material. Alternatively, cracks will tend to form at any pre-exiting stress concentrator (imperfection) in the material, leading to crack propagation.

This mechanism differs in cortical bone, which fails under both tension and compression, i.e. there are two separate fracture regions, although the tensile failure occurs first. This was demonstrated by Carter and Hayes (1977) and Carter et al. (1981) who found that under cyclic loading, *tensile* loads result in *tensile stresses* which cause failure at osteon cement lines so that the osteons debond from the surrounding interstitial bone. On the other hand, *compressive* loads result in the formation of oblique microcracks along the planes of high *shear stress* before the crack from the tensile load had extended throughout the entire specimen. The shear stress tends to initiate near blood channels (Currey and Brear, 1974), which can act as stress concentrators in bone and therefore initiate crack propagation.

The studies described above do not take into account the remodelling process, which is a critical difference between bone and standard engineering materials. This was examined by Pattin et al. (1996), who studied energy dissipation under fatigue failure. Using human femoral cortical bone specimens, they performed fatigue to fracture testing under different types of cyclic loading. They found that above specific strain thresholds, tensile-loaded fatigue specimens dissipate 6-7 times more energy than compressive loaded fatigue specimens when subjected to the same loading magnitude. These results suggest that bone remodelling may be favoured under tensile load, since more energy is available to activate a remodelling response. This is consistent with other studies showing that SFs occur due to tensile failure.

Failure of cortical bone specimens are also affected by other factors such as the frequency of loading (Caler and Carter, 1989) and the strain range (amplitude). However, the mean strain and maximum strain do not affect the fatigue life (Caler and Carter, 1989; Carter et al., 1981). Compared to most engineering materials, cortical bone has a poor fatigue resistance, but a longer fatigue life than trabecular bone (Carter and Hayes, 1977).

In summary, the fact that cortical bone fails in tension under cyclic loading is not surprising, as according to mechanical engineering theory, tensile loads cause fatigue crack propagation in ductile materials (although bone is neither ductile or brittle). However, it is apparent that bone differs from most mechanical structures in that it demonstrates failure from both tensile and compressive components of a cyclic load, although the tension load will cause failure before the compressive component. Under each of these load types, the mode of failure is different. The bone specimen tests described above can describe the behaviour of cortical bone under load; however, they do not factor bone remodelling, which will influence the number of cycles to failure. Additionally, the applied loading to bone is likely to reduce when a crack initiates as continued loading becomes painful for the individual, consequently leading to a reduction in physical activity.

5.4 Fatigue failure in cortical bone *in-vivo*

Using patient X-rays and clinical examinations, Devas (1975) was probably the first to hypothesise that the tibial SFs which occur in athletes and military recruits, i.e. oblique SFs at the junction of the mid and distal thirds of the tibia, are the result of bending forces subjecting the site to excessive tension. This is a similar mechanism to the Oakes Type I MTSS (Oakes, 1988) mentioned earlier, where he proposed that the gastrocnemius and soleus muscles caused bending moments in the tibia, subsequently resulting in injury at the smallest tibial cross-sectional profile.

Lanyon et al. (1975) bonded a strain gauge rosette to the anteromedial aspect of the tibial midshaft of a 35-year-old human male, measuring the principal strains in the bone (i.e. the maximum and minimum strains, which are the most tensile and the most compressive strains respectively). When the subject was running with shoes, the maximum tensile strain, which occurred during the push-off phase, was greater than the maximal compressive strain, and the tensile strain was in-line with the long axis of the bone. This finding suggests that tibial SFs which occur at the midshaft are due to tensile forces causing tensile stress, and is consistent with the cortical bone specimen experiments mentioned earlier by Carter and Hayes (1977) and Carter et al. (1981), who found that tensile loads result in tensile stresses, which then cause failure at osteon cement lines.

The principal strains from the Lanyon et al. (1975) study were converted into principal stresses by Carter (1978). Carter found that the longitudinal stress on the anteromedial aspect of the tibial midshaft during running was primarily compressive at the heel-strike stage, while during the push-off stage, the longitudinal stress was highly tensile. On the other hand, the transverse and shear stresses were found to be small throughout the entire running gait. This suggests that if bone does fail under tensile stress when subjected to cyclic loading, then loads from the push-off stage are a significant contributor to the development of microcracks which lead to a tibial SF.

Milgrom et al. (1999) attached strain gauges directly to the mid-diaphysis of the medial cortex of the tibia in five male and three female subjects and measured strain magnitude and strain rates. They found that, in general, both strain magnitude and strain rate increased due to muscular fatigue, but values were not presented for different stages of the gait cycle. Similarly, Burr et al. (1996) conducted a study where strain gauges were attached to the medial tibial cortex at both the tibial midshaft and 2 cm distal to the first gauge in two male subjects, although data was only presented for the midshaft. Strains and strain rates where shown to be higher when running than walking, but the phase of the gait cycle producing these strains was again not presented.

5.5 Fatigue failure in cortical bone in animals

A number of experimental studies on rabbit tibiae have been performed to determine the aetiology of stress fractures. In humans, it is ethically difficult to instrument bone then load it until fatigue or injury; however, this is possible in animals.

As mentioned in Section 5.2, Li et al. (1985) conducted an experiment where rabbits were induced to run and jump for approximately 2 hours per day by being subjected to a pulse via an electric cage, where the frequency and period of the pulse was controlled. Radiographic and histological changes in the bone were examined over a 60-day period after sacrificing the exercising rabbits at various stages during the test. Two rabbits were also sacrificed from a control group, the first at the beginning and the second at the conclusion of the experiment. From the radiographs, Li et al. (1985) found that there was a progressive periosteal reaction in 18 of the 20 rabbits, whereas the remaining tibiae showed soft tissue swelling with no radiographical changes (changes were found in 16 tibial mid-shaft, 3 distal and 1 upper third). Osteoclastic reabsorption was evident as early as the seventh day after exercise commenced, but cracks were not visible until the tenth day after loading. The histological analysis demonstrated that cracks developed on the cement lines of the Haversian systems, particularly on the anterior and medial aspects of the tibia, and that fracture lines were subsequently formed by convergence of adjacent cracks from the Haversian systems.

The experiment by Li and colleagues provided *in-vivo* verification of the early cortical bone specimen tests under cyclic loading performed by Carter and Hayes, which were discussed earlier under Section 5.3. Carter and Hayes found that tensile failure occurs first under cyclic loading, and that the tensile stresses caused failure through osteon debonding at the cement lines. Li et al. (1985) did not specify which types of cracks (longitudinal, transverse or oblique) occurred in the different locations of the tibiae. However, they did observe that most cracks occurred in the midshaft, which is consistent with other research to date on tensile stresses and tensile failure at this site.

Burr et al. (1990) applied cyclic loads to the hind limbs of 31 rabbits; one limb was subjected to compressive loads while the other limb acted as a control. The loads were applied using a specifically designed apparatus designed to apply cyclic loading of 1.5 times the body weight of the rabbit to simulate running. SFs were successfully produced in 68% of the rabbits within 6 weeks of loading and were verified by scintigraphy. Burr and colleagues stated that 89% of the SF were in the midshaft (implying that 11% were distal) and 74% were anteromedial; however, it was not clear how many of the midshaft SFs were anteromedial. As rabbit bones are quite small, it would have been difficult to visualise exact locations using scintigraphy. In addition, the rabbits were not under anaesthetic; hence their muscles could involuntary contract. This means that the loading applied to the tibia was not purely compressive as the involuntary contractions apply other loads to the bone such as bending.

Burr's group followed-up the above work with another rabbit experimental study analysing strain rate versus strain magnitude. Strain gauges were bonded to the midshaft and mid-distal third of the medial, lateral and posterior aspects of the tibia, but not the anterior border. The authors concluded that SFs were a result of increased strain rate at the mid-distal third of the tibia; however, the data presented showed that both strain rate and strain magnitude were higher in this location than in the midshaft. Hence, it could not be deduced from the results whether strain magnitude or strain rate is most likely to be associated with tibial SFs, or if both parameters in combination are significant.

6. Computer models of the tibia

More recently, computer models such as Finite Element (FE) models have been developed to examine the stresses in the tibial bone. FE models are advantageous in that the stresses can be analysed in any region of the bone modelled, loading and other boundary conditions can be readily controlled, and unlike human and animal experiments, a large number of loading conditions can be analysed.

In Section 5.5, a rabbit experimental model developed by Burr et al. (1990) was discussed. Burr and colleagues subsequently developed an FE computer model of the rabbit tibia (Burr, 1997; Burr 2001) where compressive loading only was applied. However, there were a number of discrepancies with this model. For example, the model did not have any other loads from the musculature applied other than compression, yet it is probable that the tibia was subjected to other loads such as bending in the rabbit experiments. Additionally, the results of the FE model showed that high compressive stresses occurred on the anterior border of the tibia, yet from clinical research and knowledge of fracture types at this site, SFs on the anterior border are a result of tensile failure due to tensile or bending forces. Lastly, to produce compression on the anterior border, the applied compressive load would need to be significantly anterior to the centroidal axis of the tibia, particularly as the tibia is bent anteriorly and the rabbit leg is partially flexed. However, this is not consistent with the load position being applied to the heel in the experiment.

Using an MTSS patient, Franklyn (2004) developed a human tibial FE model to examine the relationship between ground reaction forces, bone geometry and maximum principal stress (Figure 8). The model was analysed similar to a 'free-body' analysis in engineering, where a section of the tibia was modelled, and the forces acting on the free body (tibial model) were applied. The forces were derived from gait analysis data of ground reaction forces which were then mathematically transposed to the equivalent forces acting on the free body. The major muscle forces were included. The model was then validated using *in-vivo* strain gauge data available in the literature such as the data from Lanyon et al. (1975), although this validation was not extensive due to the lack of *in-vivo* cyclic loading data available in the literature for all regions of the tibia.

The model was analysed using different time steps in the running gait cycle. It was found that the highest magnitude of principal stress was tensile, disperse, located on the external surface of the cortical bone on the medial tibial midshaft and occurs during the push-off stage of the gait cycle. This high stress region was due to a specific combination of high transverse and compressive loads during the latter part of the gait cycle. These findings are all consistent with previous work where bone fails in tension, and the push-off stage of the gait cycle has been shown to result in maximal tensile strain at the midshaft during running (Lanyon et al., 1975). Additionally, cracks have been shown to initially develop on the exterior cortical surface, which is also consistent with mechanical theory, which predicts stresses are greatest on the external surfaces.

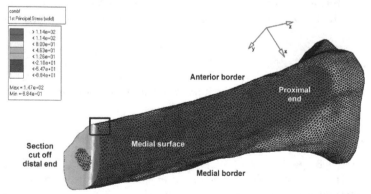

Fig. 8. Tibial FE model of an MTSS patient sectioned at the midshaft. Maximum principal stresses on the medial surface are diffuse and originate from the exterior surface (Franklyn, 2004).

Franklyn (2004) also conducted a preliminary analysis on load versus bone geometry in the FE model to replicate the stress pattern typical of a tibial SF. It was found that a localised SF pattern could not be produced by altering the loads alone, but only by changing the geometry. These results suggest that bone geometry is more influential than loading conditions in the development of tibial SFs and indicate that graded training programmes may be the most effective countermeasure for SF prevention.

7. Conclusion

Current knowledge of the aetiology and mechanics of tibial SF and MTSS development has come from a combination of clinical research, cohort studies, *in-vitro* cortical bone specimen experiments and *in-vivo* tests on both humans and animals. More recently, FE computer models have been used to better understand the relationship between tibial bone geometry, applied loads and stress distribution in the cortical bone.

Although there has been considerable research on the mechanisms behind these injuries, they are still not fully understood. However, a number of conclusions are evident. SFs of the tibial midshaft, which are longitudinal or transverse, arise from tensile and bending loads respectively. These loads produce tensile stresses which cause osteons to debond from the surrounding tissue, resulting in cracks between and through Haversian systems. On the other hand, SFs of the mid-distal junction are oblique; hence they could be due to shear stress and subsequent lamellae buckling from compressive loads, or from tensile stresses in an oblique plane due to torsional load. Clinical findings suggest tensile failure occurs at this site; hence torsional load appears to be a more likely mechanism.

Cortical bone geometry is significantly different between injured patients and non-injured control subjects. It is probable that the bone geometry alters due to impact loading rather than being inherent, but longitudinal studies are needed to determine if bone geometry alters prior to the injury or as a result of the injury. These types of studies may lead to the development of reliable prediction tools for tibial stress injuries.

Despite some common aetiology and mechanisms between tibial SFs and MTSS, it is unlikely that they are one injury on a continuum. However, it is evident that more research is needed in this area, as prevention of these debilitating injuries remains a problem which can affect successful sporting and military careers as well as the large recreational athletic population.

8. Acknowledgements

The authors would gratefully like to thank Jeff Copeland for comments and proofreading this work.

9. References

Adami S., Gatti D., Braga V., Bianchini D. & Rossini M. (1999). Site-specific effects of strength training on bone structure and geometry of unltradistal radius in postmenopausal women. *Journal of Bone and Mineral Research*. Vol 14, No 1, pp. 120-124.

Allen M. J. (1996). Shin pain. In: Hutson M. A. ed. *Sports Injuries. Recognition and Management* (2nd edition). Oxford University Press, pp. 151-154.

AMA: American Medical Association (1966). Committee on the Medical Aspects of Sports, Subcommittee on classification of sports injuries. Standard Nomenclature of Athletic Injuries. Chicago. p 126.

Beck T. J., Ruff C. B., Mourtada F. A., Shaffer R. A., Maxwell-Williams K., Kao G. L., Sartoris D. J. & Brodine S (1996). Dual-energy X-ray absorptiometry derived structural geometry for stress fracture prediction in male U.S. marine corps recruits. *Journal of Bone and Mineral Research.* Vol 11, No 5, pp. 645-653.

Beck T. J., Ruff C. B., Shaffer R. A., Betsinger K. Trone D. W. & Brodine S. K (2000). Stress fracture in military recruits: Gender differences in muscle and bone susceptibility factors. *Bone.* Vol 27, No 3, pp. 437-444.

Bennell K.; Matheson G; Meeuwisse W & Brukner P. (1999). Risk Factors for Stress Fractures. *Sports Medicine.* Volume 28, Number 2, pp. 91-122.

Bergman A. G. & Fredericson M. (1999) MR imaging of stress reactions, muscle injuries, and other overuse injuries in runners. *MRI Clinics in North America.* Vol 7, No 1, pp. 151-174.

Bernstein A., Childers M. A., Fox K. W., Archer M. C. & Stone J. R (1946). March fractures of the foot: Care and management of 692 patients. *American Journal of Surgery.* Vol 71, No 3, pp. 355-362.

Bernstein A. & Stone J. R (1944). March fracture: A report of three hundred and seven cases and a new method of treatment. *The Journal of Bone and Joint Surgery.* Vol 26, No 4, pp. 743-750.

Bertram D. R. (1944) "Stress" fracture of bone. *British Journal of Radiology.* Vol 17, No 200, pp. 257-258.

Brukner P. (1998). Stress Fractures of the Upper Limb. *Sports Medicine,* Volume 26, Number 6, pp. 415-424.

Brukner P., Bennell K. & Matheson G. (2000). Stress Fractures. Blackwell Science.

Burr D. B. (1997). Bone, exercise and stress fractures. *Exercise and Sports Science Reviews.* Vol 25, pp. 171-194.

Burr D. B. (2001). Rabbits as an animal model for stress fractures. In: Burr D. B. and Milgrom C. (Eds.). *Musculoskeletal Fatigue and Stress Fractures.* Boca Raton, CRC Press, Ch 14, pp. 221-232.

Burr D. B., Forwood M. R., Schaffler M. B. & Boyd R. D. (1995). High strain rates are associated with stress fractures. *Transactions of the Orthopaedic Research Society.* Vol 20.

Burr D. B., Milgrom C., Boyd R. D., Higgins W.L., Robin G. & Radin E. L. (1990). Experimental stress fractures of the tibia. Biological and mechanical aetiology in rabbits. *The Journal of Bone and Joint Surgery.* Vol 72-B, No 3, pp. 370-375.

Burr D. B., Milgrom C., Fyhrie D., Forwood M., Nyska M., Finestone A., Hoshaw S., Saiag E. & Simkin A. (1996). In vivo measurement of human tibial strains during vigorous activity. *Bone.* Vol 18, No 5, pp. 405-410.

Caler W. E. & Carter D. R. (1989). Bone creep-fatigue damage accumulation. *Journal of Biomechanics.* Vol 22, No. 6/7, pp. 625-635.

Carlson G. D. & Wertz R. F. (1943). March fracture, including others than those of the foot. *Radiology.* Vol 43, pp. 48-54.

Carter D. R. (1978). Anisotropic analysis of strain rosette information from cortical bone. *Journal of Biomechanics.* Vol 11, No 4, pp. 199-202.

Carter D. R., Caler W. E., Spengler D. M. & Frankel V. H. (1981). Fatigue behaviour of adult cortical bone: The influence of mean strain and strain range. *Acta Orthopaedica Scandinavica*. Vol 52, No 5, pp. 481-490.

Carter D. R. & Hayes W. C. (1977). The compressive behaviour of bone as a two-phase porous structure. *The Journal of Bone and Joint Surgery*. Vol 59, No 7, pp. 954-962.

Craig D. I. (2008). Medial Tibial Stress Syndrome: Evidence-Based Prevention. *Journal of Athletic Training*, 43(3):316–318.

Crossley K., Bennell K. L., Wrigley T. & Oakes B. W. (1999). Ground reaction forces, bone characteristics, and tibial stress fracture in male runners. *Medicine and Science in Sports and Exercise*. Vol 31, No 8, pp. 1088-1093.

Currey J. D. & Brear K. (1974). Tensile yield in bone. *Calcified Tissue Research*. Vol 15, No 3, pp. 173-179.

Deutsch A. L., Coel M. N. & Mink J. H. (1997). Imaging of stress injuries to bone. Radiography, scintigraphy and MR imaging. *Clinics in Sports Medicine*. Vol 16, No 2, pp. 275-290.

Devas M. (1975). *Stress Fractures*. Churchill Livingstone, New York.

Etherington J., Harris P. A., Nandra D., Hard D. J., Wolman R. L., Doyle D. V. and Spector T, D. (1996). The effect of weight-bearing exercise on bone mineral density: A study of female ex-elite athletes and the general population. *J. Bone & Mineral Research*, Vol 11, No 9, pp. 1333 – 1338.

Evans F. G. (1957). *Stress and Strain in Bones. Their Relation to Fractures and Osteogenesis*. Charles C. Thomas.

Feydy A., Drape J.-L., Beret E., Sarazin L., Pessis E., Minoui A. & Chevrot A. (1998). Longitudinal stress fractures of the tibia: Comparative study of CT and MR imaging. *European Radiology*. Vol 8, No 4, pp. 598- 602.

Franklyn M. (2004). Tibial stress injuries in athletes: Mechanical analyses and computer modelling. PhD Thesis, Monash University, Australia.

Franklyn M., Oakes B., Field B., Wells P. & Morgan D. (2008). Section modulus is the optimum geometric predictor for stress fractures and Medial Tibial Stress Syndrome in both male and female athletes. *Am J Sports Med*. Vol 36, No 6, pp. 1179-1189.

Fredericson M., Bergman A. G., Hoffman K. L. & Dillingham M. S (1995). Tibial stress reaction in runners: correlation of clinical symptoms and scintigraphy with a new magnetic resonance imaging grading system. *American Journal of Sports Medicine*. Vol 23, No 4, pp. 472-481.

Gaeta M., Minutoli F., Scribano E., Ascenti G., Vinci S., Brushetta D., Magaudda L. & Blandino A. (2005). CT and MR imaging findings in athletes with early tibial stress injuries: Comparison with bone scintigraphy findings and emphasis on cortical abnormalities. Radiology. Vol 235, No 2, pp. 553 – 561.

Giladi M., Milgrom C., Simkin A. and Danon Y. (1991). Stress fractures: Identifiable risk factors. *The American Journal of Sports Medicine*. Vol 19, No 6, pp. 647-652.

Giladi M., Milgrom C., Simkin A., Stein M., Kashtan H., Margulies J., Rand N., Chisin R., Steinberg R., Aharonson Z., Kedem R. & Frankel V. H. (1987). Stress fractures and tibial bone width: A risk factor. *The Journal of Bone and Joint Surgery*. Vol 69-B, No 2, pp. 326-329.

Hinterman B & Nigg B. M. (1998). Pronation in runners. Implications for injuries. *Sports Medicine*. Vol 26, No 3, pp. 169-176.

Holder L. E. and Michael R. H. (1984). The specific scintigraphic pattern of "shin splints in the lower leg": Concise communication. *Journal of Nuclear Medicine*. Vol 25, No 8, pp. 865-869.

Hullinger C. W. (1944) Insufficiency fracture of the calcaneus: Similar to march fracture of the metatarsal. *The Journal of Bone and Joint Surgery*. Vol 26-A, No 4, pp. 751-757 (1944).

Hutchins C. P. (1913). Explanation of spike soreness in runners. *Am.Phys. Ed. Rev.* 18:31–35.

Jarvinen T. L., Kannus P. & Sievanen H. (1999). Have the DXA-based exercise studies seriously underestimated the effects of mechanical loading on bone? Journal of bone and Mineral Research. Vol 14, No 9, pp. 1634-1635.

Johnell O, Rausing A, Wendeberg B, et al. (1982). Morphological bone changes in shin splints. *Clinical Orthop.* 167: 180–184.

Johnson L. C. (1963). Morphologic analysis in pathology in bone biodymanics. In: Frost H. M. (Editor) *Bone Biodynamics*. Little, Brown and Co, pp. 535-549.

Keaveny T. M. and Hayes W. C. (1993). Mechanical properties of cortical and trabecular bone. *Bone*. Vol 7, pp. 285-344.

Kiuru M. J., Niva M., Reponen A. & Pihlajamaki H. K. (2005). Bone stress injuries in asymptomatic elite recruits. American Journal of Sports Medicine. Vol 33, No 2, pp. 272- 276.

Lanyon L E., Hampson W. G. J., Goodship A. E. & Shah J. S. (1975). Bone deformation recorded in vivo from strain gauges attached to the human tibial shaft. *Acta Orthopaedica Scandinavica*. Vol 46, No 2, pp. 256-268.

Li G., Zhang S., Chen G., Chen H. & Wang A. (1985). Radiographic and histologic analyses of stress fracture in rabbit tibias. *The American Journal of Sports Medicine*. Vol 13, No 5, pp. 285-294.

Lieberman C. M. & Hemingway D. L. (1980). Scintigraphy of shin splints. *Clinical Nuclear Medicine*. Vol 5, No 1, p. 31.

Macleod M. A. (1999). Shin Splints are symptoms, not a diagnosis. Letters, Authors reply to letters from the Editor, *British Medical Journal*. Vol 318, p. 1560.

Macleod M. A., Houston A. S., Sanders L. & Anagnostopoulos C. (1999). Incidence of trauma related stress fractures and shin splints in male and female army recruits: Retrospective case study. *British Medical Journal*. Vol 318, No 7175, p. 29.

Magnusson, H. I., Ahlborg, H. G., Karlsson, C., Nyquist, F., Karlsson, M. K. (2003). Low Regional Tibial Bone Density in Athletes with Medial Tibial Stress Syndrome Normalizes after Recovery from Symptoms. *Am J Sports Med* Vol 31, pp 596-600

Magnusson, H. I., Westlin, N. E., Nyqvist, F., Gardsell, P., Seeman, E., Karlsson, M. K. (2001). Abnormally Decreased Regional Bone Density in Athletes with Medial Tibial Stress Syndrome. *Am J Sports Med* Vol 29, pp 712-715.

Matheson G. et al. (1987). Stress fractures in athletes. A study of 320 cases. Am J Sports Medicine. Vol 15, No 1, pp 46-58.

Martin R. B., Gibson V. A., Stover S. M., Gibeling J. C. & Griffin L. V. (1997). Residual strength of equine bone is not reduced by intense fatigue loading: Implications for stress fracture. *Journal of Biomechanics*. Vol 30, No 2, pp. 109-114.

Matin P. (1988). Basic principles of nuclear medicine techniques for detection and evaluation of trauma and sports medicine injuries. *Seminars in Nuclear Medicine*. Vol 18, No 2, pp. 90-112.

Michael R. H. and Holder L. E. (1985). The soleus syndrome: A cause of medial tibial stress (shin splints). *Am. J. Sports Med*. Vol 13, No. 2, pp. 87-94.

Milgrom C., Finestone A., Ekenman I., Larsson E., Nyska M., Millgram M., Mendelson S., Simkin A., Benjuya N. & Burr D. (1999). Tibial strain rate increases following muscular fatigue in both men and women. *Orthopaedic Research Society, 45th Annual Meeting*, February 1-4, p. 234, California.

Milgrom C., Giladi M., Simkin A., Rand N., Kedem R., Kashtan H., Stein M. & Gomori M. (1989). The area moment of inertia of the tibia: A risk factor for stress fractures. *Journal of Biomechanics*. Vol 22, No 11/12, pp. 1243-1248.

Moen M. H., Tol J. L., Weir A., Steunebrink R. & De Winter T. C. (2009). Medial tibial stress syndrome. A critical review. *Sports Medicine*. Vol 39, No 7, pp. 523 - 546.

Mubarak S.T., Gould R, Lee Y.F., Schmidt D.A. and Hargens A.R. (1982). The medial tibial stress syndrome (a cause of shin splints). *Am Journal Sports Med*. Vol 10, 201-205.

Murrihy S. (2009). Localisation of Tibial Bone Geometry and Bone Mineral Density Differences in Female Athletes with Tibial Stress Injuries. BMedImaging Thesis.

Myburgh K. H., Hutchins J., Fataar A. B., Hough S. F. & Noakes T. D. (1990). Low Bone Density Is an Etiologic Factor for Stress Fractures in Athletes. *Annals of Internal Medicine*. Vol 113, No 10, pp. 754 - 759.

Oakes B. W. (1988). Tibial pain or shin soreness ("shin splints")–its cause, differential diagnosis and management. In: Draper J, ed. *Second Report on the National Sports Research Program*. Canberra, Australia: Australian Sports Commission; 1986:47-51.

Oakes B. W. (1993). Weak inverters and foot pronation in MTSS subjects. Unpublished data.

Oakes B. W. & Franklyn M. (1998). Bone mineral density in tibial stress fracture and MTSS patients. Unpublished data.

Pattin C. A., Caler W. E. & Carter D. R. (1996). Cyclic mechanical property degradation during fatigue loading of cortical bone. *Journal of Biomechanics*. Vol 29, No 1, pp. 69-79.

Pomeranz S. J. (2011). Instructional lectures on MRI. Australian MRI workshop course lecture notes on assessing chronic bone injury. June 11-15, 2011, Melbourne, Australia.

Reeder M. T., Dick B. H., Atkins J. K. & Pribis A. B. (1996). Stress fractures: Current concepts of diagnosis and treatment. *Sports Medicine*. Vol 22, No 3, pp. 198-212.

Robling A. G., Burr D. B. & Turner C. H. (2001). Recovery periods restore mechanosensitivity to dynamically loaded bone. *The Journal of Experimental Biology*. Vol 204, Part 19, pp. 3389-3399.

Rorabeck C. H., Bourne R. B. & Fowler P. J. (1983). The surgical treatment of exertional compartment syndrome in athletes. *The Journal of Bone and Joint Surgery*. Vol 65-A, No 9, pp. 1245-1251.

Seibert J. A. (1995). One hundred years of medical diagnostic imaging technology. *Health Physics*. Vol 69, No 5, pp. 695-720.

Wallensten R. (1983). Results of fasciotomy in patients with medial tibial syndrome or chronic anterior-compartment syndrome. *The Journal of Bone and Joint Surgery*. Vol 65-A, No 9, pp. 1252-1255.

Permissions

The contributors of this book come from diverse backgrounds, making this book a truly international effort. This book will bring forth new frontiers with its revolutionizing research information and detailed analysis of the nascent developments around the world.

We would like to thank Kenneth R. Zaslav MD, for lending his expertise to make the book truly unique. He has played a crucial role in the development of this book. Without his invaluable contribution this book wouldn't have been possible. He has made vital efforts to compile up to date information on the varied aspects of this subject to make this book a valuable addition to the collection of many professionals and students.

This book was conceptualized with the vision of imparting up-to-date information and advanced data in this field. To ensure the same, a matchless editorial board was set up. Every individual on the board went through rigorous rounds of assessment to prove their worth. After which they invested a large part of their time researching and compiling the most relevant data for our readers. Conferences and sessions were held from time to time between the editorial board and the contributing authors to present the data in the most comprehensible form. The editorial team has worked tirelessly to provide valuable and valid information to help people across the globe.

Every chapter published in this book has been scrutinized by our experts. Their significance has been extensively debated. The topics covered herein carry significant findings which will fuel the growth of the discipline. They may even be implemented as practical applications or may be referred to as a beginning point for another development. Chapters in this book were first published by InTech; hereby published with permission under the Creative Commons Attribution License or equivalent.

The editorial board has been involved in producing this book since its inception. They have spent rigorous hours researching and exploring the diverse topics which have resulted in the successful publishing of this book. They have passed on their knowledge of decades through this book. To expedite this challenging task, the publisher supported the team at every step. A small team of assistant editors was also appointed to further simplify the editing procedure and attain best results for the readers.

Our editorial team has been hand-picked from every corner of the world. Their multi-ethnicity adds dynamic inputs to the discussions which result in innovative outcomes. These outcomes are then further discussed with the researchers and contributors who give their valuable feedback and opinion regarding the same. The feedback is then collaborated with the researches and they are edited in a comprehensive manner to aid the understanding of the subject.

Apart from the editorial board, the designing team has also invested a significant amount of their time in understanding the subject and creating the most relevant covers. They scrutinized every image to scout for the most suitable representation of the subject and create an appropriate cover for the book.

The publishing team has been involved in this book since its early stages. They were actively engaged in every process, be it collecting the data, connecting with the contributors or procuring relevant information. The team has been an ardent support to the editorial, designing and production team. Their endless efforts to recruit the best for this project, has resulted in the accomplishment of this book. They are a veteran in the field of academics and their pool of knowledge is as vast as their experience in printing. Their expertise and guidance has proved useful at every step. Their uncompromising quality standards have made this book an exceptional effort. Their encouragement from time to time has been an inspiration for everyone.

The publisher and the editorial board hope that this book will prove to be a valuable piece of knowledge for researchers, students, practitioners and scholars across the globe.

List of Contributors

Candice Jo-Anne Christie
Department of Human Kinetics and Ergonomics, Rhodes University, South Africa

Judy Kruger
Department of Environmental and Occupational Health, Rollins School of Public Health, Emory University, USA

Juan Carlos de la Cruz-Márquez, Adrián de la Cruz-Campos, Juan Carlos de la Cruz-Campos, María Belén Cueto-Martín, María García-Jiménez and María Teresa Campos-Blasco
University of Granada, Department of Physical Education and Sport, Spain

Luis Casáis and Miguel Martínez
Faculty of Education and Sport Sciences, University of Vigo, Spain

Rufus A. Adedoyin and Esther O. Johnson
Department of Medical Rehabilitation, Obafemi Awolowo University, Ile-Ife, Nigeria

Sylwia Mętel, Agata Milert and Elżbieta Szczygieł
Institute of Physiotherapy Faculty of Health Care, Jagiellonian University Medical College in Krakow, Poland
Department of Physiotherapy, Faculty of Health and Medicine, Andrzej Frycz Modrzewski Krakow University, Poland
Department of Physiotherapy, Faculty of Motor Rehabilitation, The University School of Physical Education in Krakow, Poland

Jeffrey R. Thormeyer, James P. Leonard and Mark Hutchinson
Department of Orthopaedic Surgery, University of Illinois, Chicago, USA

Da-Hon Lin
Department of Orthopedic Surgery, En Chu Kong Hospital, Taipei, Taiwan

Chien-Ho Janice Lin
Department of Neurology, University of California Los Angels, CA, USA

Mei-Hwa Jan
School and Graduate Institute of Physical Therapy, National Taiwan University, Taipei, Taiwan Yeong-An Clinic, Orthopedics & Rehabilitation, Taipei, Taiwan

Yeong-Fwu Lin
Yeong-An Clinic, Orthopedics & Rehabilitation, Taipei, Taiwan
Graduate Institute of Biomedical Engineering, National Yang-Ming University, Taipei, Taiwan

Jiu-Jenq Lin
School and Graduate Institute of Physical Therapy, National Taiwan University, Taipei, Taiwan

Cheng-Kung Cheng
Graduate Institute of Biomedical Engineering, National Yang-Ming University, Taipei, Taiwan

Patrick O. McKeon
University of Kentucky, USA

Tricia J. Hubbard and Erik A. Wikstrom
University of North Carolina at Charlotte, USA

Ian Horsley
Regional Lead Physiotherapist, English Institute of Sport, Manchester, UK

Thanos Badekas, Evangelos Evangelou and Maria Takvorian
Department of Foot and Ankle Surgery, Metropolitan Hospital, Athens, Greece

M. Franklyn
Department of Mechanical Engineering, The University of Melbourne, Melbourne, Australia

B. Oakes
Cheltenham Sports Medicine Clinic, Cheltenham, Melbourne, Australia